Essentials for Occupational Health Nursing

Arlene Guzik,
DNP, ARNP-BC, COHN-S, FAAOHN
President and Owner, Business Health Resources, Inc.
Dunedin, Florida, USA
Assistant Medical Director and Vice President of Operations,
Lakeside Occupational Medical Centers
Largo, Florida, USA

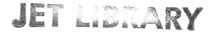
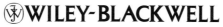

⟲WILEY-BLACKWELL
A John Wiley & Sons, Inc., Publication

This edition first published 2013 © 2013 by John Wiley & Sons, Inc

Wiley-Blackwell is an imprint of John Wiley & Sons, formed by the merger of Wiley's global Scientific, Technical and Medical business with Blackwell Publishing.

Editorial Offices
2121 State Avenue, Ames, Iowa 50014-8300, USA
The Atrium, Southern Gate, Chichester, West Sussex, PO19 8SQ, UK
9600 Garsington Road, Oxford, OX4 2DQ, UK

For details of our global editorial offices, for customer services and for information about how to apply for permission to reuse the copyright material in this book please see our website at www.wiley.com/wiley-blackwell.

Library of Congress Cataloging-in-Publication Data

Guzik, Arlene.
    Essentials for occupational health nursing / Arlene Guzik.
      p. ; cm.
    Includes bibliographical references and index.
    ISBN 978-0-8138-0689-1 (pbk. : alk. paper) – ISBN 978-1-118-51762-8 (epdf/ebook) – ISBN 978-1-118-51766-6 (mobi) – ISBN 978-1-118-51767-3 (epub)
I. Title. [DNLM: 1. Occupational Health Nursing. WY 141]
    610.73'46–dc23
                                                    2012040683

A catalogue record for this book is available from the British Library.

Wiley also publishes its books in a variety of electronic formats. Some content that appears in print may not be available in electronic books.

Cover design by Buffy Clatt

Set in 9/11pt Palatino by SPi Publisher Services, Pondicherry, India
Printed and bound in Malaysia by Vivar Printing Sdn Bhd

Disclaimer

1   2013

DEDICATION

To John and Master Toby.
For your patience and support.
I thank you.

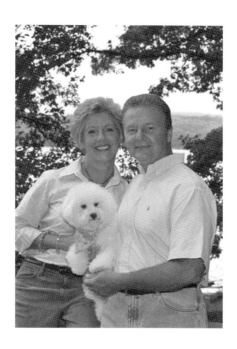

Contents

Preface

This story was once told to me years ago and it has continued impress upon me the importance of an "upstream approach" to safety.

There was once a small town, with few hundred residents who all knew one another. Folks who were born in this town generally stayed in the town for most of their lives. Everyone knew everyone. One big happy community . . . until one day.

A picnic was being held in the town park. Most everyone was there.

All were laughing and having fun, until someone shouted

"There is a body floating down the stream!"

Everything stopped. No one knew what to do. Panic ensued.

Some people jumped in the stream in attempt to save the victim.

To no avail. The stream was flowing swiftly. Few knew how to swim well.

No one knew CPR.

The precious life of a community member was lost.

The town folks were devastated.

They could never let something like this happen again in their town.

So a community meeting was called the following week. Nearly everyone came.

Plans ensued. Swimming lessons were planned. CPR training would be offered.

The town commission approved a budget for a trained rescue squad, a rescue vehicle, and the best rescue equipment. A community disaster plan was put in place.

Plans were coordinated with the neighboring city's hospital emergency department for transfer of victims. Thousands of dollars were invested in saving future victims.

Nothing was considered too expensive if it saves a life.

Time went on and another picnic was held. Everyone was having a great time.

But sure enough that afternoon, someone shouted

"There is a body floating down the stream!"

The plan would be put to its first test. Everyone jumped to action.

"Call the squad and bring in the equipment!!"

Rescuers jumped into the stream with ropes and rafts and made the rescue.

The body was brought to shore. CPR was initiated.

The rescue squad arrived and transported the victim to the neighboring city's ER.

The life was saved!!!

This called for a celebration!

"Let's have another picnic!"

Yes, a picnic to celebrate their success at saving the drowning victim.

Everyone came. This time there was a parade. There were bands.

Everyone was singing and dancing in celebration of their success.

Until someone shouted

"There is a body floating down the stream!"

Again, all jumped to action to take their role in rescuing yet another victim.

When suddenly, someone stopped to ask:"How are all these bodies getting in the stream in the first place"?

This story has continued to have significance throughout my career, not only in the aspect of safety, but in the aspects of health and well-being, as well. Although people do not generally work to have their behavior changed or their health improved, the workplace is an excellent place to establish individual and population-based efforts, not only for safety, but also for health and productivity enhancement. These efforts take place at the micro-level, focused on the workers (the picnic), to discover specific problems or issues requiring attention. But the beauty of occupational health is that efforts also are aimed at the macro-level (upstream), focused on the broad, global improvements in health, safety, and productivity of the business . . . the population.

As you read through this book, remember that you can make a difference in a little way and in a really big way. As nurses, we have been educated to address our interventions on individuals, families, and groups. As an occupational health nurse, one of the best outcomes of your efforts will be to make a difference, not only for the health and well-being of individuals and groups, but also for the health and well-being of the business.

Let's take a trip upstream . . .

Foundations for Practice

1

"The mission of occupational health nursing is to assist individuals and workplaces in achieving higher levels of personal and workplace health and safety."

(Guzik, 2005)

Nursing professionals have long been important assets in various aspects of healthcare, including hospitals, public and community health settings, military and educational settings, and in industrial and workplace settings. Occupational health nursing was originally known as "industrial nursing," evolving during the Industrial Revolution. Throughout the years, occupational health nursing has taken on a variety of roles, and the scope of practice has expanded considerably, giving rise to opportunities for nurses to care for workers in various workplace settings.

Occupational health is a small healthcare specialty that was initially devoted to the prevention and management of occupational and environmental injury, illness, and disability. The specialty has grown to encompass other dimensions of healthcare, including the promotion of health and productivity along with the support for a safe workplace. The specialty of occupational health is focused on policy and issues relevant to health and safety by devoting attention to individuals and groups in the workplace.

Occupational health nursing is the nursing practice that provides for and delivers clinical service to workers and workplaces. Occupational health nurses (OHNs) also provide health education, case management, and safety programs. The practice of occupational health is focused on promotion and restoration of health, prevention of illness and injury, and protection from work-related hazards.

Registered nurses provide an array of services to business and industry and fill diverse roles in occupational health, including those of clinician, educator, case manager, corporate director, and consultant (AAOHN, 2007).

Essentials for Occupational Health Nursing, First Edition. Arlene Guzik.
© 2013 John Wiley & Sons, Inc. Published 2013 by John Wiley & Sons, Inc.

The first record of occupational health nursing in the United States dates back to 1888. The profession has since evolved with the growth of industry and service and today provides a valued role in the workplace. According to the findings from the 2008 National Sample Survey of Registered Nurses Health Resources and Services Administration of the U.S. Department of Health and Human Services (2010), approximately 7.8% of all licensed registered nurses are working in public and community health, including occupational health.

The use of healthcare professionals has long been supported, and these professionals have demonstrated value in supporting the health and safety of the workplace and the workforce. With today's workforce becoming increasingly diverse, these demographic changes result in new safety and health issues. As a result, workers are more likely to have increased risks of work-related diseases and injuries. With the shift from industrial to service-related occupations, changes are occurring in the way work is organized and accomplished. This may result in the need for longer work shifts, more hours worked than in the typical workweek, workweeks with longer days but fewer days per week, increased need for shift work, and increased use of part-time and temporary workers. In addition, new chemicals, materials, processes, and equipment are being implemented that may pose new and additional risks to worker health (U.S. Department of Labor, 2010).

OCCUPATIONAL HEALTHCARE PROFESSIONALS

Many types of healthcare professionals work in occupational health. The physician specialty of occupational medicine dates back to the 1500s when the dangers of mining and diseases of miners were of great concern (Gochfeld, 2005). The specialty of occupational health has continued to evolve and is now focused on the recognition and prevention of injury and disease and the promotion of health. Occupational medicine arises from the principles of general medicine yet adds three dimensions of expertise: industrial hygiene, epidemiology, and toxicology (Gochfeld, 2005).

According to the American College of Occupational and Environmental Medicine (ACOEM, 2011), physicians working in occupational health "enhance the health of workers through preventive medicine, clinical care, disability management, research, and education." In recent years, the role of the physician continues to change as greater emphasis is placed on health promotion and wellness in the workplace. The role of the physician has expanded, contributing new scientific research and new clinical guidelines for healthcare, and public health initiatives focused on the workforce and on the health of the environment (ACOEM, 2011).

In large businesses, physicians may hold administrative roles, and they are involved with developing company-based healthcare policy and procedures. These physicians may also provide oversight for company health, safety, and disability programs. Physicians in occupational health may work in private practice, offering clinical services such as physical examinations, drug testing, injury management, and medical monitoring services. Private physicians may also provide consultative services to workplaces to assist in the design and development of health and safety policies and procedures.

Occupational health physicians may also be employed by government agencies or in academic settings that focus on research, consultation, or education related to occupational health.

The physician's assistant (PA) also has a role in occupational health. The PA working in occupational health, supervised by a physician, and is able to provide a broad range of healthcare services, such as diagnosis, treatment, and health promotion activity. The scope of practice for the PA is determined by the medical practice statutes specific to the state in which the PA is practicing (AAPAOM, 2010). The PA is able to practice autonomously within the scope of practice and authority delegated by the supervising physician.

The licensed practical nurse (LPN) also may hold a role in occupational health. LPNs are educated at the technical or vocational level, and their functions are generally performed under the direction of a registered nurse, a licensed physician, or a licensed osteopathic physician. The LPNs' duties must fall within the scope of practice of the state in which they are licensed to practice.

The role of the LPN in occupational health may include first aid response and the administration of treatments and medications. AAOHN recommends that LPNs be assigned only those duties and responsibilities that their skills, knowledge, and competencies warrant as defined within their state licensure and that LPNs work exclusively in health organizations under the supervision of a registered professional OHN who can provide professional supervision (AAOHN, 2003). By using professional judgment, the registered nurse must determine the appropriate activities to delegate and must consider the associated professional responsibility and liability when overseeing the activities of assistive personnel.

The registered professional nurse holds a predominant position in occupational health in a variety of roles. The American Nurses Association's Nursing's Social Policy Statement (2003) states that the profession of nursing encompasses the "protection, promotion, and optimization of health and abilities, prevention of illness and injury, alleviation of suffering through the diagnosis and treatment of human response, and advocacy in the care of individuals, families, communities, and populations." This definition encompasses the scope of practice for the role of the OHN. Figure 1.1 depicts the relationship of the OHN within the company and within the community.

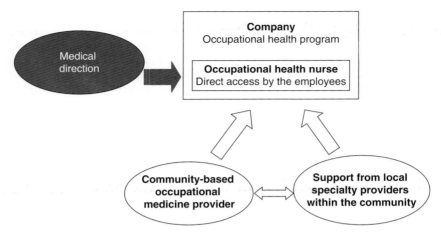

Figure 1.1 Occupational health services program.

Case in Point

The fire alarm sounds. "Code red" is announced over the speaker system, indicating a fire in the research and development department of the plant. The emergency response team is deployed to the area, and 911 is called. Evacuation procedures begin. The OHN retrieves the emergency response kit, arrives at the scene, and establishes a triage area for assessment of injured workers. The emergency response team assists with evacuation of workers to a safe area, providing a quick assessment of any worker who has incurred an injury. These workers are directed to the OHN. The OHN assesses each individual and identifies emergency or first aid needs. The OHN is assisted by members of the emergency response team to attend to the immediate needs of the injured workers. Oxygen is applied to those with respiratory symptoms. First aid is rendered for those who have abrasions, burns, or other physical injuries.

Firefighters and EMS services arrive at the scene. Firefighters are deployed to contain and obliterate the fire within the structure. EMS workers take over the assessment, treatment, and transfer of the injured workers. It is time for the OHN to intervene at a different level.

The nature of the work in this facility involves hazardous chemicals. The OHN gathers material safety data sheets (MSDS) in order to appropriately identify the involved chemicals. However, after a discussion with a facility manager, it is noted that additional risk may be posed due to the fact that this is a government research and development facility. As a result, the nature of the chemicals under development involve unknown factors. There is now additional risk considered in relation to potential exposures that may lead to both short-term and long-term health effects.

The OHN places a call to the consultant medical director who specializes in occupational health. The medical director, working at the community-based occupational health clinic, also serves as the primary treating provider and referral

---

resource for the company's occupational injuries and illnesses. A plan is established for evaluation of exposed workers based on the nature of the chemicals and associated health risks. This is determined by review of the MSDS, taking into consideration the other chemicals under development. The concern now is not only for the workers that were in the plant at the time of the explosion, but also for other types of workers who responded to the scene, including EMS and firefighters.

The plan includes a consistent evaluation of each affected worker, addressing immediate needs, but also considers the potential for future health effects from the associated chemical exposure. Other health team members, including nurse practitioners, physician assistants, and licensed practical nurses employed by the clinic, become involved. Medical evaluation and appropriate testing is conducted at the clinic and includes chest x-rays, pulmonary function tests, and laboratory testing for the specific chemicals or toxins involved. The OHN from the affected company works closely with the occupational health team members at the clinic to review the findings of the health evaluations of their workers. Each case is managed appropriate to the level of exposure, the physical findings, and health needs of each individual worker. The OHN manages each case until it is brought to closure, facilitating a return to work for each worker.

The occupational health physician and clinic are involved to a greater extent, considering the health effects of a multitude of workers and the surrounding community. A coordinated effort is undertaken with both company and public health officials to assess the level of risk associated with this event. The occupational health physician is now not only concerned about the health of the individual workers at the affected company, but also with the health of the community. A public health initiative is developed that will consistently address potential health risks to individuals in the community.

As a part of the disaster debriefing efforts, the company's OHN and medical director work with company officials to address the major contributing cause of the disaster. In addition, attention is focused on prevention of future occurrences that would have an impact on the health and safety of the work place. The OHN plays a key role in this initiative.

THE OCCUPATIONAL HEALTH NURSE

The American Association of Occupational Health Nurses (AAOHN) specifies the following qualifications for the OHN: (1) graduation from an accredited professional nursing program; (2) current license to practice as a registered professional nurse in the state(s) of employment; (3) minimum of 2 years' experience in a primary care setting, such as public/community health or ambulatory, emergency, or critical care; and (4) bachelor's degree as the preferred educational preparation (AAOHN, 2012a).

The role of the OHN includes health teaching and counseling, safety education, the promotion of wellness and education in regard to the maintenance of health, and prevention of illness. The greatest number of OHNs work as clinicians, in clinical roles, and are involved with direct worker contact. In addition, OHNs hold administrative roles as program managers and disability managers within their employer organization. Another subset of OHNs work as case managers and consultants. Some may work for worker's compensation or disability insurance companies, healthcare consulting companies, or as a self-employed independent contractors. A smaller subset of OHNs work in education or research (Thompson, 2010).

Clinician

The duties of the OHN may include first aid and emergency response, along with the administration of medications and treatments as prescribed or authorized by a duly licensed practitioner authorized under the laws of his or her respective state of practice. The role of the OHN may also include the supervision and teaching of other personnel in the performance of any of the above acts. These personnel may include licensed practical nurses and emergency response team members.

As a clinician in occupational health, the OHN not only assesses the health of individuals, but also holds a significant role in assessing the health of the work environment and the health of workers as a group. The responsibilities of this role are conducted through health assessments, physical examinations, medical monitoring, and through direct nursing care. The OHN also strives to deliver health promotion programs that focus on the needs of groups within the workplace. Based on the identification of need, therapeutic plans for intervention are established and implemented with a focus on enhancing the overall health of the worker as well as the workplace.

As a clinician, the OHN also serves as adviser or counselor to individuals in the workplace. The OHN has the ability to address occupational as well as non-occupational health issues, focusing on physical as well as psychosocial needs. The OHN uses a wealth of resources to meet the health needs of the worker and the workforce.

A significant aspect of the role as clinician includes health education. The OHN may prepare health education programs and establish outreach services that support the needs of the worker within the overall health benefits program of the company. The OHN has the opportunity to teach not only workers, but also management about aspects of personal, workplace, and public health and safety.

Manager or Administrator

There is a role for the OHN as a business leader. The OHN has the opportunity to implement strategies that will maximize employee productivity and reduce costs for the company. The OHN may serve to educate management on the impact of worker's health issues, absences, and disability that adversely effect production, staffing, budgeting, and profitability. The OHN plays a key role in assisting with the development of corporate policies and procedures that may have a positive impact on worker health, safety, and productivity, thus maximizing the bottom line (Randolph, 2004).

According to the AAOHN Position Statement on Delivery of Occupational and Environmental Health Services, OHNs should strive to develop and implement a comprehensive health program that promotes better employee health, decreases health-related cost, improves employee morale, increases productivity, decreases absenteeism, and facilitates continuity of care (AAOHN, 2004). Therefore, the OHN's primary responsibilities should focus on the following:

- Promoting a safe and healthy workforce and workplace
- Identifying health problems and hazards in the workplace and developing health and safety programs, benefits, and interventions focused on reducing risk and hazard
- Assuring that health and safety programs are in compliance with federal, state, and local regulations
- Assessing and monitoring health status and interventional outcomes for employees
- Serving as a resource for employees and for the employer regarding the selection of appropriate and cost-effective healthcare resources
- Monitoring outcomes as a measure of effectiveness

Case Manager

The OHN routinely coordinates and manages the healthcare of workers. The role of case manager initially began when OHNs managed the care and treatment of workers injured on the job, coordinating the treatment, follow-up, referrals, and emergency care for injuries and illnesses. The role has since become more comprehensive with the coordination, management, and consultation regarding nonoccupational issues, which encompasses aspects related to group health, medical leaves of absence, and disability benefits. In addition, the OHN manages services related to rehabilitation, return-to-work, and disability management. These functions are "key to employers' healthcare quality and cost containment strategies" (Randolph, 2004).

As a case manager, the OHN coordinates healthcare services for a worker from beginning of injury or illness to return to work or optimal outcome. The goal of case management is to strive for the delivery of quality care in a cost-efficient manner. Since case management may be used for both occupational and nonoccupational health situations, the activities of case management can be conducted on-site in the workplace or by telephone.

The OHN also acts as consultant, advising on the process for evaluating and developing health and safety services in the workplace. A key role of the OHN as manager or administrator is to develop program assessment tools and conduct evaluations of the occupational health and safety program. The OHN should gather this information, identify opportunities for improvement, communicate findings to company officials, and assist in the development of future programs and services. The OHN may also act as or provide significant support to safety and industrial hygiene managers, risk managers, benefits managers, and human resources professionals.

Table 1.1 Percentage of time spent occupational health nursing.

Role Category	Percent of Time
Direct Care	
COHN	31%
COHN-S	25%
Manager/Coordinator	
COHN	23%
COHN-S	28%
Case Manager	
COHN	21%
COHN-S	19%
Educator/Advisor	
COHN	14%
COHN-S	13%
Consultant	
COHN	6%
COHN-S	10%
Other	
COHN	5%
COHN-S	5%

Source: COHN, Certified Occupational Health Nurse; COHN-S, Certified Occupational Health Nurse Specialist.

Roles and activities vary significantly based on company needs and the environment in which the OHN practices. A 2004 Practice Analysis Report (Strasser et. al., 2006) indicated the percentage of time spent by OHNs in each of five general role categories. The results of the study indicated that direct care accounted for the largest percentage of the OHN's time, and that the greatest focus of activity was on safety. See Table 1.1.

THE ADVANCED PRACTICE REGISTERED NURSE IN OCCUPATIONAL HEALTH

According to the Consensus Model for APRN Regulation: Licensure, Accreditation, Certification & Education (NCSBN,2008), "Advanced Practice Registered Nurses (Nurse Practitioners) have expanded in numbers and capabilities over the past several decades with Nurse Practitioners being highly valued and an integral part of the healthcare system."

As in the practice of registered professional nursing, the performance of advanced practice registered nursing acts are approved by each state board of nursing, which also defines the specialized education, training, and experience appropriate to the scope of practice. Nurse practitioners generally may perform acts of medical diagnosis and treatment, prescribing, and procedures based on their education and experience.

Although most of the medical care in the clinical arena in occupational health has traditionally been delivered by physicians, nurse practitioners are now filling valuable roles as clinicians. In the earliest literature addressing nurse practitioners in the occupational health setting, Grimes and Garcia (1997) analyzed the new role for nurse practitioners who applied principles of primary care in the occupational setting. The Occupational Health and Safety Administration (OSHA) first addressed the role of the nurse practitioner in the occupational health setting in 1999 in a publication that addressed the qualifications of occupational health professionals (OSHA, 1999). In this publication there was an indication that nurse practitioners, certified in occupational health as a specialty area, are capable of independently performing many health evaluation and care activities traditionally provided by physicians.

The nurse practitioner role in the occupational health setting was first addressed by AAOHN in an advisory report in 1999. The advisory report, updated in 2004 (AAOHN, 2007), addresses the various roles of the advanced practice registered nurse in the occupational health setting, including the role of healthcare provider. Opportunities for nurse practitioners have since evolved within the occupational health setting, yet little research is found in which this nurse practitioner role has been evaluated (Guzik et al., 2009).

THE DOMAIN OF OCCUPATIONAL HEALTH

Occupational health is founded on a variety of scientific principles, including public health, medicine, nursing, epidemiology, toxicology, industrial hygiene, safety, and social and behavioral sciences. As a result, it is an interdisciplinary practice. The U.S. civilian workforce employed approximately 140 million people in 2009 (U.S. DOL, 2010). Workers spend up to 50% of their waking lives at work; therefore, the workplace provides a captive audience for the promotion of health and wellness. Despite improvements in occupational safety and health over the last several decades, workers continue to suffer work-related deaths, injuries, and illnesses. The workplace, therefore, provides a unique subsector for sustaining public health initiatives.

In 1979, the U.S. Surgeon General initiated efforts to address the health of the U.S. population and published a report titled *Healthy People: The Surgeon General's Report on Health Promotion and Disease Prevention*. Since that time, the U.S. Department of Health and Human Services had led a science-based initiative defining 10-year national objectives for promoting health and preventing disease. The initiative is referred to as "Healthy People."

The *Healthy People* report establishes public health initiatives based on data from the past decade, along with current data, trends, and advances. The Healthy People 2020 goals and objectives are based on current "risks to health and wellness, changing public health priorities, and emerging issues related to our nation's health preparedness and prevention" (U.S. Department of Health and Human Services, 2010).

9

The goals include improving access to comprehensive, quality healthcare services. On-site occupational health programs staffed with an OHN support this goal by providing workers efficient access to a healthcare professional at their worksite. The OHN promotes the health and safety of people at work through prevention, early intervention, and directed referrals. With a focus on environmental health, the OHN addresses physical workplace risks and exposures, such as the use of hazardous chemicals and the potential of injury or illness, in order to reduce occupational deaths and needless disability. While supporting this Healthy People initiative, the OHN also supports the productivity of the workforce. Other goals and objectives of Healthy People call for an increase in comprehensive worksite health promotion programs, including educational programs and strategies for substance abuse and stress.

The strategies of occupational health nursing are based on the principles of evaluation, protection, promotion, and restoration of health, thus leading to an enhanced quality of life. Table 1.2 outlines the essential services of the occupational health professional in relation to public health initiatives.

The OHN is "central to the management and coordination of occupational health activities" (Rogers, 2003). The OHN must recognize the need to draw knowledge, experience, and resources from a variety of aspects and disciplines and be committed to continuing education to develop knowledge and skills within the domain of occupational health nursing. This includes basic nursing principles, clinical competence, and knowledge of the legal, regulatory, and ethical aspects impacting occupational health. Because the OHN typically practices in workplaces outside the traditional clinical venue of the healthcare environment, OHNs must also augment their value by holding a basic knowledge of management concepts and principles.

Occupational health professionals work with a variety of workers and work populations in a multitude of various work environments. This variety brings into play not only physical issues, but also social, cultural, organizational, economic, political, and interpersonal issues. The OHN must develop competence in performing activities customized to workers as well as the occupational and business environment. The OHN must develop an awareness of the impact of actions and interventions not only with the worker, but also within the greater context of the business environment.

The OHN will interact with a variety of other professionals in the work setting. These professionals include human resources and benefits professionals, safety and environmental specialists, business managers, and executive staff, including finance and legal professionals. It is therefore important that the OHN develop an understanding of the variety of perspectives that impact decisions in the workplace.

Safety and health promotion provide the foundation of an effective occupational health program. Occupational health nursing has evolved well beyond first aid treatment of injuries and emergencies to include comprehen-

Table 1.2 Essential services.

Essential Public Health Services	Essential Occupational Health Services
Monitor health status to identify community health problems.	Monitor health status of the workforce.
Diagnose and investigate health problems and health hazards in the community.	Assess health risks and hazards in the workforce and workplace.
Inform, educate, and empower people about health issues.	Increase awareness and educate workers about health and safety issues.
Mobilize community partnerships to identify and self-health problems.	Establish community partnerships for health and safety interventions.
Developed policies and plans that support individual and community health efforts.	Develop health and safety policies and procedures.
Enforce laws and regulations that protect health and ensure safety.	Ensure compliance with applicable regulations related to health and safety.
Link people to needed personal health services and ensure the provision of healthcare when otherwise unavailable.	Improve access to and facilitate the delivery health services.
Assure a competent public health and personal healthcare workforce.	Support optimum health of the workforce.
Evaluate effectiveness, accessibility, and quality of personal and population-based health services.	Evaluate the effectiveness of safety and health interventions, benefits, and services.
Research for new insights and innovative solutions to health problems.	Identify continued opportunities for improvement and enhancement of health and safety in the workplace.

Source: Public Health Functions Steering Committee. *Public Health in America*, Fall 1994. http://www.health.gov/phfunctions/public.htm (December 17, 2010).

sive health and safety programs that are focused on promotion of worker health, increased productivity, and decreased health-related cost to the employer.

"Health" is not only related to the individual worker, but also should encompass a philosophy related to healthy populations and healthy work environments. It is therefore critical that the OHN support a solid foundation for an occupational health program that supports this philosophy.

REFERENCES

American Academy of Physician Assistants in Occupational Medicine (AAPAOM). (2010). Information for PAs in occupational medicine. Retrieved from www.aapaoccmed.org/Default.aspx?pageId=770960

American Association of Occupational Health Nurses (AAOHN). (2003). Position Statement. *The licensed practical nurse (LPN) in occupational health.* Retrieved from http://www.aaohn.org

American Association of Occupational Health Nurses (AAOHN). (2004). Position statement. *Delivery of occupational and environmental health services.* Retrieved from https://www.aaohn.org/position-statements/delivery-of-occupational-and-environmental-health-services.html

American Association of Occupational Health Nurses (AAOHN). (2007). Nurse practitioners in occupational and environmental health. Retrieved from https://www.aaohn.org/component/option,com_docman/task,cat_view/gid,132/

American Association of Occupational Health Nurses (AAOHN). (2012a). Occupational and environmental health nursing: Your key to health care cost containment. Retrieved from https://www.aaohn.org/dmdocuments/Your-Key-to-Health-Care-Cost-Containment%5B1%5D.pdf

American Association of Occupational Health Nurses (AAOHN). (2012). Occupational and environmental health nursing profession fact sheet. Retrieved from www.aaohn.org/component/option,com_docman/task,cat_view/gid,129

American Association of Occupational Health Nurses (AAOHN). (2012). Standards of occupational and environmental health nursing. *Workplace Health & Safety, 60*(3), 97–103.

American Association of Occupational Health Nurses (AAOHN). (2012). The licensed practical/vocational nurse in occupational and environmental health. *Workplace Health & Safety, 60*(3), 104.

American Nurses Association. (2003). Nursing's social policy statement (2nd ed.). Silver Spring, MD: Nursesbooks.org.

American College of Occupational and Environmental Medicine (ACOEM). (2011). Scope of occupational and environmental health programs and practice. Updated March 03, 2011. Retrieved from http://www.acoem.org/Scope_HealthPrograms_Practice.aspx

Dirksen, M. E. (2001). Occupational and environmental health nursing: An overview. In M. K. Salazar (Ed.), Core curriculum for occupational and environmental health nursing (2nd ed., pp. 3–32). Philadelphia: W.B. Saunders.

Felton, J. S. (1996). Medical direction in occupational health nursing. *The American Journal of Nursing, 66*(9), 2019–2022.

Gochfeld, M. (2005).Chronologic history of occupational medicine. *Journal of Occupational and Environmental Medicine, 47*:96–114.

Goetzel, R. Z., Shechter D., Ozminkowski R. J., Marmet P. F., Tabrizi M. J., & Roemer E. C. (2007). Promising practices in employer health and productivity management efforts: Findings from a benchmarking study. *Journal of Occupational and Environmental Medicine, 49*(2), 111–130.

Grimes, D. E. & Garcia, M. K. (1997) Advanced practice nursing and worksite primary care: challenges for outcomes evaluation. *Advance Practice Nursing Quarterly, 3*(2), 19–28.

Guzik, A., Menzel, N. N., Fitzpatrick, J., & McNulty, R. (2009). Patient satisfaction with nurse practitioner and physician services in the occupational health setting. *AAOHN Journal, 57*(5), 191–197.

Hanna, J. K. (2012). Occupational health nursing around the world. *Workplace Health & Safety, 60*(6), 251–252.

Institute of Medicine, Committee for the Study of the Future of Public Health. (1988). The future of public health. Washington, DC: National Academies Press.

Institute of Medicine, Committee to Assess Training Needs for Occupational Safety and Health Personnel in the United States. (2000). Safe work in the 21st century: Education and training needs for the next decade's occupational safety and health personnel. Washington, DC: National Academies Press.

Lukes, E. (2007). Epidemiology basics for occupational health nurses. *AAOHN Journal, 55*(1), 26–31.

McCauley, L. A. (2012). Research to practice in occupational health nursing. *Workplace Health & Safety, 60*(4), 183–189.

McCullagh, M. C. (1994). Occupational health nursing education for the 21st century. Public Health Functions Steering Committee. Public Health in America. Retrieved from http://www.health.gov/phfunctions/public.htm

McCullagh, M. C. (2012). Occupational health nursing education for the 21st century. *Workplace Health & Safety, 60*(4), 167–176.

National Council of State Boards of Nursing (NCSBN). (2008). *APRN Joint Dialogue Group Report. Consensus model for APRN regulation: Licensure, accreditation, certification & education.* Retrieved from https://www.ncsbn. org/7_23_08_Consensue_APRN_Final.pdf

Occupational Safety and Health Administration (OSHA). (1999). *The occupational health professional's service and qualifications: questions and answers.* Retrieved from http://www.osha.gov/Publications/osha3160.pdf

Ramos, E. I. (2006). Occupational health nurses and case management. *Nursing Economics, 24*(1), 30–40, 3.

Randolph, S. A. *Occupational and environmental health nursing.* (2004). Retrieved from www.nsna.org/Portals/0/Skins/NSNA/pdf/Career_Randolf2.pdf

Reidel, J. E., Lynch, W., Baase, C., Hymel, P., Peterson, K. W. (2001). The effect of disease prevention and health promotion on workplace productivity: A literature review. *American Journal of Health Promotion, 15*(3), 167–191.

Rogers, B. (2003). Occupational health nursing, concepts and practice (2nd ed.). Philadelphia: W.B. Saunders.

Rogers, B. (2012). Occupational and environmental health nursing: Ethics and professionalism. *Workplace Health & Safety, 60*(4), 177–181.

Salazar, M. K. (2002). Defining the roles and functions of occupational and environmental health nurses: Results of a national job analysis. *AAOHN Journal, 50*(1), 16–25.

Strasser. P. B. (2006). Occupational health nursing: 2004 practice analysis report. *AAOHN Journal, 54*(1), 14–23.

Strasser, P. B. (2012). Occupational and environmental health nursing: The foundations of quality practice. *Workplace Health & Safety, 60*(4), 151–157.

Thompson, M. C. (2010). Review of occupational health nurse data from recent national sample surveys of registered nurses—Part I. *AAOHN Journal*, (58)1, 26–37.

U.S. Department of Health and Human Services, Centers for Disease Control and Prevention. (2010). Occupational injuries and deaths among younger workers—United States, 1998–2007. *Morbidity and Mortality Weekly Report*, 59(15), 449–455.

U.S. Department of Health and Human Services, Health Resources and Services Administration. (2010). *The registered nurse population. Initial findings from the 2008 national sample survey of registered nurses*. Retrieved from http://bhpr.hrsa.gov/healthworkforce/rnsurveys/rnsurveyinitial2008.pdf

U.S. Department of Labor, Bureau of Labor Statistics. (2009). Consumer price index calculator. Retrieved from http://www.bls.gov/data/inflation_calculator.htm

U.S. Department of Labor, Bureau of Labor Statistics. (2010). Employment status of the civilian noninstitutional population, 1940 to date. Retrieved from http://www.bls.gov/cps/cpsaat1.pdf

Professional Issues

2

"Occupational and Environmental Health Nursing is the specialty practice providing for and delivering health and safety services to employees, employee populations and community groups. The practice focuses on promotion and restoration of health, prevention of illness and injury and protection from work-related and environmental hazards."

(AAOHN, 2009)

PROFESSIONAL ISSUES

Awareness of issues surrounding professional nursing is important in defining the scope of practice and supervision in the occupational health setting. The scope of occupational health service delivery depends on the practice setting, the size of the workforce, and the number, diversity, and health characteristics of workers. The size and geographic location of the practice setting is also significant. In addition, consideration must be given to the community resources available near and around the practice setting.

The type of industry or work setting served will also dictate the scope of service, taking into consideration the types of processes and services provided at the work place. Potential health and safety risks associated with specific industries and job tasks will also dictate the need for specific interventions, medical surveillance, and workforce education and training.

In establishing an occupational health program, it is critical to understand the company philosophy and how the occupational health services relate to the overall organizational structure, process, and goals. The ability to assess specific health needs of the work population and potential hazards in the environment will drive the resources needed to establish an effective occupational health service, thus providing support for the corporate mission. Because occupational health services are not core to most company operations, it is important to develop a program built on a solid foundation of core principles related to

Essentials for Occupational Health Nursing, First Edition. Arlene Guzik.
© 2013 John Wiley & Sons, Inc. Published 2013 by John Wiley & Sons, Inc.

worker and workplace health and safety This requires diligence, communication, and consistent justification of goals and outcomes of the program.

Several resources are available for development of an occupational health program for both nurses and physicians. Two renowned associations that serve as the primary resources in the United States are the American Association of Occupational Health Nurses (AAOHN) and the American College of Occupational and Environmental Medicine (ACOEM).

AAOHN is a professional association for healthcare professionals working in or interested in the specialty of occupational health. The vision of AAOHN is to "create a positive economic impact through workers' health and well-being" that assists the occupational health nurse in supporting a productive workforce. AAOHN provides resources and support through education, research, and support for public policy by providing practice resources for occupational health nurses and through the development of strategic specialty alliances (AAOHN, 2010).

ACOEM is a professional association "dedicated to promoting the health of workers through preventive medicine, clinical care, research, and education." ACOEM's mission is to support the education of health professional and the public, support research, enhance the quality of practice, and to guide the development of public policy in order to advance the specialty of occupational and environmental medicine (ACOEM, 2010).

Both associations, along with other health and safety associations dedicated to the specialty of occupational health, provide support for the development of clinical practice, leadership development, and specialty education and research that is focused on promoting the health and safety of workers, workplaces, and the community.

MEDICAL DIRECTION

Since Registered Professional Nurses work under the supervision of a physician, medical direction for the occupational health program is important. Medical Direction for the occupational health program may be achieved through a direct relationship with a company-based medical director or may be facilitated through a contractual arrangement with a community-based physician familiar with the principles of occupational health and safety. In selecting a supervising medical director, the occupational health nurse (OHN) should define specific criteria expected from the relationship before identifying potential candidates.

In a document covering pertinent guidelines, best practices, and professional opinions, specific criteria that include skills and competencies expected of the physician practicing in occupational health are outlined (Russi et al., 2010). These criteria include interpersonal, administrative, and management skills; grounded knowledge of safety management; a willingness to interact with safety and workplace managers; knowledge of the principles of industrial hygiene and toxicology; focus on preventive and evidence-based medicine,

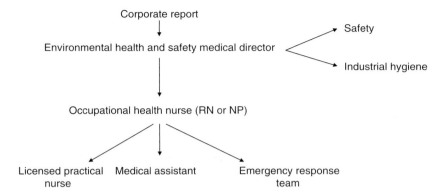

Figure 2.1 Organizational chart for company medical direction: corporate medical director.

including medical monitoring, assessment, diagnosis, and treatment of common workplace injuries and illnesses; and a strong focus on return to work and productivity. The credentials of the selected candidate for the supervising medical director role should be validated through the state board of medicine or state department of health. Required criteria include an active license to practice medicine in the specific State, medical license free of actions, disciplinary action or review, and absence of legal proceedings against the physician.

The physician, as medical director, should not be expected to provide services without fair compensation. Since the medical director's liability exposure and insurance premium may be impacted by the number of staff overseen directly and indirectly, compensation should be considered with this in mind.

The company must first decide the role of the medical director and make it worth the investment. The reporting relationship within the organization should be determined to provide clear lines of authority and responsibility. A company-based corporate medical director may hold responsibility for all aspects of environmental health and safety and will report to a member of senior management (see Figure 2.1). Commonly, the corporate medical director will report to the same member of senior management who is responsible for human resources or risk management. In a contractual arrangement, a consultant medical director would have a reporting relationship as an advisor to the company, while providing consultant supervision of the occupational health nurse, but hold no direct responsibility within the company (see Figure 2.2). A written agreement between the company and the medical director should outline the reporting relationships, terms, conditions, and expectations of performance. A sample contract for medical direction is provided in Appendix 3.

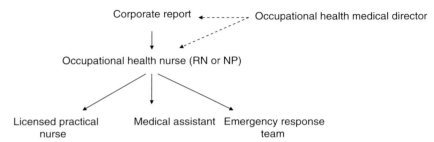

Figure 2.2 Organizational chart for company medical direction: consultant medical director.

Table 2.1 Medical direction documents.

Medical Director Agreement	Defines the role and scope of services for the program's medical director and outlines the terms and agreements of the contractual relationships.
Clinical Practice Guidelines	Defines the specific health conditions and provides guidelines for the assessment and intervention that are within the scope of practice of the OHN. Also defines the nonprescription and prescription medications that can be administered.
Prescription Release Authority	Defines the specific medication that may be ordered through the pharmaceutical supply vendor under the medical director's professional license.

A contracted medical director should perform to the level of the company's expectations and should be compensated accordingly. The medical director may be paid on an hourly basis or may be paid through a monthly retainer that is reasonable and includes compensation for on-call, on-site visits, case management meetings, and writing/approving protocols and directives. Table 2.1 outlines the required documents for medical direction and their purposes.

The medical director's performance should be evaluated regularly to establish and evaluate clear expectations according to the employment the agreement. The company should hold the medical director accountable for meeting or exceeding performance expectations. You can never "pay too much" for medical directorship. Compensation hinges on expectations and the value having a medical director brings to the occupational health and safety program.

The medical director should have an established relationship with the senior management of the company. This includes key officials and day-to-day managers of departments such as safety, human resources, industrial hygiene, engineering and facilities management, environment services, and the company's health and disability insurance carriers (ACOEM, 2008). The medical director may participate in applicable committee meetings related to occupational health and safety and should also play an active role in the development of health and safety policies and procedures.

The success of an occupational health medical director affiliation is largely dependent on the relationship with occupational health nurses and other occupational health program staff. This relationship requires a strong philosophical alignment and commands respect for the skills and opinions of all members of the occupational health team.

The greatest issues to be considered with medical directorships are:

1. **Potential liability exposure for the medical director**. Liability depends on the scope of service provided. At what level and how many occupational health staff does the medical director oversee? What is the scope of practice for the OHNs and the medical director? What does the state's Nurse Practice Act require in regard to medical direction for those under the medical director's supervision?

2. **Value added services of the medical director**. Is 24/7 phone availability required? Is the medical director willing to write and sign medical directives and practice protocols? Are the medical director willing to conduct on-site workplace walk-throughs and on-site clinic audits? Are on-site visits required, and if so, how often? What is the scope of service provided when on-site? Is the medical director willing to evaluate patients and render medical services on-site? Is he or she willing to intervene and consult with treating providers on workers' compensation cases? Is he or she willing to act as a resource to workers' compensation and disability adjusters, case managers, and defense attorneys?

3. **Value of the medical director to the company**. Consultations with the medical director can save a company from exposure in workers' compensation claims, regulatory issues, and substance testing concerns. The medical director's role is to provide medical-legal guidance to ensure due diligence and appropriate handling of health and safety issues in the workplace. If the medical director has provided guidance to save exposure on just one workers' compensation claim, the medical director may prove his or her worth.

Each state board of nursing defines the scope of practice for registered professional nurses and nurse practitioner. Nurses working in occupational health must maintain knowledge of the regulatory requirements that apply to their practice in occupational health and assure appropriate medical oversight and supervision. There are distinct differences in the scope of practice for registered professional nurses and nurse practitioners. The scope of medical director supervision must be appropriate to the occupational health team members and comply with regulatory statutes guiding the practice of professional nursing.

REGISTERED PROFESSIONAL NURSES

The registered professional nurse must work under written medical directives from the supervising physician. These directives provide standing orders, protocols, prescriptive release authority, and levels of clinical intervention that guide the clinical practice of the registered nurse. These medical directives should be reviewed and signed annually by the occupational health nurse and by the supervising medical director.

The medical directives should define the general conditions for practice including but not limited to the following:

- Prescriptive authority release with pharmacy provider
- List of authorized prescription drugs, including oxygen
- Clinical practice protocols
- Use of the supervisory medical director's license and Drug Enforcement Administration (DEA) certificate
- Role and scope of service of the supervising medical director

ADVANCE PRACTICE REGISTERED NURSES

The delivery of occupational health services by nurse practitioners may take place in various practice venues. Examples include business or workplace settings, independent practice, collaborative practice with physicians or other healthcare professionals, community-based clinics, and institutional or academic clinic-based settings (AAOHN, 2007).

Each state has differing statutory requirements for practice as a nurse practitioner. The nurse practitioner working in an occupational health setting must maintain an awareness of the legal scope of practice and the practicing state's statutory requirements for supervisory oversight. The state statutes, the practice setting in which the nurse practitioner functions, along with the scope of clinical practice, dictates the extent to which the nurse practitioner requires supervisory or collaborative oversight from the medical director. The scope of clinical practice will depend on populations served and the needs of the community or workforce population.

Nurse practitioners may practice as independent on-site providers or may function as a member of an interdisciplinary healthcare group practice.

OTHER OCCUPATIONAL HEALTH TEAM MEMBERS

The medical director may also hold responsibility for the delegation and supervision of tasks rendered by support staff in the occupational health setting. This includes licensed practical nurses, medical assistants, emergency medical technicians, and emergency response team members. The roles, duties, and responsibilities of these team members should be clearly outlined in policies and job descriptions in order to assure compliance within their scope of practice, education, and experience. The OHN, working under the supervision of the medical director, may have the authority to provide delegation and supervision of other occupational team members

Medical directives

Since a physician is typically not in regular attendance in most occupational health settings, both legal and ethical considerations dictate that the duties of the OHN concerning patient care should be established in a written set of medical directives. These medical directives should address the types of minor injuries or exposures that might be incurred by workers in the work setting and specify the level of healthcare to be rendered. Medical directives include: (1) practice guidelines and (2) prescription release authorization (see Appendix 4 and 5).

The medical directives guide the practice of professional nursing in the occupational health setting. These directives include written protocols or practice guidelines, along with standing orders, and are intended to assist the OHN and other team members in providing safe, quality healthcare to workers. Practice guidelines enable the occupational health staff to practice independently in the occupational health setting by defining the parameters of healthcare and treatment.

Medical directives strive to assure consistency, provided the same procedure is followed each time under the same set of circumstances. These written practice guidelines should cover the necessary healthcare services to be rendered in both emergency and routine situations. The practice guidelines should specify who can do what, assuring the actions match the scope of practice for each job category.

Medical directives are intended to provide legal guidance for healthcare delivery by defining the minimum requirements for safe, effective, and appropriate care. The written directives should be approved and signed by the medical director and by each OHN practicing under the medical directives. The signed medical directives should be readily available for reference in the occupational health setting, should be reviewed annually by the OHN and the medical director, and be updated as appropriate.

Standing orders are signed instructions from the medical director that describe the scope of practice under which the occupational health staff may act. They contain specific orders related to addressing symptoms or emergencies, outlining the assessment and interventions that the occupational health staff may perform, including the administration of nonprescription and prescription medications in the occupational health setting. See sample in Appendix 5.

Prescription release authorization from the medical director is also usually required by the pharmacy supplier in order to distribute prescription medications to the OHN in the occupational health setting. This form is signed by the medical director and details a list of prescription medications that may be ordered and administered by the OHN. See sample in Appendix 5.

The duty of the medical director is to give the occupational health staff all necessary and proper medical oversight. Failure to do so could be negligence on the part of the physician and could also imply that the OHN and support staff are practicing without appropriate medical direction.

LEGAL ASPECTS
In the United States, nursing practice is regulated at the state level through a standard titled "The Nurse Practice Act." Each state's Nurse Practice Act defines and regulates the practice of nursing, describing the legal scope and authority of the nurse, indicating that each nurse is directly accountable and responsible to the consumer for the quality of nursing care rendered. As a result, all staff members in the occupational health setting are responsible for practicing within the scope of practice set forth by their respective regulatory state board.

LICENSURE
All members of the occupational health team must maintain appropriate licensure and/or certification related to their scope of practice and state regulations. In the occupational health setting, the OHN often holds multistate responsibilities. In today's business environment, OHNs may work for companies with multiple corporate locations. Typically, the OHN's primary location is at the corporate headquarters, yet the OHN may have oversight for the occupational health program in multiple other locations. As a result, the OHN must have provisions for professional licensure and medical direction for those locations outside his or her primary state of residency. The OHN often conducts activities that guide and direct patient care such as performing health screenings, case management to determine the healthcare needs of employees, administering medications/vaccinations, and consulting with other healthcare professionals regarding an employee health issue. In order for the OHN to conduct these types of activities, OHNs must hold an active nursing license with each state in which they are practicing professional nursing. Activities that may not require professional license within the state would include activities that are primarily administrative in nature, such as designing healthcare programs, developing policies and procedures, and training.

Some states are members of the Nurse Licensure Compact (NLC). This compact allows nurses to hold multistate licensure. According to the National Council for State Boards of Nursing (NCSBN, 2007), the NLC permits nurses to have one license, usually in their state of residency, and to practice nursing in other compact states, both physical and virtually.

SCOPE OF PRACTICE FOR THE OHN
AAOHN (2012) defines seven specific functions involved in the practice of occupational health nursing. These functions guide the scope of practice of the OHN and serve as a foundation of practice.

1. **Health Assessment**. The OHN conducts health assessments of individuals and in groups of workers in the workplace. These assessments are facilitated through health history documentation, health risk evaluations, testing and monitoring, or physical assessments. The OHN also conducts medical surveillance evaluations with groups of workers to monitor health status through the course of employment. The OHN may also gather data from health benefits utilization statistics as a basis for health interventions, health promotion, and health education strategies.
2. **Case Management**. The OHN acts as a case manager for both occupational and nonoccupational illness and injury management. The primary focus is to assure appropriate access and use of healthcare services. The OHN also facilitates a timely return to work and appropriate reasonable accommodation as required.
3. **Health Promotion and Health Education**. The OHN develops and manages a comprehensive, multilevel health promotion program that supports the organizational objectives. The OHN bases educational and interventional activities specific to the health risks of the worker population.
4. **Counseling and Crisis Intervention**. The OHN provides individual counseling and guidance for workers. The OHN participates in managing employee assistance programs addressing the psychosocial needs of the workforce as well as with the development of policies, procedures, and educational programs related to behavioral health and substance abuse.
5. **Health and Hazard Surveillance**. The OHN conducts periodic health assessments and implements preventive services for workers based on risk. This includes the implementation of immunization programs, infection control, travel health services, and appropriate medical monitoring.
6. **Injury Prevention and Loss Control**. The OHN routinely assesses the workplace to identify potential health and safety hazards. The OHN collaborates with other occupational health professionals, such as industrial hygienists, safety professionals, ergonomics, and toxicologists, as appropriate.
7. **Work-Related Injury and Illness Management**. The OHN coordinates health and rehabilitation for workers, assuring an optimal return to work and satisfactory outcomes. The OHN collaborates with other health professionals to diagnose and treat occupational illnesses and injuries, facilitating a return to optimal health and wellness.

There are a wide range of conditions that encompass the scope of practice for the OHN, and the situations may present themselves in a variety of fashions. Workers may become injured or ill as a result of their work and require assessment and treatment from the OHN. Workers may also require monitoring for the presence of certain health conditions as a part of the medical surveillance program. Additionally, workers often seek consultation with the OHN for a wide range of private health concerns. A list of common conditions seen in the occupational health arena can be found in Table 2.2.

Table 2.2 Common conditions seen in occupational
health Services.

Emergencies
Acute chest pain
Anaphylaxis, adults
Insect sting, diffuse reaction
Insect sting, local reaction
Minor burns
Minor lacerations

Abdomen
Abdominal pain (nongynecologic and nontraumatic)
Gastroenteritis
Hemorrhoids
Indigestion
Urinary symptoms, women

HEENT
Allergic rhinitis, adults
Conjunctivitis
Corneal abrasion and foreign body
Ear ache; middle ear
Ear infection; outer ear
Ear wax: inspissated cerumen
Epistaxis (nose bleed)
Hordeolum (stye) and chalazion
Migraine headaches
Sinus congestion
Sore throat
Upper respiratory tract infection

Respiratory
Asthma
Acute attack in known asthmatic
Chronic bronchitis
Cough and chest congestion

Cardiovascular
Chest pain
Hypertension

Musculoskeletal
Ankle sprain
Back pain
Dislocations
Fractures
Gout
Knee sprain
Neck sprain

Skin
Atopic dermatitis
Dry skin
Chicken pox
Varicella

Table 2.2 (*continued*)

Contact dermatitis
Herpes zoster (shingles)
Pediculosis capitis (head lice)
Pruritis
Psoriasis
Scabies
Seborrheic dermatitis
Tinea corporis
Tinea cruris (jock itch)
Tinea pedis (athletes feet)
Urticaria
General
Anxiety
Depression
Obesity
Panic attacks
Tobacco abuse/addiction
Blood sugar management

STANDARDS OF PRACTICE FOR THE OHN

AAOHN also defines a set of standards that guides the practice of occupational health nursing. According to the standards, OHNs "collaborate with employees, employers, the occupational health and safety team, and other professionals to identify health and safety needs; prioritize interventions; develop and implement interventions and programs; and evaluate care and service delivery" (AAOHN, 2004b). OHNs should strive to build their practice on this foundation of the standards (see Table 2.3). The standards address the scope of practice by applying the use of the nursing process specifically to the specialty and also include standards that reflect outcome identification and resource management. The complete text of standards can be found at www.aaohn.org.

COMPETENCE

The Occupational Health Nurse brings a unique perspective to management and clinical roles, acting as an employee advocate while balancing the needs of the workplace (AAOHN, 2007). AAOHN has therefore defined nine specific categories of core competencies for the occupational health nurse. These competencies address the continuum of practice experience and mastery of skills and abilities that are measurable and stated in behavioral terms. An overview of AAOHN's core competencies are listed in Table 2.4. The complete text of core competencies can be obtained from AAOHN at www.aaohn.org.

AAOHN's core competencies are based on three levels (competent, proficient, expert) applied to each of the nine categories. In the first category, AAOHN considers "competence," as achieving mastery of the role as clinician, program coordinator, or case manager. The second category of "proficient"

Table 2.3 Standards of Occupational and Environmental Health Nursing (AAOHN).

Standard I. Assessment

Standard II. Diagnosis

Standard III. Outcome Identification

Standard IV. Planning

Standard V. Implementation

Standard VI. Evaluation

Standard VII. Resource Management

Standard VIII. Professional Development

Standard IX. Collaboration

Standard X. Research

Standard XI. Ethics

Source: AAOHN. (2004). Standards of occupational and environmental health nursing. Atlanta: AAOHN. www.aaohn.org.

Table 2.4 AAOHN Core Competencies for the Occupational Health Nurse.

Competency	Summary
Clinical	Demonstrates technical and clinical proficiency by using the nursing process to assess and provide treatment within scope of practice.
Case Management	Possesses the ability to conduct an objective assessment. Identifies and initiates appropriate interventions. Develops and manages case management and integrated disability management programs.
Workforce, Workplace, and Environmental Issues	Analyzes risks associated with hazards and coordinates worker health surveillance programs.
Regulatory–Legislative	Assures compliance with regulatory standards.
Management	Designs, manages, and evaluates programs and services that support business strategies that lead to cost-effective occupational health services.
Health Promotion	Assesses, plans, and evaluates health promotion and disease prevention strategies.
Education and Training	Implements and communicates outcomes and effectiveness of safety and education programs.
Research	Utilizes evidence-based strategies in identifying research opportunities.
Professionalism	Maintains scientific, regulatory, and business knowledge and serves as a role model and mentor.

Source: www.aaohn.org.

indicates that the OHN is able to predict events and has sophisticated clinical or management skills applicable to the practice. In achieving the third competency level of "expert," the OHN should hold leadership skills in developing occupational health policy, functions, and an upper management role, provides consultant services to businesses, and conducts or designs occupational health research.

PROFESSIONAL DEVELOPMENT

The occupational health nurse should be active in professional association membership, including the applicable nursing specialty of occupational health. This provides an aspect of peer networking, mentorship, and professional support for the occupational health nurse. AAOHN serves as an excellent resource for professional and program development for the OHN.

Continuing education is required to maintain licensure as well as to maintain specialty certification in occupational health. The OHN is expected to participate in continuing education that supports the continued development of skills and knowledge specific to occupational health practice.

The Occupational Health and Safety Administration (OSHA) sponsors Education and Research Centers throughout the United States. These centers are funded and dedicated specifically to support the education and research needs of occupational health professionals and provide a wide breadth of multidisciplinary topics for continued education. Degree opportunities in the specialty of occupational health are also available. Continuing education programs and certificate programs are offered related to various occupational health specialties, such as safety and industrial hygiene. The centers also offer programs that provide education specific to clinical practice, such as hearing conservation and spirometry.

The profession of occupational health demands a dynamic, life-long commitment to continuing education and professional growth. The occupational health nurse must seek opportunities for continued learning to stay abreast of changes in not only clinical aspects, but also research and regulatory aspects of the specialty as well. There are many local, state, and national conferences and workshops offered that support continued education for occupational health professionals. In today's virtual environment, the OHN is also able to seek out opportunities for continued growth and development through webinars, distance learning, and Web-based conferences.

Professional certification for occupational health nurses validates professional knowledge that is core to safe practice.

The American Board of Occupational Health Nursing (ABOHN, 2010) states that "certification is a mark of prestige," and indicates a significant personal and professional accomplishment. Certification as an occupational health nurse provides evidence that the OHN holds knowledge regarding management of occupational illnesses and injuries, regulatory requirements that affect the workplace, disease management, and health promotion strategies. Certification as an occupational health nurse "indicates mastery of a body of knowledge that is current and reflects cutting edge practice" (Salazar et al., 2002). Employers may regard certification as a mark of quality and may take this into consideration when making selection decisions to fill the position of the occupational health nurse (ABOHN, 2010).

Two specialty certification designations are available:

1. The Certified Occupational Health Nurse (COHN) is available to registered nurses holding a minimum of associate or diploma degrees. The core content of the examination is focused on validating knowledge related to direct clinical care. This certification provides value for the occupational health nurse in the clinical environment or for those who are in case management roles.
2. The Certified Occupational Health Nurse-Specialist (COHN-S) is available to registered nurses with a bachelor's degree or higher. The core content of the COHN-S examination also validates knowledge for OHNs in management, education, and consultant roles.

Additional information about specialty occupational health nursing certification is available at www.abohn.org.

PROFESSIONAL LIABILITY

Unlike traditional nursing roles, occupational health nurses often work in autonomous environments. The OHN may be the only healthcare professional on-site in the workplace. For this reason, professional competence is an expectation. Additionally, the OHN must have a network of professional and specialty resources and mentors to assist in clinic and administrative decision making.

Oakley (2008) advises that OHNs should surround themselves with clinical and professional support in order to maintain and improve specific standards of care by developing practice-focused relationships. Because most OHNs work in isolation, professional supervision and mentorship are key to successful practice.

A traditional healthcare setting often provides nurses with professional liability coverage. This is not true of most other workplace settings where OHNs establish practice. The OHNs will find themselves in workplace settings that do not have healthcare as a core aspect of operations. This includes manufacturing and industrial settings, other service industries such as hospitality, and various other workplace settings. It therefore becomes important that the OHN secure professional liability or malpractice insurance that is appropriate to the practice setting and provides coverage for the scope of practice in that setting (AAOHN, 2000). The OHN should ensure that the company's general liability insurance addresses coverage for the scope of practice of the occupational health program and team members. In addition, the OHN should secure professional malpractice insurance coverage appropriate to the scope of practice.

The occupational health nurse must maintain keen awareness of risks and liabilities associated with the scope of practice related to program development and implementation. The OHN must research and know the regulations and statutory guidelines that guide practice, maintaining an awareness of proposed legislative changes that affect the professional scope of practice or that may affect any aspect of the occupational health program. The OHN should seek guidance from risk management or legal professionals as appropriate, not only to address liability for personal practice, but also to address the impact of program development and associated liability for the company. The OHN should seek content experts and mentors to assist with decision making related to legal and professional aspects of practice.

CONFIDENTIALITY

The Health Insurance Portability and Availability Act of 1996 (HIPAA) protects any personally identifiable health information (protected health information, or PHI) from unauthorized disclosure. HIPAA applies to an employer if the employer sponsors any "health clinic operations available to employees, or provides a self-insured health plan for employees, or acts as the intermediary between its employees and healthcare providers" (U.S. Department of Health and Human Services, 2003). The OHN has the responsibility of determining if the services provided within the occupational health program fall under the definitions of a covered entity as a healthcare provider (Litchfield, 2009). The privacy rule controls how a health plan or covered healthcare provider discloses protected health information to an employer.

In a position statement on confidentiality of medical information in the workplace, ACOEM recommends that the occupational health professional must "attempt to balance the importance of the worker's need and right to keep information confidential versus the employer's need and legal right to know or the interests of other parties" (ACOEM, 2008).The occupational health nurse must be keenly familiar with all HIPAA regulations, including state-specific regulations that apply to the work setting. AAOHN recommends that all of all protected health information be controlled by the occupational health nurse. This process should include obtaining the appropriate authorization for disclosure from the worker and releasing this information only when it is appropriate for the worker's situation. In the occupational health setting, there are three levels of confidentially that require diligence in regard to HIPAA (AAOHN, 2003).

Level I information includes any information required by law. OSHA (2004) holds that the HIPAA privacy rules do not apply to required information on the OSHA 300 log and the removal of names from the log is not necessary. In addition, when information is required for public health purposes, legal proceedings, or regulatory purposes, HIPAA does not apply. For this reason, HIPAA does not apply to workers' compensation health information. This includes information related to worker exposures, illnesses, and injuries incurred in the workplace. In addition, if health information is required for emergency purposes or for purposes of national security, HIPAA does not apply.

Level II includes information obtained for the purposes of fitness for duty of the worker. HIPAA is applicable in the occupational health setting for the purposes of medical surveillance. The employer or the healthcare provider must provide written notice to the worker that the protected personal health information will be disclosed to the employer.

Level III includes all other health information. This includes all health information related to health problems that are non-work-related. This includes information related to all healthcare encounters, including mental health and related counseling.

According to AAOHN (2003), confidentiality is a "professional and ethical issue as well as a legal obligation and should be handled with a high level of professionalism." In a position statement on confidentiality of medial information in the workplace, the American College of Occupational and Environmental Medicine (ACOEM, 2008) writes "all employee health and medical records should be treated as confidential by the employer and provider."

The occupational health nurse will encounter a variety of situations where access to protected health information is of concern and is covered under HIPAA regulations. This includes, but is not limited to, medical records from worker's personal healthcare providers for non-work-related situations, return-to-work notes that may contain diagnoses or treatment information, health history information collected in the occupational health setting related to health promotion activities, healthcare benefits data, protected information attached to health benefits claims, and all personal health information gathered by the occupational health nurse in relation to incidental visits to the occupational health clinic or office.

The occupational health setting should have written policies and procedures addressing confidentiality of protected health information, including how this information is released and transmitted. The policies should address how health information is collected, stored, and who has access to the records. The policies should address a procedure for workers to file a complaint and procedures on how to handle a complaint. A medical records custodian should be identified, and preferably will be the occupational health nurse. Training should be provided to all employees who may have access to protected health information. In the occupational health clinic setting, the worker must be provided written notice of the privacy practices related to their medical records.

Protected health information should never be used to influence hiring decisions or any other decisions related to human resources or benefits and should never be disclosed to other entities without full, written permission of disclosure by the worker. Health information related to regulatory benefits of the Americans with Disabilities Act and Family Medical Leave Act should be kept separate from personnel records and in a separate locked file. And although HIPAA does not apply to workers' compensation claims, some states impose limits on what health information the employer may know. Therefore, the OHN must ensure that access to health information is in compliance with appropriate state and federal statutes.

HIPAA compliance assistance is available at http://www.hhs.gov/ocr/privacy/hipaa/understanding/summary/privacysummary.pdf.

SUMMARY

The success of an occupational health program is often dependent on management's perception of health and safety needs of the workplace and the perceived value of the occupational health professional. Physicians and nurses hold valuable roles that contribute to the success of an occupational health program. These healthcare professionals are expected to develop core competencies that meet certain qualifications, including clinical skills, behaviors, and intellectual knowledge, that support the value of the occupational health professional. Table 2.5 outlines the core competencies of both nurses and physicians in occupational health.

It is important to clearly identify who will manage the occupational health services and to whom this person reports. The opportunity to report to a high level within the organization provides direct access to members of the senior management team. This may prove valuable in minimizing conflicts of interest and keeping lines of communication open. The occupational health nurse should be included in all workplace policy-making decisions related to safety and health. Keeping senior management personally and routinely informed of program operations is of key importance in maintaining a successful occupational health program.

Table 2.5 Comparison of Core Competencies for Nurses and Physicians in Occupational Health.

Occupational Health Nurse	Occupational Medicine Physician
Clinical	Clinical
Case management	Work fitness and disability integration
Workplace environmental issues	Environmental health
Regulatory/legislative	Law and regulations
Management	Toxicology
Health promotion	Health and productivity
Education and training	Hazard recognition, evaluation, and control
Research	Disaster preparedness and emergency management
Professionalism	Public health, surveillance, and disease prevention

Source: www.AAOHN.org, www.ACOEM.org

REFERENCES

American Association of Occupational Health Nurses (AAOHN) Advisory. (2000). Managing professional risk. *AAOHN Journal, 50*(1), 166–171.

American Association of Occupational Health Nurses (AAOHN). (2003). Competencies in occupational and environmental health nursing. *AAOHN Journal, 51*(7), 290–302.

American Association of Occupational Health Nurses (AAOHN). (2004). *Standards of occupational and environmental health nursing.* Retrieved from http://www.aaohn.org

American Association of Occupational Health Nurses (AAOHN). (2007). Advisory. Nurse practitioners in occupational and environmental health. Retrieved from https://www.aaohn.org/advisories/nurse-practitioners-in-occupational-and-environmental-health.html

American Association of Occupational Health Nurses, Inc. (2007). Competencies in occupational and environmental health nursing. *AAOHN Journal, 55*(11) 442–447.

American Association of Occupational Health Nurses (AAOHN). (2007). Multistate licensure. Retrieved from https://www.aaohn.org/advisories/multistate-practice.html

American College of Occupational and Environmental Medicine (ACOEM). (2008). *Confidentiality of medical information in the workplace.* Retrieved from http://www.acoem.org/guidelines.aspx?id=3538

American Association of Occupational Health Nurses (AAOHN). (2008). *Occupational and environmental health nursing profession fact sheet.* Retrieved from http://www.aaohn.org/dmdocuments/OHN

American Association of Occupational Health Nurses (AAOHN). (2009). Code of ethics and interpretive statements. Retrieved from https://www.aaohn.org/for-your-practice-items/code-of-ethics.html

American College of Occupational and Environmental Medicine (ACOEM). (2010). Guidance for occupational health services in medical centers. http://www.acoem.org/Search.aspx?q=guide+the+development+of+public+policy+in+order+to+advance+the+specialty+of+occupational+and+environmental+medicine

American Association of Occupational Health Nurses (AAOHN). (2012). AAOHN Information. The occupational and environmental health nursing profession. Revised February, 2012. Retrieved from https://www.aaohn.org/component/option,com_docman/task,cat_view/gid,129/

American Association of Occupational Health Nurses (AAOHN). (2012). Standards of occupational and environmental health nursing. *Workplace Health & Safety, 60*(3), 97–103.

American Nurses Association (ANA). (1999). Scope and standards of home health nursing practice. Washington DC: ANA Publishing.

Beser, A. & Bayil, A. (2006). A scale for evaluating employee satisfaction with nursing care. *AAOHN Journal, 54*(10), 455–461.

Burgel, B. J. (2012). The occupational health nurse as the trusted clinician in the 21st century. *Workplace Health & Safety, 60*(4), 143–150.

Damrongsak, M. & Brown, K. C. (2008). Data security in occupational health. *AAOHN Journal, 56*(10), 417–421.

D'Arruda, K. A. (2002). Legal issues: HIPAA update: Administrative simplification and national standards. *AAOHN Journal, 50*(11), 496–498.

Dirksen, M. E. (2001). Occupational and environmental health nursing: An overview. In M. K. Salazar (Ed.), Core curriculum for occupational and environmental health nursing (2nd ed., pp. 3–32). Philadelphia: W.B. Saunders.

Health Insurance Portability and Accountability Act of 1996 (HIPAA). (2000). Federal Register. 65 FR 82462. Retrieved from http://www.hhs.gov/ocr/hipaa/finalreg.html

Konradi, D. B. (2012). Learning to think like a professional nurse: A critical questions strategy. *Journal of Nursing Education, 51*(6), 359–360.

Litchfield, S. M. (2009). HIPAA and the occupational health nurse. *AAOHN Journal, 57*(10) 399.

National Council of State Boards of Nursing (NCSBN). (2007). Nurse Licensure Compact. Retrieved from http://www.ncsbn.org/nlc.htm

Oakley, Katie. (2008). Occupational health nursing. Chichester, England: John Wiley & Sons.

Occupational Safety and Health Administration (OSHA). (2004). Letters of interpretation: Section 1904.35. In *OSHA recordkeeping handbook*. Retrieved from http://www.osha.gov/Publications/recordkeeping/OSHA_3245_REVISED.pdfOccupational Safety and Health Administration (OSHA). Access to employee exposure and medical records standard. 19 CFR § 1910.20.

OCR HIPAA Privacy. (2003). *Disclosures for public health activities*. Retrieved from http://privacyruleandresearch.nih.gov/pdf/ocr_publichealth.pdf

Public Health Functions Steering Committee. (1994). *Public health in America*. Retrieved from http://www.health.gov/phfunctions/public.htm

Rogers, B. (2012). Occupational and environmental health nursing: Ethics and professionalism. *Workplace Health & Safety, 60*(4), 177–181.

Russi, M., Buchta, W. G., Swift, M., Budnick, L. D., Hodgson, M. J., Berube, D., & Kelafant, G. A. (2010). *Guidance for occupational health services in medical centers*. Retrieved from www.acoem.org.

Salazar, M. (Ed.). (2001). AAOHN core curriculum for occupational health nursing. Philadelphia: W.B. Saunders.

Salazar, M. K., Kemerer, S. D., Amann, M. C., & Fabrey, L. J. (2002). Defining the roles and functions of occupational and environmental health nurses: Results of a national job analysis. *AAOHN Journal, 50*(1), 16–25.

Strasser, P. B. (2012). Occupational and environmental health nursing: The foundations of quality practice. *Workplace Health & Safety 60*(4), 151–157.

successful interdisciplinary collaboration.

Thompson, M. C. (2006). Legislation affecting occupational health nursing: Identifying relevant laws and regulations. *AAOHN Journal*, 54(1), 38–45.

Thompson, M. C. (2012). Professional autonomy of occupational health nurses in the United States. *Workplace Health & Safety* 60(4), 159–165.

U.S. Department of Health and Human Services. (2003). *Summary of the HIPAA privacy rule*. Retrieved from http://www.hhs.gov/ocr/privacy/hipaa/understanding/summary/privacysummary.pdf

U.S. Department of Health and Human Services. *Employers and Health Information in the Workplace*. Retrieved from http://www.hhs.gov/ocr/privacy/hipaa/understanding/consumers/employers.html

U.S. Department of Health and Human Services *Health Information Privacy for Covered Entities*. Retrieved from: http://www.hhs.gov/ocr/privacy/hipaa/understanding/coveredentities/index.html

Wachs, J. E. (2005). Building the occupational health team: Keys to successful interdisciplinary collaboration. *AAOHN Journal*, 53(4), 166–171.

Wachs, J. E. (2005). Collaboration. *AAOHN Journal*, 53(4), 158.

Workers and Workplaces

3

The workplace is a sum of its parts . . . with a focus on the promotion of health, safety, and well-being of individuals, the employer will reap the benefits of a more productive workplace.

(Guzik)

Support for a healthy workforce is the basis for occupational health. This implies that the occupational health nurse (OHN) will focus efforts on creating a healthy work environment, with an emphasis on individual health, safety, and injury prevention.

In order to support the success of the occupational health program, the OHN must know the work environment, including processes and physical demands. The OHN should collect, analyze, interpret, and communicate information related to the diversity of the workforce, along with related injuries, illnesses, risks, and hazards. This information is then used to guide the development of policies, procedures, and strategies that will lead to risk reduction and intervention activities. The emphasis is to raise awareness within the workplace among management and workers of opportunities to enhance the health of workers and safety of the workplace.

The duties of the OHN are often determined by the work setting and worker population served. OHNs "seek to prevent job-related injuries and illnesses, provide monitoring and emergency care services, and help employers implement health and safety standards" (Bureau of Labor Statistics, 2010).

Because workplace injuries and illness can often be prevented, information about where, when, how, and why workers get ill or injured on the job is needed to develop preventive and health promotion strategies. This information may be gathered from accident reports and injury logs and compared to national data for workforces in the same industrial categories. Workforce statistical data gathered through the human resources department will provide information related to the diversity of the workforce, including age, gender, and ethnicity.

Essentials for Occupational Health Nursing, First Edition. Arlene Guzik.
© 2013 John Wiley & Sons, Inc. Published 2013 by John Wiley & Sons, Inc.

In addition, data regarding health benefits utilization gathered from the company's health benefits providers may offer information regarding both occupational and non-occupational health claims.

Public health data can also be used to identify effective preventive practices for specific populations. This data may also guide the development of new and safer production processes, work practices, or improved technologies. These data enable the OHN to plan educational activities and support changes to make the workplace healthier and safer.

This approach to population-based data is founded on the principles of epidemiology, an aspect of medical science that looks at the distribution and determinants of health in specific populations. A unique aspect of occupational health is that the OHN must deal with individuals as patients while also dealing with workforce populations. Occupational health professionals hold expertise in the prevention, evaluation, and management of worker populations and associated health risks (Russi et al., 2010).

It is important to note that today's workers are increasingly a part of a global workforce, requiring OHNs to include this aspect as a part of the analysis of the workforce. It is important for the OHN to also analyze and plan to meet the needs of the international worker. Workers assigned to locations in foreign countries should be included in the OHN's assessment of the workforce. In addition, international travel is common in today's workforce. Worker assignments in foreign locations and assignment to foreign travel may present significant health risks, especially in remote, tropical, or developing countries (Burestero, 2000).

WORKFORCE CHARACTERISTICS

There are millions of people employed in the world, and many of those people hold more than one job. Our workforce is becoming much more diverse and older. The workforce also includes an increasing number of women. In the United States, there is an increasing shift from goods-producing industries to service-provider industries. Over the years, there has also been a significant increase in the use of temporary workers. We have also seen an increase in alternative work arrangements, such as working from home and virtual work environments.

With declining birth rates, the growth of the working age population, ages 15–64, will slow. Thus, the average age of the workforce is expected to rise. People are working past retirement age, and they are making up a larger share of the labor pool. The level of education of the average worker is also rising., and most jobs today are demanding higher education requirements.

According to the U.S. Census Bureau and the U.S. Administration on Aging (2010), there were approximately 39 million Americans aged 65 and over. By 2030, the number of Americans over the age of 65 is expected to rise to 70 million. It is anticipated that we will soon experience a labor shortage of about 23 million workers as a result of retiring workers who will vacate 32 million positions. In addition, there will be 20 million newly created jobs. The labor force will face the largest shortages ever seen, and businesses will be competing for top talent.

According to the U.S. Bureau of Labor Statistics (2010), total employment is projected to increase and reflect an aging and more radically diverse racial and ethnic workforce. Most new jobs will be in professional and service-related occupations. Persons aged 55 years and older are projected to make up nearly one-fourth of the labor force. Increased immigration, along with a higher growth rate among minorities, will have an influence on the increasing diversity of the workforce.

WORKFORCE POPULATIONS

For the first time in history, we have four generations represented in the workforce.

The oldest work group, often referred to as *The Matures* or *Veterans*, were born between the 1920s and the 1940s. This group represents approximately 25% of the work population. Known as the silent generation, these workers are known to be loyal, hardworking, and disciplined. They are conservative and mindful of company and societal rules. They have lived through The Great Depression and economic hardship. Having lived through World War II and the Korean War, they are patriotic. This group saw the establishment of the Social Security System and the rise of labor unions. They believe in the value of hard work, sacrifice for the common good, and loyalty to the organization. Their support for the needs of the group supersede individual needs. They have definite respect for authority and have a strong work ethic and loyalty to the organization. They do best in a very organized work environment and, as a result, may be averse to risk.

The largest group of today's workers are known as the *Baby Boomers*, born between the 1940s and 1960s. This group drives to excel and is very group oriented. They take pride in accomplishments and also have great respect for rank and title. They have lived through economic prosperity and have seen the expansion of suburbia. Baby Boomers lived through the Vietnam War, assassinations of public figures, and the civil rights movement. They also experienced the evolution of television and space endeavors. Baby Boomers grew up in a time of prosperity, change, and expansion, leaving them with a strong sense of security. They became less concerned about career issues and more concerned about family and future security. They are optimistic, team oriented, and committed to volunteerism. They compromise approximately 53% of the labor force and most likely lead the majority of businesses in the United States (Kowalski, 2004).

A third group of workers, called *Generation X*, born between the 1960s and 1980s, represent a large multicultural workforce. This is a very educated, resourceful, and entrepreneurial group. A large percentage of this group is college educated. They have lived through harsh economic conditions. Many grew up in homes where both parents were working or in single-parent homes, and they were known as *latchkey kids*. As a result, they grew very resourceful. They are computer literate, focused on personal development, independent, and take great initiative. They think globally. This is a very

37

spiritual group, focused on quality of life. They are loyal to people, but not necessarily to the employer. This generation has been marked by unrest and disappointment in leaders, causing anxiety around health, safety, job, and financial security.

A fourth group of workers born between 1980s and 2000s are known as *Generation Y*. This group is technically proficient, having grown up in the age of technology. This ethnically diverse population includes worldly, highly educated, and civic-minded individuals. They have a strong sense of integrity and value. They are optimistic. Because of the advances in technology and the enormous number of conveniences, this generation is frequently flooded with choices, often driving their ambition and achievements. Information is at their fingertips because of their proficiency in surfing the Internet. Yet because of this, their choices and decisions may often be made without the benefit of wisdom and skill gained through experience.

Managing generational workforces is often a challenge. The OHN should have a working knowledge of the differences and characteristics of each group of workers.

The Matures are a stable and detail-oriented group. Their work is thorough. They are loyal and hardworking. Despite these assets, they may be perceived as a liability due to their reluctance to change. Because they are uncomfortable with conflict, they may be reticent to challenge the system and unwilling to look for opportunities for improvement.

Baby Boomers are service oriented and driven to go the extra mile. They are good at relationships and willing to please. They live to work. Baby Boomers also are uncomfortable with change and conflict and therefore unwilling to cause unrest. They are focused on process and not necessarily on outcome.

Generation X is known as being adaptable and independent. They are not intimidated by authority. They are technologically literate and very creative. They work to live, meaning the quality of their personal lives may be more important than work. They are often impatient and inexperienced. They are criticized as being cynical and having poor people skills.

Generation Y is loyal and optimistic. They are able to multitask, and they are fast thinking and technologically savvy. Because of their lack of real-world experience, they have a need for supervision and structure. With a strong focus on technology, they may have poor people and service skills.

MANAGING DIVERSITY
Issues are often generation specific. The OHN must learn to modify the tactics of communication in order to be effective in managing and training this diverse workforce.

The OHN must be flexible to incorporate feedback from all workers and capitalize on the strengths of all generations and cultural differences.

Although the characteristics of workers show significant differences, there are common concepts that must create the underpinning of effective management

Table 3.1 Training and development.

Generations	Matures	Boomers	Gen X	Gen Y
Traditional learning resources	Machines	Television	Computers	Internet
Strategies for effective training	Take plenty of time.	Use team-building exercises.	Provide access to different types of information.	Provide more structure and supervision.
	Give them the big picture.	Focus on challenges.	Focus on balance.	Focus on customer service and interpersonal skills.
	Emphasize long-term goals.	Focus on the near future.	Help them train for another job.	Clearly communicate expectations.
	Let them share their experience.	Focus on their role.	Provide resource lists.	Let them know what they do matters.

and training. Table 3.1 outlines strategies for effective training for diverse populations. Although the strategies for training should be modified to meet the diversity of the workforce, work performance expectations should not differ for these different work groups. Every worker should be held to the standard outlined for the job. Accommodations should not be made that compromise the integrity of the organization or diminish the effectiveness of the organization's mission. Each worker is expected to support the mission of the organization. All workers should comply with policies and procedures set forth by the organization.

Despite their differences, commonalities may be found among the different generational groups. Typically, everyone wants to succeed and everyone wants to feel valued. Workers want to be kept informed about matters that concern them in the workplace. Workers want clear communication about the expectations of their employer.

Although the generational work groups may vary in their work style and expectations, their reaction to change, challenges, and organizational politics may also be different. This may create a collision of values, expectations, ambitions, and attitudes. Situational style of leadership should be employed, using strategies that bring out the best in each worker and capitalize on their individual and generational interests. The OHN should use a variety of tactics, such a special projects, committee work, team-building efforts, technology skills, and network groups as part of training efforts.

Training and development should capitalize on the use of coaching and mentoring situations among the generational groups. The OHN should provide opportunities that include independent study as well as group learning experiences. One important consideration in a multigenerational workforce is that the workers may learn from each other through an experiential learning process.

WORKPLACES
Most U.S. workplaces employ fewer than 500 workers, and these small businesses represent 98% of all U.S. business enterprises. Yet, many of these workplaces fail to have formal health and safety programs in place. The need for a formal occupational health program is based on the employer's evaluation of the nature of its business, the potential for hazard, the physical demands of the job functions, and its geographical location (Balge & Krieger, 2000).

Standard Industrial Codes
The standard industrial classification (SIC) system is used to classify workplaces by type of activity. These classifications are used for the purpose of data collection and analysis (USOMB, 2010). The assignment of an industrial code is based on the primary activity of the business. The activity is determined by the primary product produced or distributed or the primary services rendered. Table 3.2 outlines some major industrial classifications.

The Standard Industrial Classification (SIC) system defines categories of workplaces with common characteristics (OSHA, 2010). Common categories include the following:

- Division A: Agriculture. This category includes all forms of agriculture, including farming, livestock, and forestry. Also included in this category are fishing and hunting trades.
- Division B: Mining. This category includes mining for coal, metals, oil, and gas. It also includes quarry mining and mining for nonmetal minerals.
- Division C: Construction. Construction includes building and general contractors, along with contractors of special trades.
- Division D: Manufacturing. This division includes the manufacturing of food, tobacco, textiles, and apparel, along with lumber, furniture, paper, and chemicals. Also included are fabrication of metal products, stone, and clay.

Table 3.2 Standard industrial classifications.

Administrative	Public Administration
Agriculture, Forestry, Fishing	Retail trade
Construction	Services
Finance, Insurance, Real Estate	Transportation, Communication, Utilities
Management	Utilities
Mining	Wholesale Trade

Source: Occupational Safety and Health Administration (OSHA). U.S. Department of Labor. http://www.osha.gov/pls/imis/sic_manual.html. 2010

- Division E: Transportation, Communication, Utilities. This category includes railroad and public transport, along with transportation by water and air. Also included are pipelines for gas, sanitary services, and electric utilities. Communication includes radio and television broadcast, telegraph, and cable services.
- Division F: Wholesale Trade. Wholesale trade includes trade for durable and nondurable goods.
- Division G: Retail Trade. Includes building and hardware, general merchandise, and automotive trade. It also includes food, apparel, furniture and furnishings, along with dining establishments.
- Division H: Finance, Insurance, Real Estate. This division includes banking, credit and commodities brokers, along with real estate and investment.
- Division I: Services. In this category are lodging, entertainment, and personal services, along with business, engineering, and automotive services. Also included in this category are healthcare, legal, and educational services.
- Division J: Public Administration. Includes executive, legislative, and judicial government, including economic and national security affairs.

Additional definitions of workforce characteristics can be found in *The Dictionary of Occupational Titles* (USDOL, 2003). This information categorizes workers into specific job types related to particular industries. The DOL assigns a unique description code to each occupation within a specific industry.

The settings related to the above classifications each provide unique experiences and challenges for the occupational health program. The environment of the workplace is changing rapidly, with increased technology and globalization. This impacts the demographic, social, and technological forces within the workplace. The occupational health nurse must make observational assessments focused on inspection of the work performed and job hazard analysis. This includes the assessment of physical, biological, and airborne hazards, including repetition and mechanical stressors.

Despite these differences, the Occupational Safety and Health Act of 1970 (OSH Act) states that employers are responsible for providing a workplace "free from recognized hazards that are causing or are likely to cause death or serious physical harm." The employer must provide a mechanism to identify potential occupational hazards and implement effective hazard management. The OHN can play a key role in meeting this expectation.

In considering the development of a safety and health program, the employer should take into consideration a number of factors. According to the Occupational Safety and Health Administration (OSHA, 2010), the decision should take into consideration the number and types of hazards in the workplace, along with the distance and access to community-based healthcare facilities. The decision is also based on the level of management support, seriousness of the hazards, and the need for training and education of workers.

When considering the services of an OHN, the following should be taken into account:

1. Is the workplace a large corporation, or do they have an affiliation with a large corporation with geographical branches. Larger corporations are most likely to have a strong occupational health and safety program. As a result, they will tend to implement a more structured approach to occupational health services in the company's remote geographical locations.
2. If the workplace is not a part of a larger corporation, what resources are currently available for occupational health and safety?
3. What is the geographical layout of the workplace? How many buildings or sites are there?
4. What is the physical location of worksite? Is it located in an urban, suburban, or rural environment?
5. Is there efficient access to adequate medical services in the community?
6. What are the hazardous exposures that are most likely to occur?
7. What are the job-oriented and worker-oriented activities? Do these activities involve machines, tools, or equipment that may put workers at risk?
8. What is the context of the work performed? Is manual labor involved? What technology is available? And what human resources are required?
9. What physical demands or mental processes are required as essential functions for the job?
10. What is management's expectation for production and quota-related performance?
11. What is the social climate of the workplace? Is it worker friendly? Is it a labor union environment?
12. What is the relationship of workers with management? Is it a participative environment? Does management value its workers, and do the workers value the company?
13. What is the predominant style of communication and decision making?
14. What is the anticipated future and the projected rate of growth for the company?

Business justification for an OHN is dependent on the nature of the business activity, potential for hazardous workplace exposures and injuries, physical demands of the jobs, geographic location of the business, and available community resources. Organizations with more than 250 employees and workplaces with relatively high occupational illness and injury rates are more likely to employee an OHN. Most common employer-based sites with OHNs include manufacturing, service providers, transportation, communication, and utilities. A workplace involved in high-hazard work is more likely to be able to justify the cost of services of an OHN versus the workplace involved in low-hazard work (Salazar, 2001).

Practice settings for occupational health are as various as the many types of workplaces. Beyond the clinical setting, the OHN may also be employed by insurance and governmental/regulatory agencies to provide utilization review, case management services, consultation, education, and research. Specific functions are determined by a number of factors, including the nature of the work in the associated hazards, the number of employees, the organizational structure, and the organization's administrative and financial support.

The workplace management must be supportive of all efforts related to the occupational health program, and there must be a commitment to provide appropriate resources and support. The OHN must then collaborate with management to develop cost-effective health and safety programs specific to the workplace population.

FUTURE TRENDS IN OCCUPATIONAL HEALTH AND RESEARCH

According to The Bureau of Labor Statistics, working-age adults spend more than one-third of their day at work or on work-related activities (see Figure 3.1). The changing environment of the workplace and the increasing diversity of the workforce demand different approaches to education and training. One must prepare to meet the heterogeneous needs of the workforce, including gender perspectives, cultural diversity, and literacy challenges. The increasing use of part-time and temporary workers and the use of subcontractors for specialized work will continue to impact the workforce. Telecommuting is increasingly common, with workers working from home or from remote locations. The workplace is also influenced by increasing immigration and the development of multinational corporations that impact of the cultural formation and behaviors affecting workers.

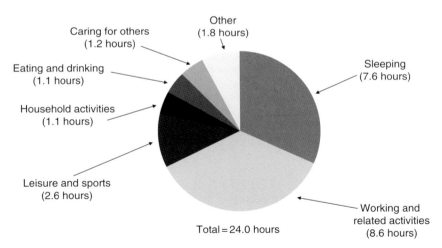

Figure 3.1 Time use on an average work day for employed persons ages 25 to 54 with children. Data include employed persons on days they worked, ages 25 to 54, who lived in households with children under 18. Data include nonholiday weekdays and are annual averages for 2010. *Source*: U.S. Department of Labor, Bureau of Labor Statistics, American Time Use Survey. http://www.bls.gov

Table 3.3 Workforce demographics and effect on business.

Changing Workplace Demographics	Effects on Occupational Health Nursing and Business
Aging workforce	• Increased worker fatigue • Increased chronic illnesses of workers • Increased healthcare costs
People working longer	• Aged people entering workforce • Postponed worker retirement • Forced retirement • Worker's decreased ability to perform essential functions • Increased on-the-job injuries • Grandparents with parental responsibilities requiring financial support to care for children
More women in the workforce	• Family issues increasingly important, more than work • Childcare obligations requiring absence from work • One-parent families resulting in absences
Workers working second and third jobs	• Decrease allegiance to single employer • Refusing overtime • Employees not afraid to resign because they have supplementary income
Increased diversity • Women • Asian and Hispanic • Multiple other nationalities	• Multilingual environment • Multicultural issues, including healthcare • Differences in work ethic • Training challenges
More immigrants • Either high or low education levels	• Challenges regarding education and cultural diversity
Electronic environment • Increased demand for computer skills • Virtual workforce	• E-mail, Internet, pagers, cell phones • Increasing use of Net meetings and conferencing • Workers working from home or remote locations
Increased cost of benefits	• More chronic illness • Increasing use of pharmaceuticals • Employee paying increased share of benefits cost • Employees opting out of benefits
Increased demand for nurses • Varied opportunities	• Critical nursing shortage • Lack of commitment on part of younger nurses • Outsourcing of nursing services

A strong focus on family, resulting in the demand for virtual work environments and flex time, impacts the workplace. Workers working second and third jobs also create an influence. U.S. workers being deployed abroad to countries with different workplace standards make it important for the OHN to be aware of international issues related to child labor, women's health, and workplace health and safety.

The aging workforce, literacy concerns, and cultural diversity will all have an impact on safety, workers' compensation and disability issues. The development of health benefits programs should include components that speak to the generational and cultural needs of the workforce. There must be a greater understanding of individual needs and respect for individual differences by creating choices and accommodating diversity. Table 3.3 outlines the expected changes in workforce demographics and the effects on occupational health nursing and business.

Interventions related to health, wellness, safety issues require consistent and clear communication, education, and training. Wellness strategies should identify specific programs that will appeal to these differences. Safety interventions should include strategies to reach each generation and meet literacy challenges. There is a growing need for continued advances in science and research regarding worker health and productivity. There is a continued need for integrated efforts between clinicians, educators, researchers, and politicians related to public policy development and funding for future research. There must be a balanced concerned for advances in science, technology, and protection for worker health and safety.

The overview of the 2010–2020 projections published by the Bureau of Labor Statistics projects significant changes in the face of tomorrow's workers and workplaces. The labor force is projected to continue to grow older (Figure 3.2).

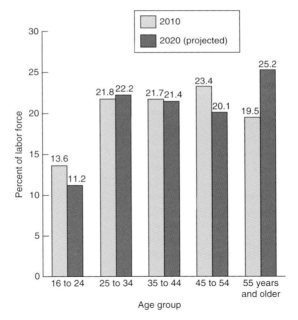

Figure 3.2 Percent of labor force, by age group.
Source: U.S. Department of Labor, Bureau of Labor Statistics, Division of Industry Employment Projections. http://www.bls.gov

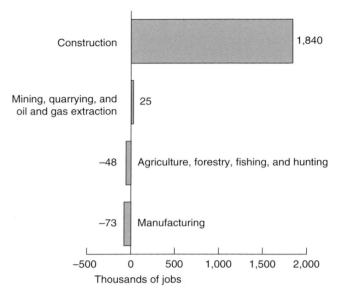

Figure 3.3 Numeric change in wage and salary employment in goods-producing industries, 2010–2020 (projected).
Source: U.S. Department of Labor, Bureau of Labor Statistics, National Employment Matrix.
http://www.bls.gov

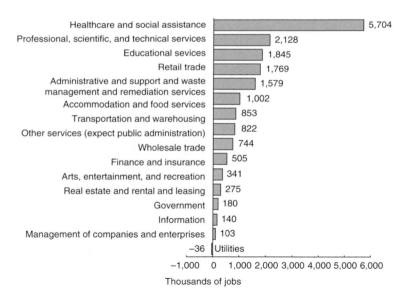

Figure 3.4 Numeric change in wage and salary employment in service-providing industries, 2010–2020 (projected).
Source: U.S. Department of Labor, Bureau of Labor Statistics, BLS National Employment Matrix.
http://www.bls.gov

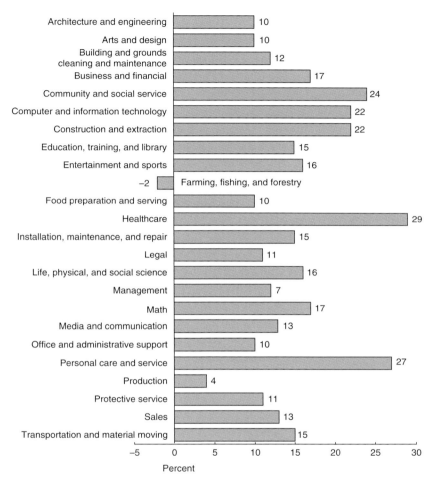

Figure 3.5 Percent change in total in employment, by major occupational group, 2010–2020 (projected). *Source*: U.S. Department of Labor, Bureau of Labor Statistics, BLS Division of Occupational Outlook. http://www.bls.gov

Goods-producing industries are projected to provide an increase in construction-related jobs mirrored by a significant loss of jobs in manufacturing (Figure 3.3). Service industry jobs are projected to increase mostly for accommodation and food services, as well as education and professional services. Healthcare-related jobs are projected to increase significantly (Figure 3.4). Job growth among occupations is projected to vary widely (Figure 3.5), and the OHN must stay abreast of these significant changes. Work

47

settings that were common to occupational health services may dwindle, resulting in changes in need for OHN services. Therefore, the OHN must maintain an awareness of business trends and be prepared to face the challenges of role change as the landscape of America's workforce evolves.

REFERENCES

Balge, M. A. & Krieger, G. R., Eds. (2000). Substance abuse. *Occupational health and safety* (3rd ed., pp. 409–430). Chicago: National Safety Council.

Burastero, S. (2000). Travel health and remote work programs. In M. A. Balge & G. R. Krieger (Eds.), *Occupational health and safety* (3rd ed., pp. 249–276). Chicago: National Safety Council.

Goetzel, R. Z., Guindon, A. M., Turshen I. J., & Ozminkowski, R. J. (2001). Health and productivity management establishing key performance measures, benchmarks and best practices. *Journal of Occupational and Environmental Medicine, 43*(1), 10–17.

Knave, B., & Ennals, R. (2002). International trends in occupational health research and practice. *Industrial Health, 40*, 69–73.

Kowalski, K. (2004). *Managing four generations.* Presentation at IPMA-HR Conference. Phoenix, Arizona.

Leggett, D. (2007) The aging work force—Helping employees navigate midlife. *AAOHN Journal, 55*(4), 169–175.

Levine, S. (1993). *The leader in you: How to win friends, influence people, and succeed in a changing world.* New York: Simon & Schuster.

Marinescu, L. G. (2007). Integrated approach for managing health risks at work—The role of occupational health nurses. *AAOHN Journal, 55*(2), 75–87.

Pelletier, B., Boles, M., & Lynch, W. (2004). Change in health risks and work productivity over time. *Journal of Occupational and Environmental Medicine, 46*(7), 746–754.

Russi, M., Buchta, W., Swift, M. Budnick, L. Hodgson, M. Berube, D. Kelafant, G. (2010). Guidance for Occupational Health Services in Medical Centers. Retrieved from http://www.acoem.org/uploadedFiles/Public_Affairs/Policies_And_Position_Statements/Guidelines/Guidelines/MCOH%20 Guidance.pdf

Salazar, M. (2001). *Core curriculum for occupational and environmental health nursing* (2nd ed.). Philadelphia: W.B. Saunders.

U.S. Department of Labor. Bureau of Labor Statistics. (2010–2011). Tomorrow's jobs. Overview of the 2008–2018 projections. *Occupational outlook handbook* (2010-2011 ed.). Retrieved from http://www.bls.gov/oco/oco2003.htm

U.S. Department of Labor (USDOL). (2003). *Dictionary of occupational titles* (4th ed.). Retrieved from http://www.occupationalinfo.org

U.S. Department of Labor. (1970). OSH Act. Retrieved from www.osha.gov/pls/oshaweb/owasrch.search_form?p_doc_type=OSHACT

U.S. Department of Labor, Bureau of Labor Statistics. U.S. Census Bureau and the U.S. Administration on Aging. *SIC manual.* www.bls.gov/oco/ocos083.htm

U.S. Department of Labor, Bureau of Labor Statistics. (2009). *Employment projections: 2008–2018 summary*. Retrieved from http://www.bls.gov/oco/oco2003.htm http://www.osha.gov/pls/imis/sic_manual.html

U.S. Office of Management and Budget (UOMB). (2012). *Standard industrial classification manual*. Retrieved from http://www.census.gov/eos/www/naics/index.html

Stencel, B., Hans, B., Hanson, H. (2005). Web presentation: *Communicating across the generations*. University of Wisconsin-Extension, Department of Community Resource Development.

Program Development

4

The rationale for occupational health services is to ensure that an employer's workforce is medically qualified, fit, and available for work through the evaluation, protection, promotion, and restoration of worker health and safety.

The Occupational Safety and Health Act, Section 5 (A)(1) [Section 5(a)(1)] states that each employer shall provide "a place of employment which is free from recognized hazards that are causing or are likely to cause death or serious physical harm" to workers. Businesses are impacted by nearly $170 billion in expenses related to occupational injuries and illnesses. These costs erode company profits. Effective management of occupational health and safety can reduce injury and illness costs by 20 to 40% (OSHA, 2010). Several factors are then critical to the successful implementation of an occupational health program.

MANAGEMENT COMMITMENT

The effectiveness of an occupational health and safety program largely depends on the management's involvement in the program. This requires a strong philosophical approach that is consistent with the overall organizational goals and objectives. These goals and objectives should be well aligned across divisions and departments. For example, the development of strategies of the occupational health program should be supported by the departments of human resources, safety, finance, and operations.

Management must commit to providing the resources for program development and implementation, as well as commit to sustaining the program going forward This commitment includes a sufficient budget for capital, technical, operational, and human resource support. Management should clearly set expectations within the organization for assigned expertise and authority, as well as for a process for ongoing program evaluation. The following are core elements for success:

- Effective leadership
- Active participation and support from all levels

Essentials for Occupational Health Nursing, First Edition. Arlene Guzik.
© 2013 John Wiley & Sons, Inc. Published 2013 by John Wiley & Sons, Inc.

- A strong focus on prevention and control
- Worker education and training
- Ongoing evaluation of program effectiveness

Management should be visibly involved in the design, implementation, and evaluation of the occupational health program. This includes active involvement in establishing the workplace health and safety philosophy, participating in developing policies and procedures, and establishing the expectation that workers understand and support this philosophy. A critical aspect of support includes the fact that management must commit the necessary resources for an effective program. This includes human capital as well as financial support.

Management must also support worker involvement at all levels of the organization and support active participation of workers on safety and health committees and problem-solving groups. Management must also support the need for worker education, training, and protection. A commitment to regulatory compliance, including safety, health, and environmental regulations, is necessary for an effective occupational health program.

The occupational health nurse (OHN) is often identified as the most appropriate person to manage the occupational health program. As a result, the OHN must assume responsibility and accountability for developing an effective program. Additional philosophical support from management will include the extent and nature of providing healthcare services on site. Since healthcare usually is not a core operational aspect of most companies, management must decide the extent of healthcare services that will be provided and the associated financial and liability risk. Additional program components that should be considered include wellness and health promotion initiatives and disability management strategies. A strong philosophical approach to medical confidentially must also be defined. The OHN typically holds responsibility for health record administration. Procedures related to access to health information must be addressed at the inception of the occupational health program.

The most effective outcomes of an occupational health program are hinged on a comprehensive, holistic approach to program development. This approach stretches across multiple departments in the organizational structure. If strategies and initiatives are misaligned, the program will fail to demonstrate effective outcomes.

Strategies for Success
The OHN should use the following strategies:

- Be keenly aware of the philosophy of top leadership and plan occupational health services that support the overall organizational mission and goals
- Whenever possible, strive to have a consistent reporting structure for both health and safety programs
- Plan an approach that integrates the services of health, safety, workers' compensation, and disability management

---

Case in Point

The OHN reports to the vice president of human resources and the department manager reports to the vice president of operations. The OHN may hold responsibility for managing occupational injuries and notices a rise in injuries from a certain department. As a part of incident investigation, the OHN identifies an opportunity to reduce incidents that arise from unsafe operations resulting in worker injury in a particular department within operations. The OHN decides to propose a strategy to reduce incidences that lead to those injuries by improving safety. The strategy requires a financial investment in personal protective equipment (PPE) for the workers. This most likely will lead to reduced incidences of risk and injury. There will be fewer injuries, and this could result in lower workers' compensation costs. Since this is one of the performance expectations of the OHN, it surely seems a great idea.

When the OHN approaches the operations manager with the strategy, there is strong resistance. The bottom line is that there is not enough money in the operations manager's budget to support the purchase of the PPE and provide the appropriate worker training. If the operations manager spends money on the unbudgeted PPE, this means the department will be over budget, and the operations manager will be held accountable. And besides, it's not just about the purchase of the PPE. Workers will need to spend time in training sessions to learn the appropriate use of the PPE. This will result in reduced productivity of the department. Since the use of PPE will not have any direct influence on increasing productivity, efficiency, or output, it becomes difficult for the operations manager to explain the budget variance to the vice president of operations and the manager is hesitant to approach his boss about the situation. This scenario identifies an inconsistent philosophy related to improving safety and reducing injuries between the OHN and the operations manager.

Let's consider an alternative that is a result of a consistent philosophy.

- Because of top management's expectation that there will be support for a safe and healthy workforce, the operations manager realizes this is a great opportunity. The OHN and the operations manager then devise a plan to address both the vice president of human resources and the vice president of operations with the plan. They develop a plan of action for purchasing the PPE and training workers on the use of PPE. They have included associated costs, not only for the equipment, but also for the expected cost impact of training on operations. The plan also includes the expected return on investment (ROI) as a result of reduced frequency of incidents and injuries, including medical costs and lost productivity. They are able to demonstrate the cost-benefit analysis that leads to significant saving in workers' compensation claims experience.

- Develop written policies and procedures on all aspects of the health and safety programs
- Establish a strong stay-at-work philosophy that support worker productivity

WORKPLACE ASSESSMENT

Once the company philosophy is clear, and before making changes in the safety and health operations, the OHN should gather information about the current culture and practices that are part of the organization. Assessment strategies should focus on identifying the atmosphere of organizational politics and strategies (Rogers, 2003).

The physical location of the workplace is critical to the planning process. Where is the workplace located? Is it close to community resources, such as hospitals and urgent care centers? What is the average travel time to the emergency departments or the average response time for EMS? Are the workers working in close proximity, or are they dispersed over a larger geographic location or several buildings? How many workers are employed? Is there rapid employee turnover? Is there expected growth of the company?

The OHN must know the audience and decision makers within the organization. Is the company an independent workplace, or is it a remote unit or subsidiary of a larger corporation? Large corporations often have corporate occupational health and safety programs that provide a host of resources to the smaller, remote units. In addition, there may be a corporate medical director or nurse manager who assists in establishing the corporate philosophy and strategies. As a result, the smaller work unit must comply with corporate plans and programs.

Because occupational health programs impact several aspects of the organization, it is important to know the key players that will be involved in decisions. Executive management sets the tone for expectations; however, legal and financial aspects must also be considered. Others having stake in the program may include risk management, safety, human resources, and labor unions. The OHN must also identify program partners outside the organization, such as workers' compensation, group health insurers or third-party administrators, and legal counsel, that may serve to influence change or be impacted by change.

The formal structure of the organization is usually straightforward; however, most organizations have an internal culture that integrates relationships between workers. This culture establishes an informal mechanism for working relationships, communication, and decision making. Communication within organizations takes place in both formal and informal forms. It is important for the OHN to recognize that there is value in both forms that can be used to communicate health and safety strategies.

Recognition of the leadership styles that pervade the organization is also important. Change is often disruptive and may create discomfort at all levels of the organization and therefore requires strong leadership (Daft, 2004). The OHN will be more successful in initiating and implementing change when management and workers are willing to commit. Clear communication through both formal and informal channels may prove to be a valuable strategy.

The OHN must also assess the physical structure and condition of the workplace and the existing supplies and resources available to the safety and health program, recognizing both acceptable and unsafe or unhealthful work practices. The assessment should include checking on the use of any hazardous materials, observing employee work habits and practices, and discussing safety and health problems with employees (OSHA, 2005). There are low-hazard workplaces, such as service industries, and there are more hazardous work conditions, such as industrial and construction settings. Thus the nature of the workplace regarding work activity, physical demands, geographic locations, and hazardous exposures set the tone for the development of occupational health and safety strategies. Facilities and equipment should be evaluated with regard to regulatory compliance and inspection schedules. A workplace inspection checklist (see Table 4.1), along with other resources, is available at www.cdc.gov/niosh/docs/2004-135 (NIOSH, 2004). The checklist can be customized by adding or deleting items that particularly apply to the worksite.

Specific health and safety needs of the worker population must also be assessed. Observing how workers work and interact in the workplace provides information about how the work is accomplished and may also provide insight regarding the need for change. This type of interaction also allows workers to get to know the OHN and may foster a sense of respect and support. Interviews with employees or focus groups may also assist in gathering pertinent information.

Addressing immediate needs is important; however, the focus of an effective occupational health program is based on long-term strategies that support and sustain the health and protection of the workforce. An assessment of the workplace should include a comprehensive health and safety survey intended to identify potential risks and hazards. The workplace assessment should include an analysis of current safety and health-training activities, work practices, and existing policies and procedures. Worker job descriptions should be reviewed to identify physical job demands, potential risks, and associated health and safety training needs.

The OHN should gather information related to incident and accident data. Special attention should be given to identification of recurring incidents, accidents, and injury types and severity in relation to specific operations, departments, and locations. Review first aid cases, OSHA recordable cases, and workers' compensation claims with attention to the impact on cost and losses in productivity. Comparing the company's insurance rating with others in the same industry will provide data that may support the need for improvement. Data gathered from the human resources department regarding worker absences and disability benefit utilization may prove valuable. Group health benefits data can also provide important information

Table 4.1 Workplace inspection checklist.

Self-inspections should address safety and health issues in the following areas:

- **Processing, Receiving, Shipping and Storage**—equipment, job planning, layout, heights, floor loads, projection of materials, material handling and storage methods, training for material handling equipment.
- **Building and Grounds Conditions**—floors, walls, ceilings, exits, stairs, walkways, ramps, platforms, driveways, aisles.
- **Housekeeping Program**—waste disposal, tools, objects, materials, leakage and spillage, cleaning methods, schedules, work areas, remote areas, storage areas.
- **Electricity**—equipment, switches, breakers, fuses, switch-boxes, junctions, special fixtures, circuits, insulation, extensions, tools, motors, grounding, national electric code compliance.
- **Lighting**—type, intensity, controls, conditions, diffusion, location, glare and shadow control.
- **Heating and Ventilation**—type, effectiveness, temperature, humidity, controls, natural and artificial ventilation and exhausting.
- **Machinery**—points of operation, flywheels, gears, shafts, pulleys, key ways, belts, couplings, sprockets, chains, frames, controls, lighting for tools and equipment, brakes, exhausting, feeding, oiling, adjusting, maintenance, lockout/tagout, grounding, work space, location, purchasing standards.
- **Personnel**—training, including hazard identification training; experience; methods of checking machines before use; type of clothing; PPE; use of guards; tool storage; work practices; methods for cleaning, oiling, or adjusting machinery.
- **Hand and Power Tools**—purchasing standards, inspection, storage, repair, types, maintenance, grounding, use and handling.
- **Chemicals**—storage, handling, transportation, spills, disposals, amounts used, labeling, toxicity or other harmful effects, warning signs, supervision, training, protective clothing and equipment, hazard communication requirements.
- **Fire Prevention**—extinguishers, alarms, sprinklers, smoking rules, exits, personnel assigned, separation of flammable materials and dangerous operations, explosion-proof fixtures in hazardous locations, waste disposal and training of personnel.
- **Maintenance**—provide regular and preventive maintenance on all equipment used at the worksite, recording all work performed on the machinery and training personnel on the proper care and servicing of the equipment.
- **PPE**—type, size, maintenance, repair, age, storage, assignment of responsibility, purchasing methods, standards observed, training in care and use, rules of use, method of assignment.
- **Transportation**—motor vehicle safety, seat belts, vehicle maintenance, safe driver programs.
- **First Aid Program/Supplies**—medical care facilities locations, posted emergency phone numbers, accessible first aid kits.
- **Evacuation Plan**—establish and practice procedures for an emergency evacuation, e.g., fire, chemical/biological incidents, bomb threat; include escape procedures and routes, critical plant operations, employee accounting following an evacuation, rescue and medical duties and ways to report emergencies.

Source: www.cdc.gov/niosh/docs/2004-135

to use to develop health and wellness strategies. Insurance carriers, local safety councils, trade associations, and state agencies may provide valuable data for benchmarking purposes.

Table 4.2 provides examples of categories of data that can be gathered as part of the workplace assessment.

Table 4.2 Categories of workplace assessment data.

Health of Workers	Safety	Workers' Compensation	Productivity
Group Insurance	**Incident Review**	**Cost Analysis**	**Days Away from Work**

Conduct a health benefit claims review. Analyze claims by:
• Volume
• Cost
• CPT code
• Specialty service
Analyze total claims by:
• Employee
• Dependents
• Age
• Pharmacy utilization
	Conduct an analysis of:
	• Reported incidents:
	  ◦ Frequency
	  ◦ Severity
	  ◦ Cost impact
	  ◦ Near misses
	• By department
	• By shift
	• By month
	• By day of the week
		Conduct a claims analysis for:
		• Frequency of claims
		• Claims by department
		• Average claim costs
		  ◦ Medical
		  ◦ Lost time
		  ◦ Litigation
		• Modified work days
		• Lost work days
			Review attendance rosters for:
			• Absences
			• Sick days
			  ◦ Personal
			  ◦ Family-related
			• FMLA protected days

Employee Surveys	**Employee Surveys and Worksite Walk Throughs**	**Satisfaction Survey**	**Disability Benefits**
Determine interest in: • Onsite services • Health screenings • Health education Inquire about use of healthcare provider services: • Date of last healthcare visit • Nature of the visit • Associated diagnoses • Lost work days due to illness • Date of last physical examination • Perceived barriers to healthcare	Assess knowledge of safety procedures: • Surveys • Interviews • Observe workers' adherence to safety processes and use of personal protective equipment • Observe management's compliance with safety processes and procedures	Conduct a survey of workers to determine: • Satisfaction with incident-reporting process • Satisfaction with medical services • Satisfaction with return-to-work and transitional work programs	Insurance claims: • Time off under short-term disability • Time off under long-term disability

---

Case in Point

The OHN conducts a workplace assessment without input from management or workers. A review of health benefits utilization from group health data shows that there are a large number of workers with diabetes. Careful consideration is taken to develop a plan for establishing a wellness program that includes specific health education strategies related to diabetes. A great plan is developed for a diabetes management education program and coordination with a local community health system. The plan includes a series of educational sessions provided by nutritionists and diabetes educators at the workplace. Announcements are posted throughout the workplace, including the date, time, and topics of the educational sessions. The first session is approaching, and the OHN starts talking to workers about their plans to attend. There is resistance from workers. The workers are concerned about confidentiality of their personal health information. They don't want their coworkers or their supervisors to know they have diabetes. If they show up at the educational session, surely everyone will know. There is also resistance from supervisors. They refuse to allow workers time away from their jobs to attend the educational sessions. The result: No one shows up at the first session. The OHN has now expended a lot of time, effort, and the resources of both the company and the health system on a project that has had a poor outcome.

Strategies for Success:

- The OHN should include workers and management in the assessment and planning process. This often takes place through the development of a wellness committee that comprises management and workers at all levels throughout the organization.
  - Ask what type of health education sessions workers would be interested in attending. Conduct written surveys to receive more objective information related to the interest of the workers. Develop priorities and programs based on the results of the surveys.
- Address issues and concerns of confidentiality in the planning process. If workers are concerned about attending the sessions, what are the alternative resources for sharing this information in a different format that does not require physical attendance?
- Obtain a decision from management as to whether workers are able to attend the educational sessions on work time. If so, specifically how much time will be allotted? In addition, supervisory staff must be made aware that this initiative is supported by upper management and their support is critical to the success of the program.
  - If workers are not permitted to attend the educational sessions on work time, what arrangements can be made to hold the sessions over the lunch period or on off-duty time.
- Include the members of the wellness committee as ambassadors throughout the workplace to stimulate interest and encourage attendance. Part of the promotion includes the message that you don't need to have diabetes in

order to attend. The sessions will also address risk factors and ways to reduce the risk of developing diabetes. It may also be helpful for those who have family members with diabetes.

- Assess the availability of alternatives. What resources are available for access to Web-based educational sessions and material? Is there a budget for educational material that can be dispersed throughout the workplace in various forms, such as brochures and posters? Is there access to community-based educational sessions sponsored by the local health system? How can the group health insurance provider play a role in providing worker and family access to health education?

DEVELOP A PLAN

After careful assessment, the next step in the process is to develop a plan for implementing the occupation health program. This includes the development of goals and objectives that meet the need of workers and the workplace. The OHN must formulate goals, objectives, and associated action plans that will serve as a road map for development of the program or project. The plan should identify major changes or improvements that will enhance the health and safety of the workplace.

The goals of an occupational health program should be broad, encompassing a wide range of need. The development of an occupational health program should be based on four common strategies for occupational health services (see Table 4.3):

- **Evaluation** of worker health and safety
- **Protection** of worker health and safety
- **Promotion** of work health and safety
- **Restoration** of worker health and safety

Table 4.3 Occupational health program strategies.

Evaluation	Protection	Promotion	Restoration

• Employment physicals
• Drug screens
• Fitness for duty evaluations
• Injury assessments
• First aid treatment
• Medical surveillance testing
• Biological and environmental monitoring
• Medical treatment
	• Regulatory compliance
	  ◦ OSHA
	  ◦ Workers' compensation
	  ◦ Family medical leave
	  ◦ Americans with Disabilities Act
	• Safety management
	• Hazard protection
	• Surveillance requirements
		• Wellness
		• Screenings
		• Education
		• Vaccinations
		• Disease management
		• Resource and referral
		• On-site primary care services
		• Employee assistance programs
		• Ergonomics
		• Safety awareness
			• Facilitating return to work
			• Absence management
			• Disability case management
			  ◦ Workers' compensation
			  ◦ Short and long term disability
			• Medical accommodations

It is also essential that the goals of the occupational health and safety program be consistent with the corporate mission and goals, supported from the top of the organization, and become a part of the corporate strategic plan. For instance, a goal may be intended to support the efforts of the human resources department in recruiting and retaining workers. The goals may also be targeted to areas of operations in order to support productivity and fitness for duty. The goals may be related to specific components of the occupational health program, such as safety, case management, disability management, or health promotion and assessment.

Specific objectives related to each goal must then be identified. These objectives should also be based on the occupational health and safety assessment. They must also be flexible and negotiable in regard to their relationship and interaction with other departments and initiatives within the company. Each objective should be accompanied by specific measurable outcomes that will be used to evaluate the results. There should be defined metrics that will be used for program evaluation. This may include costing health services in relation to financial investments in the program and determining a return on that investment. The measures may also include metrics related to increased productivity as a result of improved health and safety in the workplace. Sample goals, objectives, and outcome measures are provided in Table 4.4.

Part of the plan includes establishing a budget. There are two parts to establishing a budget: expected revenue and associated expenses. For each aspect of the occupational health program an estimated value and cost-benefit must be derived. It is difficult to approach management and ask for financial support for an occupational health program if the financial return on investment cannot be demonstrated. In relation to the occupational health budget, the term *revenue* is used in a broad sense. In the most traditional occupational health setting, the program is not a revenue-generating department. It does not serve to generate direct income for the company. The revenue or value of an occupational health program is demonstrated primarily through cost savings and increased productivity. It is therefore quite important, when asking for financial support for program development, to clearly outline the return on investment. The OHN must be able to articulate and demonstrate value in relation to the cost of the program.

An established plan will serve additional purposes. Of utmost importance, the plan should define the size and type of facility required for successful operation of the occupational health services. The plan may serve to outline the number of occupational health nurses and personnel necessary to execute the plan. It should also outline specific equipment and capital needs related to the program. Additional resources may be needed for the implementation of the occupational health program, and the plan should include resources for the development of written policies and procedures, resources for the treatment of first aid and emergencies, examination and testing areas, and facilities for substance testing.

Table 4.4 Sample occupational health program goal statements.

Goals	Objectives	Expected Outcome Measures
To provide efficient access to quality healthcare in a cost-effective manner	• To establish an on-site occupational health clinic	• Employees visit the clinic for health-related issues ◦ Number of visits/ utilization • Reduction in workers' compensation costs
To reduce risk and improve safety of the workplace	• To implement a formal process for evaluation of incidents that may lead to injuries and illnesses • To develop written procedures and educate workers on the process for reporting incidences and near misses	• Reduction in number of incidents • Reduction in number and severity of work-related injuries and illnesses • Reduction in workers' compensation claim costs
To support a productive workplace through minimizing disability and the development of a stay-at-work philosophy	• To provide a formal process of case management for both occupational and nonoccupational claims • To establish transitional work plans to accommodate health-related restrictions	• Reduced days away from work ◦ Occupational ◦ Nonoccupational • Reduced cost related to absences and disability
To maintain worker support and satisfaction with health and safety initiatives	• To develop a health and safety committee that will assist in the development, implementation, and evaluation of health and safety program initiatives	• Workers are better informed and educated on health and safety policies and procedures • Increased participation of workers in health and safety programs
To enhance the ability to recruit and retain quality employees in an environment of increasing competition	• To develop a company-wide wellness and health promotion initiative • Open an on-site primary care clinic • Open an on-site fitness center	• Participation of workers in health promotion activities

The location of for the occupational health facility hinges on the types of services that will be provided. The facility should be located near the area of most risk, have quick access, and ensure a confidentiality. It is also determined by the size of the company, number and health characteristics of the workers, types of processes and services conducted, the number of shifts to be covered, and the potential health and safety hazards (Russi et al., 2010).

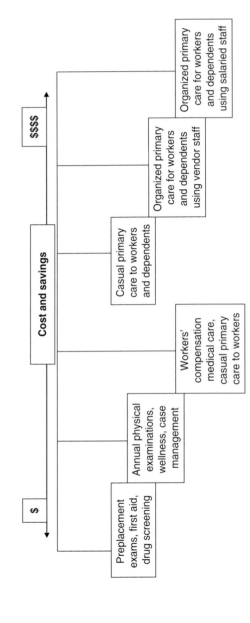

Figure 4.1 Occupational health services continuum.

Program components must be determined in advance. AAOHN (2009) defines the following program components that are essential for a successful occupational health program:

- *Health assessments.* Performing health histories and physical examinations, medical surveillance testing, periodic physical examinations.
- *Case management.* Coordinating the care of ill and injured workers, facilitating referrals, facilitating return to work, and monitoring outcomes.
- *Health promotion and health education.* Conducting medical testing, providing educational programs, developing health services on-site.
- *Counseling and crisis intervention.* Developing employee assistance programs and a drug-free workplace.
- *Health and hazards surveillance.* Maintaining awareness of required regulations, conducting biological and environmental monitoring, observing trends, and making appropriate referrals.
- *Injury prevention and loss control.* Creating safety awareness, conducting safety audits, inspections, and incident investigations. Developing policies, procedures, and strategies.
- *Work related injury and illness management.* Providing first-line intervention for the provision of first aid and treatment of emergencies, minor illnesses, and minor injuries. Assuring appropriate follow-up and continuous care as appropriate.

Figure 4.1 displays the broad continuum of occupational health services that can be rendered in an on-site occupational health facility. From a traditional occupational health service to the establishment of an organized company-based primary care clinic, there are endless possibilities for health services. A single-unit facility staffed by one OHN typically provides limited healthcare services, health promotion initiatives, and case management. This would entail a lower financial investment for the company and may yield a lower return on investment. As the type of services moves along the continuum, the investment in resources increases and usually demonstrates a significantly higher return on investment for the company. Rogers (2003) defines four types of program models:

- One nurse, one health services unit on-site
- Multiple nurses, one health services unit on-site
- Multiple nurses, multiple health service sites
- Consortium, shared occupational health services by a coalition of companies

One size does not fit all. The OHN must develop a plan that meets the needs of workers and workplaces in a most cost-efficient manner. Program planning and development should consider the impact on the organization as a whole and include a long-term strategy. The use of professional and community

Table 4.5 Professional resources related to occupational health.

Resource	Description	Web Site
American Association of Occupational Health Nurses (AAOHN)	The American Association of Occupational Health Nurses, the primary professional association for occupational health nurses and other healthcare professionals serving the workplace. AAOHN is "dedicated to advancing and maximizing the health, safety, and productivity of domestic and global workforces by providing education, research, public policy, and practice resources for occupational and environmental health nurses."	www.aaohn.org
American College of Occupational and Environmental Medicine (ACOEM)	ACOEM is the nation's largest medical society dedicated to promoting the health of workers through preventive medicine, clinical care, research, and education. ACOEM focuses efforts on enhancing "the health and safety of workers, workplaces, and environments."	www.acoem.org
American Industrial Hygiene Association (AIHA)	AIHA is a professional association for scientists and engineers with emphasis on health and safety of workers, workplaces in the community. AIHA is "devoted to the anticipation, recognition, evaluation, prevention, and control of those environmental factors or stresses arising in or from the workplace that may cause sickness, impaired health and well-being, or significant discomfort among workers or among citizens of the community."	www.aiha.org
America Society of Safety Engineers (ASSE)	ASSE, the oldest professional safety society, is "committed to protecting people, property, and the environment, providing key information and action on occupational safety, health and environmental issues and practices." Members focused on creating a safer, healthier workplace and developing safer products in order to prevent workplace injuries and illnesses.	www.asse.org
National Safety Council (NSC)	The National Safety Council is committed to the prevention of "injuries and deaths at work, in homes and communities, and on the roads through leadership, research, education and advocacy." Initially established to focus on workplace safety, the NSC has expanded focus to also include transportation safety and safety of homes and communities.	www.nsc.org

Table 4.5 (*Continued*)

Resource	Description	Web Site
Occupational Safety and Health Administration (OSHA)	The Occupational Safety and Health Administration's admission is to "ensure safe and healthful working conditions for working men and women by setting and enforcing standards and by providing training, outreach, education, and assistance." OSHA publishes a set of regulatory standards applicable to specific workplaces and work hazards.	www.osha.gov
National Hearing Conservation Association (NHCA)	The mission of the NHCA is to "prevent hearing loss due to noise and other environmental factors in all sectors of society." NHCA provides an avenue for education and exchange of information that promotes the development of "improved and more effective occupational hearing conservation programs."	www.hearingconservation.org
The Centers for Disease Control and Prevention (CDC)	The CDC is one of the major operating components of the Department of Health and Human Services created to provide the "expertise, information, and tools that people and communities need to protect their health—through health promotion, prevention of disease, injury and disability, and preparedness for new health threats."	www.cdc.gov
National Institute for Occupational Safety and Health (NIOSH)	The National Institute for Occupational Safety and Health (NIOSH) is the federal agency "responsible for conducting research and making recommendations for the prevention of work-related injury and illness." The efforts of research and practice, NIOSH serves to "generate new knowledge in the field of occupational safety and health and to transfer that knowledge into practice for the betterment of workers."	www.niosh.gov

resources is essential in the development of the plan. These resources can strengthen the foundation of the plan from a professional and regulatory standpoint and provide the support needed for justification for certain aspects of the plan. Table 4.5 provides a list of professional resources for use during program planning. These resources cover a broad scope of professional issues applicable to the development and maintenance of a successful occupational health program.

SELLING THE PLAN

The written plan and associated budget must be documented in terms that are very understandable to members of the senior management team, those who make decisions related to the allocation of financial resources for the company. The plan may also be scrutinized by the company's legal department in regard to the potential associated corporate and medical liability. For this reason, the plan should be outlined in steps related to priority, based on immediate need and return on investment. The OHN must be willing to make adjustments to the plan based on changing priorities or the availability of company resources. The OHN must also recognize the need to revise the plan to correspond with changes in the workplace (Daft, 2004). A sample program proposal is provided in Table 4.6.

So, who do you sell it to? And how do you sell it? Start by knowing your audience. Find out who will be the key decision makers. To find out who may be consulted along the way to render an expert opinion regarding the scope services and associated financial and legal risks. Key decision makers may include:

- Executive managers
- Risk managers
- Corporate attorney
- Chief financial officer
- Safety manager
- Human resources manager
- Operations managers
- Workers
- Third parties

  - Health benefit and workers' compensation insurers or third-party administrators
  - Workers' compensation defense attorneys
  - Labor relations

The OHN should champion the plan for success. Formal and informal meetings should be arranged with influencers and decision makers. Sit with workers in the break room to discuss the plan. Hold focus group sessions to gather opinions at the grassroots level. Take the opportunity to not only discuss the plan, but also request feedback from their particular perspective. Identifying obstacles and challenges at the beginning allows the OHN to make revisions to the plan based on input from influencers and decision makers. If allocation of finances seems to be a challenge, seek other cost-effective alternatives that may lead to the same intended outcome. Have a back-up plan in place.

IMPLEMENT THE PLAN

The hard work is done. The seeds have been planted. Now comes the fun. It is great to watch your efforts come to fruition.

Table 4.6 Sample occupational health program proposal.

Service	Current Function	Current Resources	Proposal	Proposed Cost	Additional Resources	Projected Annual Savings
To increase services in the occupational health clinic to offer physical examinations and limited primary care services	Provide emergency, first aid, and evaluations of work-related injuries/illnesses Preplacement physical examinations are outsourced to the community-based occupational health clinic All other medical services are referred to the community occupational health clinic or to the worker's primary care provider	Occupational health clinic with three examination rooms and associated medical equipment One full-time registered nurse One full-time receptionist/clerk.	To expand the scope of services to include: • Preplacement fitness for duty evaluations • Annual wellness exams • Limited primary care services	$118,000 Anticipated number of preplacement physical examinations: 120	Full-time nurse practitioner: $80,000 Full-time medical assistant: $35,000 Medical director fee: $3,000 Total annual cost: $118,000	Company savings: $75,000 Includes: • Eliminated the use of community-based occupational health clinic for preplacement exams • Limited primary care services lead to reduction in worker sick days and days away from work, resulting in increased productivity Worker savings: • No copay for visit at company-based clinic • Early detection of health risks through wellness initiatives and appropriate referral for intervention
Workers' compensation medical care	Worker in need of medical treatment beyond the scope of the OHN are referred to the community occupational health clinic OHN provides case management	Same as above	Provide a limited scope of treatment for worker's compensation injuries. Those cases in need of radiology or specialist services will be referred to a preferred provider network	$0	As above	>$55,000* Includes: • Reduced medical cost preclaim • Reduced use of outside medical services • Reduced claim experience

(Continued)

Table 4.6 (*Continued*)

Service	Current Function	Current Resources	Proposal	Proposed Cost	Additional Resources	Projected Annual Savings
Conduct all drug screening on-site at the occupational health clinic	Currently provided by the community occupational health clinic at $25 per drug screen. Current annual cost: $3,000	Same as above	All urine drug screening will be conducted in the on-site occupational health clinic. Use of instant drug screen kits for preplacement testing Guarantees immediate reporting to human resources of negative results.	Instant urine drug screen kits • $7 each Anticipated annual use: 120 Additional lab and medical review cost for confirmation of nonnegative results • $15 each Estimated annual use: 6 TOTAL: $930.00	As above	$2,070
TOTAL ANNUAL INVESTMENT						$118,930
TOTAL ANNUAL SAVINGS						$132,070
NET RETURN ON INVESTMENT						$ 13,140

*Does not include reduced cost of worker's time away from job for medical treatment.

Determine priorities. Take a stepwise approach based on your action plan. Decide what needs to be accomplished and who will be involved in the implementation process. For each step of the implementation process there should be assigned responsibility and accountability. An effective safety and health program enables input and participation from every worker, making safety and health the responsibility of every individual. (Russi et al., 2010).

Facilitating change in the workplace is not easy, but if the groundwork has been laid and there has been involvement from workers at all levels within the organization, the change is accepted much easier than if careful planning and involvement of workers had not been involved.

Case in Point

The OHN comes up with a great plan. The plan includes expanding the services in the occupational health clinic to include treatment of work-related injuries and illnesses using the services of a nurse practitioner. The intended objective is to reduce workers' compensation costs. An action plan is developed that includes associated human and financial resources required for the enhanced services. The plan predicts a significant return on investment. The OHN garners support at all levels within the organization. The plan is implemented; the nurse practitioner is hired and begins treating worker injuries on-site in the occupational health clinic. The injured workers seem to be happy with the increase in services in the occupational health clinic. The plan has increased efficient access to quality healthcare services on-site, reducing workers' need to travel to a community-based occupational health clinic for evaluation and treatment.

Within a few months, the OHN is summoned to a meeting with the risk manager. It seems that the company's workers' compensation insurance carrier is concerned that the on-site treatment of workers is in violation of the state's workers' compensation statutes, requiring that workers be given a choice of treating facilities. In addition, the company's workers compensation defense attorney has raised question about the scope of services being provided at the occupational health clinic. Specifically, there is concern about the ability to defend claims from workers who were treated on site.

Strategies for Success

An additional step in the planning process to include input and garner support from third parties would have been beneficial. Because of the associated regulatory and legal issues surrounding the treatment of injured workers, support from those who manage and defend the claims is critical.

- The OHN should ensure that the program plan is grounded in compliance with applicable regulatory statutes. It is important to be armed with assurance of regulatory compliance in the event the program is challenged. A program development checklist is provided in Appendix 6.

- Outside influencers hold the ability to sabotage the efforts of an occupational health and safety program if they are unable to clearly see the intended benefits and outcomes related to not only the company, but also to them.
- The OHN should seek input and garner support from program partners outside the organization as well as inside the organization.

REFERENCES

American Association of Occupational Health Nurses (AAOHN). (2003). Competencies in occupational and environmental health nursing: Practice in the new millennium. *AAOHN Journal, 51,* 290–302.

American Association of Occupational Health Nurses (AAOHN). (2004a). AAOHN code of ethics and interpretive statements. Atlanta, GA: AAOHN.

American Association of Occupational Health Nurses (AAOHN). (2004b). Standards of occupational and environmental health nursing. Atlanta, GA: AAOHN.

American Association of Occupational Health Nurses (AAOHN). (2009). Occupational and environmental health nursing: Your key to cost containment. Atlanta, GA: AAOHN.

American Association of Occupational Health Nurses (AAOHN). (1995). Guidelines for an occupational health & safety service. Atlanta, GA: AAOHN.

American Association of Occupational Health Nurses (AAOHN). (2001). Compensation & benefits study: A statistical survey of job profiles, salaries, and benefits (3rd ed.). Atlanta, GA: AAOHN.

Daft, R. (2004) Organization theory and design. Mason, OH: Thompson Learning.

Dirksen, M. E. (2001). Occupational and environmental health nursing: An overview. In M. K. Salazar (Ed.), Core curriculum for occupational and environmental health nursing (2nd ed., pp. 3–32). Philadelphia: W.B. Saunders.

Felton, J. S. (1996). Medical direction in occupational health nursing. *The American Journal of Nursing, 66*(9), 2019–2022.

National Institute for Occupational Safety and Health (NIOSH). (2004). NIOSH Publication No. 2004-135. *Does it really work?* Retrieved from http://www.cdc.gov/niosh/docs/2004-135/whatDoesMean/default.html

National Safety Council. (2000a). *Case studies in safety and productivity.* Retrieved from http://www.nsc.org or call 1-800-621-7619.

Occupational Safety and Health Administration (OSHA). (2005). Small business handbook: Small business safety and health management series. OSHA 2209-02R 2005. Washington, D.C.: OSHA.

Occupational Safety and Health Administration (OSHA). (2010). Safety and Health Add Value to Your Business. Retrieved from http://www.osha.gov/Publications/safety-health-addvalue.html

Prossin, A. (1985). Developing and occupational health program: The team approach. *Canadian Family Physician.* 10, 1911–1915.

Rogers, B. (2003). Occupational health nursing, concepts and practice (2nd. ed.). Philadelphia: W.B. Saunders.

Russi, M., Buchta, W., Swift, M. Budnick, L. Hodgson, M. Berube, D. Kelafant, G. (2010). Guidance for occupational health services in medical centers. Retrieved from http://www.acoem.org/uploadedFiles/Public_Affairs/Policies_And_Position_Statements/Guidelines/Guidelines/MCOH%20Guidance.pdf

Salazar, M. K. (Ed.). (2003). AAOHN core curriculum for occupational health nursing. Philadelphia: W.B. Saunders.

Salazar, M. K., Kemerer, S. D., Amann, M. C., & Fabrey, L. J. (2002). Defining the roles and functions of occupational and environmental health nurses: Results of a national job analysis. *AAOHN Journal*, *50*(1), 16–25.

Scant, P. & Dillman, D. P. (1994). How to conduct your own survey. New York: John Wiley and Sons.

Schulte, P. & Pandalai, S. P. (2011). A comprehensive approach to workforce health. NIOSH. Retrieved from http://blogs.cdc.gov/niosh-science-blog/2011/12/workforce/

Smith. G. S. (2001). Public health approaches to occupational injury prevention: Do they work? *Injury Prevention*. 7 (Suppl 1). Retrieved from http://bmj-injuryprev.highwire.org/content/7/suppl_1/i3.full

Strasser, P. B., Maher, H. K., Knuth, G., Fabrey, L. J. (2006). Occupational health nursing 2004. Practice analysis report. *AAOHN Journal*, *54*(1), 14–23.

Scant, P. & Dillman, D. P. How to conduct your own survey. (1994b). New York: John Wiley and Sons.

National Safety Council. (2000). *Case studies in safety and productivity*. Retrieved at http://www.nsc.org or call 1-800-621-7619.

The National Committee for Injury Prevention and Control. (1989). Injury prevention: meeting the challenge. *American Journal of Preventive Medicine*, *5*(3).

American Evaluation Association. Business and Industry Topic Interest Group of the American Evaluation Association. Retrieved at http://www.e-valuate-it.com/aea-bi-tig/resources.asp

RESOURCES

Institute for Work and Health. http://www.iwh.on.ca/

Guide to evaluating the effectiveness of strategies for preventing work injuries: how to show whether a safety intervention really works. NIOSH Publication No. 2001–119.

OSHA PUBLICATIONS

A single free copy of the following materials can be obtained from the OSHA, Area or Regional Office, or contact the OSHA Publications Office, U.S. Department of Labor, 200 Constitution Avenue, NW, N-3101, Washington, D.C. 20210, or call (202) 693-1888, or fax (202) 693-2498.

Access to Medical and Exposure Records. OSHA Publication No. 3110.

All About OSHA. OSHA Publication No. 2056 (Spanish language version, No. 3173).

Asbestos Standard for General Industry. OSHA Publication No. 3095.

Consultation Services for the Employer. OSHA Publication No. 3047.

Control of Hazardous Energy (Lockout/Tagout). OSHA Publication No. 3120.

Emergency Exit Routes Quick Card. OSHA Publication No. 3183.

Employee Workplace Rights. OSHA Publication No. 3021 (Spanish language version, No. 3049).

Employer Rights and Responsibilities Following an OSHA Inspection. OSHA Publication No. 3000 (Spanish language version, No. 3195).

Hand and Power Tools. OSHA Publication No. 3080.

How to Plan for Workplace Emergencies and Evacuations. OSHA Publication No. 3088.

It's the Law Poster. OSHA Publication No. 3165 (Spanish language version No. 3167).

Job Hazard Analysis. OSHA Publication No. 3071.

Model Plans & Programs for the OSHA Bloodborne Pathogens and Hazard Communications Standard. OSHA Publication No.3186

Occupational Safety and Health Act. OSHA Publication No.2001.

OSHA Inspections. OSHA Publication No. 2098.

Personal Protective Equipment. OSHA Publication No. 3151.

Servicing Single-Piece and Multi-Piece Rim Wheels. OSHA Publication No. 3086.

Facilities and Resources

5

Occupational Health Nursing:
Helping the rich and the poor.
Sharing knowledge and providing understanding.
Creating a haven in the workplace for comfort and care.

(Guzik)

The occupational health nurse practices in a variety of settings, and the extent of services provided depends on the size, complexity, and operations of the workplace. Common types of occupational health program settings include the following:

- **Large industry**. This setting generally hosts greater than 1,000 workers in a single location. There is often a corporate medical director, sometimes holding a senior executive level position with the company, who provides guidance and direction for the occupational health and safety program. The company usually has a fully equipped on-site occupational health clinic. The occupational health nurse (OHN) conducts health assessments, health interventions, and substance testing related to worker fitness for duty. In addition, the OHN often has case management responsibilities for both occupational and non-occupational disability management and is in charge of facilitating a return to work for injured and ill workers. In this setting, the OHN often works among a variety of occupational health professionals, including other nurses and physicians, industrial hygienists, and safety specialists.
- **Medium-sized companies**. Workplaces with 500–1,000 employees usually have structured occupational health programs. The size and extent of the program depends on the nature of the work. Workplaces with 250 or more employees in a work setting that has potential risk or need of health surveillance or training can often justify the need for an OHN. The OHN's role may vary in scope depending on the needs of the workforce. If the OHN's role is strictly administrative, including case management, the OHN may work in an

Essentials for Occupational Health Nursing, First Edition. Arlene Guzik.
© 2013 John Wiley & Sons, Inc. Published 2013 by John Wiley & Sons, Inc.

office environment. If clinical services are rendered, the typical setting is usually comprised of a clinical examination area and an area for medical supply storage. In this setting, the OHN attends to workers who become ill or injured on the job. The scope of service includes the provision of first aid and emergency treatment. The OHN is trusted with a limited formulary of prescription medications that can be administered under the direction of written protocol with a consultant medical director. The OHN is also trusted to administer over-the-counter (OTC) medications for certain health conditions, as well. To a great extent, OHNs in this setting are also responsible for case management, specifically for workers' compensation cases, those workers who have become injured or ill on the job. Health promotion and consultation also comprise a large part of the OHN duties since the OHN often becomes a very trustworthy resource for workers in regard to their personal health conditions.

- **Small companies**. Small companies may employee OHNs on a part-time basis. Rather than being directly employed by the company, the OHN may provide consultative services on a contractual basis as an independent contractor. The occupational heath program is sometimes structured around the use of a variety of community health resources and support, since supportive resources within the company are usually limited.
- **Healthcare system and community-based occupational health clinics**. Community health systems or clinics often strive to offer occupational health services to companies in their local communities. OHNs may be employed along with other occupational health professionals that provide a variety of occupational health services for client companies. In this setting, the OHN has access to a vast range of medical and ancillary support programs and services, including medical specialists, wellness experts, physical therapist, nutritionists, etc. As a result, the OHN may call on these experts to support the needs of the occupational health program.

The remainder of this chapter focuses on the resources necessary to establish and maintain an on-site occupational health program within a business or industry. The operational resources include an adequate budget, facilities, equipment, and supplies necessary to operate the occupational health program (Rogers, 2003). The type, location, and size of the facility for the occupational health program depends on the scope of services rendered.

The approach to establishing occupational health services was covered in the previous chapter and includes the following:

- Identify the target market
- Decide what services will be offered and develop a plan
- Develop a program budget
- Employ competent staff
- Establish the appropriate facility, equipment, and supplies
- Provide service to the expected standard
- Evaluate the effectiveness of the program

BUDGET ISSUES

If clinical services are rendered, medical equipment must be purchased or leased. Careful consideration must be given to the frequency of use of specialty occupational health equipment since it is sometimes quite costly and requires approval for capital expenditure. Cost justification for purchase of the equipment should be clearly defined. A list of common capital expenditures is included in Table 5.1. There must be a system for regular maintenance, calibration, and documentation of the quality of the equipment. Since this equipment is usually used to conduct testing required by regulatory standards, such as hearing conservation and respiratory protection, quality, calibration, and validation of accuracy of the equipment is critical Therefore, it is recommended that all equipment used or purchased meet the standards of regulatory requirements.

THE OCCUPATIONAL HEALTH FACILITY

An on-site occupational health clinic should be strategically located near the majority of workers in order to provide efficient access. The hours of operation for the occupational health services should be considered based on the number of employees, work schedules, and the types of services provided. The hours of operation may also fluctuate based on the needs of the workforce and the need for occupational health testing or training on various shifts and days of the week. The size of the facility depends on usage and the types of services provided.

If the workplace involves multiple buildings, worker access to the site of occupational health services is important. Parking near the clinic should be adequate. Parking lots and the entrance to the facility should be handicap accessible. There should be clear signage acknowledging the presence of the occupational health clinic and first aid station. The facility should present a clean, professional, and well-maintained appearance.

The facility itself, including restrooms, should be handicap accessible. Fire extinguishers should be clearly visible, and there should be clearly defined fire exits. There should be documented evidence of a fire inspection within the last 24 months.

The waiting area should be well ventilated with ample seating, usually two seats per number of appointments per hour. Restrooms should be clean and in good repair. The facility should be well lit, neat, clean, and organized. Patient education material should be strategically placed in waiting areas and in examination rooms.

There should be an adequate number of exam rooms for the volume of use. The exam rooms should be neat, clean, and organized and provide adequate privacy. Sinks should be available for hand washing. The exam rooms should be stocked with supplies to meet first aid needs and other intervention. Table 5.2 provides a list of common supplies stocked in the occupational health exam room.

Table 5.1 Capital supplies and equipment.

Area	Quantity
Waiting Area	
Chairs	6
Patient education material display	1
Reception Area	
Desk	1
Office chair	1
Computer	1
Printer	1
File cabinet	1
General/office supply storage cabinet	1
OHN Office	
Desk	1
Office chair	1
Chair	1
File cabinet	1
Computer	1
Exam Room (each)	
Exam table	1
Chair	1
Exam stool	1
Step stool	1
Supply storage cabinet	1
General	
Medication storage cabinet	1
Medical supply storage cabinet	1
Refrigerator, medication	1
Refrigerator, specimen	1
Medical Equipment	
Otoscope/ophthalmoscope	1
Sphygmomanometer, various size cuffs (adult, adult large, adult extra-large)	1 each
Titmus vision tester	1
Snellen eye chart	1
Near vision chart	1

Table 5.2 Exam room inventory.

Item	Quantity
2 × 2 gauze, nonsterile	1 pkg
2 × 2 gauze, sterile	10 packs
4 × 4 gauze, nonsterile	1 pkg
4 × 4 gauze, sterile	10 packs
Absorbent pads	10
Elastic wrap bandage (2″, 4″, 6″)	2 each
Kling Flexicon bandages (2″, 4″, 6″)	2 each
Latex-free foam wrap (2″, 4″, 6″)	2 each
Adhesive bandages, assorted sizes	1 box
Cotton balls	1 bag
Cotton-tip swabs, nonsterile	12
Cotton-tip swabs, sterile	12
Tongue blades, nonsterile	12
Tongue blades, sterile	12
Lubricant jelly	12
Antibiotic ointment	12
Alcohol swabs	1 box
Normal saline, 500 ml	1
Emesis basin	1
Tissues	1 box
Exam drapes	12
Exam gowns	12
Nonsterile gloves, S, M, L, XL	1 box each
Exam table paper	3
Tape, micropore or paper	2
Otoscope tips	1 pkg
Sharps container	1
Various patient education handouts	

Written emergency response protocols should be in place. The facility should be equipped with emergency supplies, including pharmaceuticals and oxygen (see Table 5.3). The presence of an automatic external defibrillator (AED) has become a common fixture in many work settings, sometimes located in the occupational health facility or in an area of the workplace that poses the most risk and demand for use of the AED.

Table 5.3 Clinic emergency supplies.

Item	Quantity
Automatic external defibrillator	Optional
Ambu bag, with mask	1
Oxygen cannula	6
Oxygen mask with tubing	2
Oxygen	1 tank
Benadryl, 25 mg PO	6 single dose packages
Epinephrine (EpiPen)	2
Aspirin, 85 mg	2 single dose packages
Nitroglycerine, 0.4 mg	1 bottle

Procedure:

1. Emergency supplies are to be kept in a designated area that is readily accessible in the event of an emergency. They should be kept in a case that is clearly labeled "Emergency Supplies" be easily transportable.
2. All staff in the occupational health clinic should be trained to know where the supplies are stored.
3. Supplies are to be checked monthly using the "Emergency Equipment and Supply Monthly Checklist."
4. Check expiration dates on all supplies and plan to replace those nearing expiration date.
5. Check oxygen tank for level and refill as necessary.

MONTHLY CHECKLIST	Jan	Feb	Mar
Automatic external defibrillator.	Checked daily. See log.		
Ambu bag, with mask			
Oxygen cannula			
Oxygen mask and tubing			
Oxygen tank			
Benadryl, 25 mg PO			
Epinephrine, (EpiPen)			
Aspirin, 85 mg			
Nitroglycerine, 0.4 mg			

LICENSURE

Licensure and certification of the occupational health facility should be clearly displayed. This includes occupational business licenses, if applicable. In some states, a healthcare facility license is required. If laboratory services are provided on-site, a Clinical Laboratory Improvement Amendments (CLIA) waiver certificate should be displayed. If pharmaceutical services are rendered, a state-specific pharmacy license may be required. Facilities that include basic x-ray services will be required to obtain state radiology license. The OHN should also determine the need for biohazardous waste certification and the provision of disposal of waste in compliance with state laws.

The licenses of professional healthcare providers, including physician, nurses, and x-ray technicians should also be clearly displayed. Specialty certifications for other occupational health staff should also be on display. Examples include medical assistant certification, drug-screening certification, breath alcohol technician certification, hearing conservation certification, etc. Special training certificates indicating professional board certification for the medical and nursing staff can also be displayed.

SUPPLIES

The occupational health facility should provide an adequate supply of standard basic clinic supplies. The extent of clinical supplies depends on the scope of services rendered in the occupational health clinic. Typical first aid supplies such as adhesive bandages, compression bandages, ice bags, and antibiotic ointment should be considered. Other medical supplies, such as splints and crutches will depend upon the levels of medical and nursing services rendered. It is prudent to have the review and signature of the medical director endorsing the supplies that will be stocked in the clinic. An inventory of common supplies is provided in Table 5.4.

PHARMACY

There should be a clearly defined process of dispensing medication that assures accountability. This includes both OTC and prescription pharmaceuticals. All pharmaceuticals must be properly labeled when dispensed, and patient information handouts should be available.

Stock medications should be organized in a properly controlled manner, and all medications should be checked regularly for expiration dates and replenished accordingly. There should be a process for medical error and adverse reaction reporting. Some states require a specific pharmacy license for the occupational health clinic, and if so, the occupational health clinic may subject to pharmacy inspections. Therefore organization and control of the pharmaceuticals stocked in the workplace is of great importance.

A variety of OTC and prescription pharmaceuticals can be stocked in the occupational health clinic. The need for these medications depends on the extent of services provided by the OHN and other occupational health staff. A list of common OTC and prescription medications is provided in Table 5.5. There are certain legal requirements for the OHN to be able to order and stock prescription medications. Most often, prescription medications include vaccines appropriate to the needs of the workforce and prescription medications that would be administered in the event of an emergency. In order for the OHN to order and stock prescription medications, a written authorization is required from the medical director. The pharmaceutical supplier most often also requires

Table 5.4 Clinic supply inventory.

Alcohol prep pads	1 box
Alcohol	1 bottle
Ammonia capsules	1 box
Antibiotic ointment, single foil packs	1 box
Bandages, adhesive	1 box each
• 1 × 3	• Digit, large
• 2 × 2 patch	• Digit, small
• 2 × 3	• Knuckle
• 4-wing	• Spot
Bandage, elastic (2″, 3″, 4″, 6″)	1 box each
Basin, bath	1 each
Basin, emesis	1 each
Biohazard spill kit	1
Biohazard waste bags	1 box
Burn gel packs	1 box
Butterfly closures	1 box
Chlorine bleach	½ gallon
Cold/heat packs	1 case
Cotton balls	1 small bag
Cotton tip applicators, 6″, nonsterile	1 box
Cotton tip applicators, 6″, sterile	1 box
Crutches, adult	1
Crutches, adult XL	1
Disinfectant CaviCide spray	1 can
Dressing, nonadherent, 3 × 3	1 box
Eye pad, oval, small	1 box
Eye patch, adhesive	1 box
Eye wash, 4 oz	2 bottles
Garbage bags, biohaz waste, red	To fit trash can
Gauze rolls, 2″, 4″, 6″	1 bag each
Gauze sponges	
• 2 × 2 sponges, nonsterile	1 bag
• 2 × 2 sponges, sterile	1 box
• 4 × 4 sponges, nonsterile	1 bag
• 4 × 4 sponges, sterile	1 box
Germacidal solution, instrument	1 gallon
Gloves, exam, latex-free, nonsterile, medium	1 box
Gloves, exam, latex-free, sterile, sz. 7	1 box
Hydrocortisone cream, 1% single packs	1 box
Hydrogen peroxide	1 bottle

Table 5.4 (*Continued*)

Lubricant jelly foilpack	1 box
Needles, sterile 18 ga., 1″	1 box
Needles, sterile, 25 ga., 1″	1 box
Needles, sterile, 23 ga., 1.5″	1 box
Oxygen emergency cylinder	1 each
Oxygen nasal cannula	2 each
Oxygen non-rebreather mask	1 each
Paper, exam table	1 case
Penlight, blue tip	3 per pkg
Pillowcase, standard disposable	1 case
Scalpel w/#11 blade	1 box
Scissors, bandage 5″	1
Sharps container, 5 quart	1
Skin prep adhesive pads	1 box
Sodium chloride, .9%, 250 cc.	1 bottle
Steri-strips, 1/4 × 1.5″	1 box
Sting swabs	1 box
Sundry jars	4
Surgical prep pads	1 box
Surgical prep solution	1 bottle
Surgical scrub brush	1 box
Suture removal kit, disposable	2 each
Syringe, 10 cc, leur lock, w/o needle	1 box
Syringe, 20 cc, leur lock, w/o needle	1 box
Syringe, 3 cc, 23 ga., 1″ needle	1 box
Syringe, 50 cc, Asepto	1 box
Syringe, 5 cc, leur lock w/o needle	1 box
Tape, micropore, 1″, 3″	1 box each
Tongue depressors, nonsterile	1 box
Tongue depressors, sterile	1 box
Tubegauze, #2, and cage	1 box
Wrap, self-adherent, 2″, 4″, 6″	**2 each**

Soft Splints
Wrist wrap
Knee wrap
Ankle wrap
Sling
Finger splints, assorted

(*Continued*)

Table 5.4 (*Continued*)

Equipment

Anatomical chart reference

Audiometer and soundproof booth (optional)

Chair

Exam stool

Exam table

Lamp, goose neck w/magnifier

Oto/ophthalmoscope, w/desk charger

Pillow

Scale, balance

Spirometer (options)

Snellen eye chart

Sphygmomanometer

Stethoscope

Thermometer

Titmus vision tester (optional)

Trash can, infectious waste

Tubegauze applicator #2

Wall-mounted needle disposal
and glove dispenser
(combination unit)

Wheelchair, adult

Additional Office Supplies

Bookcase

Cell phone/beeper

Chair, office

Charts and posters, various educational

Computer

Desk organizer

Desk, lockable

Fax, confidential

File folders for employee medical files

File cabinet, lockable 4 drawer

Hole puncher

Phone

Printer

Reference manuals, various

Stapler

Tape dispenser

Table 5.5 Common OTC and prescription medications.

Over-the-Counter Medications

Antacid such as aluminum hydroxide or magnesium hydroxide

Anti-diarrheal such as bismuth or diphenoxylate/atropine

Antiemetic

Antihistamine such as diphenhydramine

Anti-inflammatory such as ibuprofen, acetaminophen, naproxen sodium

Aspirin

Cough suppressant such as guaifenesin

Topical antibiotic cream

Topical antifungal cream

Topical anti-inflammatory such as hydrocortisone cream

Prescription Emergency Medications

Epinephrine auto-injector

Silver sulfadiazine cream

Nitroglycerin 1/150 gr.

Prescription Vaccines

Tetanus diphtheria toxoid

Hepatitis A

Hepatitis B

Varicella

Flu

a copy of the medical license and Drug Enforcement Administration (DEA) license of the medical director before prescription medications are released to the OHN. As a result, the medical director holds liability for the appropriate storage, control, and use of these medications in the workplace. Appendix 4 provides a sample prescription authority by the medical director.

Over-the-Counter Medications

There is a long tradition in occupational health of OHNs dispensing OTC medications to workers. In addition, there is tradition of stocking OTC medications in first aid stations throughout the workplace, permitting open access to these medications by workers. It is also common to have OTC medications stocked in emergency response kits throughout the workplace. Although this practice poses little risk, there are important issues of liability that must be considered. The OHN is responsible for assuring that the OTC medications in every location have not passed their expiration date. This requires that an inventory of medications and their locations must be kept and that a schedule of inventory control be maintained. The OHN should also establish a clear policy and procedure regarding who has access to OTC medications and under what conditions.

Certain liabilities and cautions surrounding access to OTC medications in the workplace exist that must be acknowledged. Workers may self-diagnose incorrectly and self-administer inappropriate OTC medication for their condition. Overdoses of OTC medication, although not common, do occur. Serious health conditions can result from overuse and frequent use of certain medications, as well. This is commonly seen in the use of anti-inflammatory and analgesic medications that can lead to gastrointestinal, liver, and kidney problems. Overuse can lead also to dependence, even with OTC medications. Drug allergies and drug interactions, although subtle, may also occur.

The distribution of OTC medications by nurses is guided by state nurse practice acts. The Food and Drug Administration (FDA) and state-specific pharmacy regulations also guide the distribution and sale of OTC medications (Litchfield, 2010). As a result, there are liability issues surrounding the dispensing of OTC medication in the workplace. The plan to provide OTC medications in the workplace requires the following due diligence.

1. Check the nurse practice act in your specific state for statements regarding medication administration and dispensing.
2. Check state-specific pharmacy laws and requirements.
3. Discuss issues of company liability with management and the medical director.
4. Conduct a cost-analysis of and consider alternative dispensing models.
5. Develop a written policy and procedure for providing and dispensing OTC medications in the workplace.

Common alternative models used to dispense OTC medications in the workplace have been proposed by Humphrey and Gruber (2008).

Self-Service

A traditional model used by many employers is the use of self-serve boxes. The employer orders OTC medications in bulk, usually prepackaged in single doses, usually 100–250 doses per box. This model is often used by companies that do not employ an OHN. The box of medications may be stocked in first aid stations around the workplace, and workers have free access to this medication. Common medications include analgesics, anti-inflammatories, decongestants, antihistamines, antibiotic ointment, and anti-inflammatory creams. This model depends on the worker to self-diagnosis and self-treat. The worker is responsible for the type of medication selected and the amount self-administered. The company holds liability in this model to assure the integrity of the medications and to assure the medications are within the expiration date. The company also holds potential liability should the worker ingest too much medication or have a serious reaction to the medication while at work. Additionally, this model is expensive because workers have open access to bulk supplies of medication without a method of accountability.

Clinic Dispensing by the OHN

The workplace with an established occupational health clinic provides an option for dispensing by a licensed healthcare practitioner. In this model, the workers present to the clinic and are assessed by the OHN. The OHN, working under written guidelines from the medical director for medication dispensing, assumes the responsibility for dispensing the type and amount of OTC medication appropriate for the worker's healthcare condition. The OHN is then responsible for medication inventory and control and appropriate documentation of assessment and intervention in the worker's health record. This provides more accountability for the medication inventory by a licensed professional while maintaining a record of medication use by workers. The disadvantage of this system is that it requires workers to take time from the job to visit the clinic, and access to medication is limited to the time the clinic is open.

On-site Pharmacy

Large companies with organized health clinics on-site may also provide an on-site pharmacy. In this model, workers not only have access to licensed nurses and physicians, but they also have access to on-site pharmacists to assist with medication dispensing. Because this model is expensive and requires regulatory licensing, most employers find it difficult to justify the cost of an on-site pharmacy.

Vending Machines

The used of vending machines to dispense OTC medications in the work place has become the model of choice for most worksites. Vending machines allow workers direct access to OTC medications without the need to see a healthcare practitioner. In this model, the OHN and company officials make the decision regarding the type of medications to stock in the vending machines and the cost of the medications to workers. Workers then assume responsibility for self-diagnosis and self-treatment. Access to OTC medications then is not limited. The worker is responsible for the type of medication selected and the amount self-administered. The employer may choose to subsidize the cost of the medication to make it more affordable for workers. The employer can choose to manage the vending machine operations by stocking and retrieving revenue generated from the sale of OTC medication. However, a most common method is to outsource the service to vendors who provide this service on a contractual basis. The vendor then holds responsibility for stocking the medication and assuring integrity of the medication. The occupational health clinic will still serve as a resource for employees who seek assistance with assessment and treatment of health conditions by the OHN.

The AAOHN *Advisory on Over-the-Counter Medications* (2008) lists the follow alternatives to the use of OTC medications in the workplace:

• Eliminate the use of over-the-counter medications
• Use a vending machine for over-the-counter medications

- Develop an employee self-administered medication system
- Develop nursing guidelines with standing orders or protocols to direct the use of OTC medications in the workplace

AAOHN (2008) also suggests the following actions on the part of the OHN to assure safety of the use of OTC medications in the workplace. The OHN should conduct an evaluation of common OTC medications requested or used in the workplace. Consideration regarding what OTC medications should be stocked should be based on the effect of the medications on worker productivity and safety. Avoid access to medications that have sedating side effects, such as anti-histamines. The use of sedating medications may increase risk of incident or injury with workers in safety-sensitive positions. Because of the side effect of drowsiness, worker productivity may also be affected. OTC medications containing alcohol and caffeine also have potential adverse effects on worker performance and should be avoided. The OHN should also evaluate the use of OTC medications that have the potential for drug interactions with common prescription medications. The OHN should be familiar with and should assure worker access to medication information related to all available OTC medications. This information should clearly indentify the ingredients, indications, side effects, contraindications, and potential drug interactions. In addition, the OHN should have emergency supplies and medications on hand in the occupational health clinic to intervene in the event of medication reactions.

The OHN should also have a mechanism and procedures for disposing of expired and unwanted pharmaceuticals. Outdated and unwanted pharmaceuticals should be quarantined to avoid inappropriate use. There may be regulations and guidelines that are state-specific for disposal of pharmaceuticals. The OHN should do the following:

- Contact the state's department of environmental protection, department of pharmacy, or department of health to obtain regulations related to medication disposal.
- Establish a pharmacy management plan for return of pharmaceuticals through a "return distribution" vendor. The pharmacy supplier may be able to recommend resources for this purpose.
- Follow specific instructions on the drug label for disposal of specific medications.
- Consider the use of community drug take-back programs.

STAFFING

Staffing of the occupational health facility should be adequate for volume. The staff should be properly trained and/or certified. CPR certification of the occupational health staff is recommended, and staff should be competent in emergency response.

Staff should be courteous, professional, and have the ability to communicate adequately with a wide variety of workers. In order to communicate with workers who do not speak English, there should be a provision for translation. Patient education and safety training material should be available in the languages common to the workforce. The staff should display a positive demeanor and attitude and have the ability to convey an understanding of the principles and concepts of occupational health and safety.

The dress code for the OHN depends on the scope of services provided. In a traditional health clinic model, the OHN may wear business casual attire, and sometimes a lab jacket. If the OHN is involved in direct patient care that requires response to injuries and emergencies, a dress code consistent with that of a health care clinic, including a scrub uniform, would be appropriate. If the role of the OHN is to be integrated with workers in their work environment, the OHN must dress appropriate to the demands and comply with all regulatory requirements for personal protection. This may include the need to wear steel-toed shoes, hearing or eye protection, hard hats, etc.

LABORATORY

Provisions for storage and disposal of biohazardous waste should be in place. The facility should have an exposure control plan that is familiar to all staff. The occupational health facility may also be subject to regulatory inspections for biohazardous waste. Inspection records should be maintained on-site in the occupational health facility. Some states also require a certificate of exemption if the facility does not fall under the requirements of this regulation. There should be adequate supplies to support the concept of universal precautions, including personal protective equipment such as goggles, masks, gowns, and gloves.

CLIA establishes quality standards for all laboratory testing to ensure the accuracy, reliability, and timeliness of test results. Healthcare offices that perform certain on-site laboratory tests, (including blood sugar and cholesterol tests, urine dips, etc.) are required to hold a CLIA waiver certificate. As defined by CLIA, waived tests are categorized as "simple laboratory examinations and procedures that have an insignificant risk of an erroneous result." (CDC, 2006). If these tests are performed in the occupational health clinic, the OHN must comply with obtaining a certificate of waiver for the clinic. A certificate must be obtained through the specific state agency and renewed every 2 years. In doing so, the facility is required to abide by the manufacturers' instructions for performing the waived tests, and the facility is subject to regulatory inspections by the state agency.

If drug screening services are conducted in the occupational health clinic, issues of regulatory compliance for the restroom facilities must be addressed. Chapter 10 outlines the principles of a drug-free workplace.

X-RAY

X-ray facilities are not common in most occupational health clinics unless the clinic provides evaluation and treatment by physicians, nurse practitioners, or physician assistants. If the occupational health clinic has a basic x-ray suite, the state radiation license must be posted in an obvious location near the x-ray equipment. A state radiation inspection compliance notice should also be posted. Most states require also that a "pregnancy warning" be posted in the x-ray suite in a place that is clearly visible to the patient.

STANDARDS, POLICIES, PROCEDURES

The development of written policies and procedures provide structure for the occupational health program. Written policies and procedures should be in place regarding the process of admitting and discharging a patient, as well as standards for health visit documentation. There should also be written policies and procedures for substance testing and clinical services. The access to these clinical standards and protocols assures consistency of treatment among providers and assures the treatment is based on evidence-based guidelines. The occupational health facility policies and procedures should also include a process for error reporting and complaint resolution. The medical director should review and approve all clinic policies and procedures.

SERVICES

The occupational health program has the potential for providing a wide variety of services. The scope of services provided in an on-site occupational health clinic is dependent on a variety of factors, such as specified job duties and priorities for OHN, space, needs of the workforce, and the specific mission to be accomplished. Healthcare services could include administering vaccines, conducting on-site health surveillance, providing wellness initiatives, and providing other laboratory services.

The OHN may provide after-hours call-in response to on-the-job injuries and illnesses. This provides workers access to an occupational health professional who can provide telephone assessment and guidance for treatment. This often reduces the need for costly emergency room visits by the injured worker. Additionally, the OHN may also provide response for drug or alcohol screening, including after-hours calls.

AFTER-HOURS APPOINTMENTS

Hours of operation of the occupational health facility should be clearly displayed. Instructions for communicating with the occupational health nurse after hours should be clearly communicated and posted in all departments. The workforce and management should be well informed of the availability of 24-hour coverage. There should to be specific written guidelines on how to contact the OHN after hours and how calls are managed.

FORMS

Forms used in the occupational health clinic should be consistent with standards for forms used in the healthcare industry. These include, but are not limited to, patient registration forms, privacy acknowledgment forms, consents for treatment, health history and physical examination forms, work status forms, and patient education forms. Forms that are used by the occupational health staff should be drafted to be specific to the use of the facility and should undergo legal review and approval. Figure 5.1 provides a flow chart for development, review, and approval of clinic forms.

HEALTH RECORDS

Employers have both a legal and ethical obligation concerning maintenance and confidentiality of the health information related to their workers. Federal regulations require that health records related to medical surveillance be kept for 30 years after the last date of employment, and the employer is under obligation to disclose such information under certain circumstances. The purpose of OSHA Standard 1910.1020(a) is "to provide employees and their designated representatives a right of access to relevant exposure and medical records; and to provide representatives of the Assistant Secretary a right of access to these records in order to fulfill responsibilities under the Occupational Safety and Health Act. Access by employees, their representatives, and the Assistant Secretary is necessary to yield both direct and indirect improvements in the detection, treatment, and prevention of occupational disease." (OSHA, 2011) Therefore the occupational health clinic must have a process in place that grants appropriate access to employee health records.

Medical record keeping is an essential requirement and should not only comply with regulatory requirements, but also should be consistent with the standard for healthcare documentation for the professional. Records are integral part of nursing care, and accurate record keeping is a "mark of a skilled and safe practitioner." (Oakley, 2008).

Policies and procedures should be in place regarding health record availability to the employer, regulatory agencies, to the benefits guarantor, or any other outside source. The company should also have any written policy and procedure regarding confidentiality of health records that is compliant with the federal regulations of the Health Insurance Portability and Accountability Act (HIPAA). The policy and procedure should require a written release from the worker before records are released for any purpose. The OHN may be confronted with situations in which the employer, worker's supervisor, human resources official, or corporate attorney request access to a worker's health record. For this reason, the occupational health nurse should be adept in communicating expectations and regulations addressing requests to disclose personal health information and fulfill such requests with assurance of compliance with confidentiality standards and regulations (AAOHN, 2004). There should be a process for both active chart storage and inactive chart storage that assures efficient access to records when needed while always keeping health records protected from public access.

The health record should always be complete and legible. Health records should be well organized in chronological order and in a consistent format. All entries in the health record, including each page of the health records, should include the patient's name, date, and unique identifier, such as employee

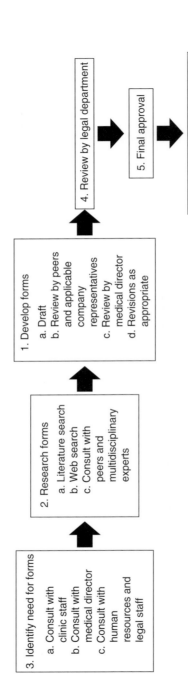

Figure 5.1 Development of forms.

number, date of birth, or last four numbers of the Social Security number. Allergies should be prominently noted, and the health record should include contact information in the event of emergency The documentation of each patient encounter should include the reason for the encounter, applicable history, assessment and intervention, and plan of care. The record should also indicate discharge instructions and return-to-work status. The return-to-work status should include clearly defined limitations or physical restrictions related to the essential functions of the job.

Outlines for documentation of various health services visits can be found in Appendix 7.

COMPUTER TECHNOLOGY

An electronic health record (EHR) system provides a solid foundation for the occupational health program to record both occupational and non-occupational encounters. The EHR must meet HIPAA privacy standards assuring that access to personal health records is not available to company officials or to health benefits and workers' compensation guarantors. The EHR should be able to provide a record of both occupational and non-occupational health encounters.

The ideal components of an occupational health EHR include the ability to record the following:

- Individual demographic information
- Individual health history, including past health and surgical history
- Individual health status, including current health problems, active medication list, and a list of medication and environmental allergies
- Immunization records
- Appointment scheduling
- Records of physical examinations
  - Preplacement exams
  - Regulatory exams
  - Fitness-for-duty exams
  - Wellness exams
- Substance testing results
  - Urine/hair/saliva tests
  - Breath alcohol tests
  - Blood alcohol tests
- Medical surveillance data
  - Audiometric results
  - Laboratory and diagnostic test results
  - Pulmonary function test results
- Duty status history
- First report of incident/injury tracking
- Claims reporting/submission
- OSHA 300 Log
- Case management documentation

Written policies and procedures should be in place regarding who has access to the EHR and should address a specific process for access to health information. Anyone holding access to the EHR must have a unique identifier passcode. The monitor should be strategically placed in a location that limits visual access to the screen by others while in use. A system for regular backup of data should be in place, and the policy should address standards for electronic transmission of health information, as well as procedures for destruction of health information (AAOHN, 2004). The EHR should support all requirements for regulatory compliance while offering efficient access to health information for individuals and workforce populations. This enables the OHN to track individual health status along with the ability to track trends among worker populations.

AUDITS

Facility quality and compliance is critical, and the OHN is the primary individual accountable for assuring the integrity of the facility and its operations. Routine audits should be performed that address compliance with regulatory requirements, healthcare facility standards, and practice standards. Internal self-audits should be conducted at least quarterly with focus on facility compliance, service delivery, and staff performance. This audit includes a checklist of regulatory items and chart review.

An exhaustive clinic and operations audit should be conducted annually. This audit is a deep dive into not only the operations of the clinic, but also a multidisciplinary approach that involves all stakeholders within the company. Stakeholders involved with the occupational health services include the clinic staff, human resources and benefits professionals, safety and risk managers, and operations managers. The purpose of this type of audit is to validate the quality of service delivery that is being provided in the clinic, not only by looking within the clinic, but also through the eyes of the external stakeholders. The outcome of this type of audit will also provide guidance and recommendations for establishing consistency across multiple company-based clinics and assessing satisfaction of stakeholder relationships with clinic staff. The outcome of an exhaustive audit is aimed at enhancing and maximizing the quality and delivery of service that meets the needs of all stakeholders. The exhaustive audit is most times completed by an independent third-party consultant who can conduct the audit in an objective, nonbiased fashion. The advantage of using an independent consultant is to obtain professional guidance based on the expert's broader perspective and to invite recommendations for improvement from an industry-wide perspective. The role of this consultant is not only to evaluate the clinic services, but also to introduce strategies that facilitate the coordination of interdepartmental relationships and to maximize the value of clinic and vendor services. The intended outcome of the project is to increase the confidence of workers and management in the value of their occupational health services.

SUMMARY

The OHN holds the potential to provide a wide range of occupational health services at the workplace and is therefore obligated to establish services that meet the health and regulatory needs of the workplace. Oftentimes the employer is uncertain about the scope of services that can or should be provided or may not always be aware of the specific health and safety needs that could or should be addressed. A "things to consider" checklist is provided in Appendix 8 that will provide basic guidance for clinic start-up.

Faced with regulatory and ethical obligations, the OHN must strive to meet the needs of the workforce by providing services that are of value to the employer while meeting the specific health needs for the workers. Because on-site occupational health services are provided in an environment that is outside the typical healthcare milieu, the OHN must develop a quality product while maintaining standards and compliance with health regulations consistent with a healthcare practice and environment. It is the OHN's responsibility to convey these standards by educating management and workers on the moral, ethical, and regulatory aspects of healthcare services in relation to the business environment.

REFERENCES

American Academy of Family Physicians. (2005). *OTC drugs: Getting the most from your medicine*. Retrieved from http://familydoctor.org/851.xml

American Association of Occupational Health Nurses AAOHN. (1996). *Code of ethics and interpretive statements*. Atlanta, GA: AAOHN.

American Association of Occupational Health Nurses AAOHN. (1999). *Standards of occupational and environmental health nursing*. Atlanta, GA: AAOHN.

American Association of Occupational Health Nurses AAOHN. (2003). *Position statement: Confidentiality of employee health information*. Atlanta, GA: AAOHN.

American Association of Occupational Health Nurses (AAOHN) Advisory. (2004). *Confidentiality of employee health information*. Atlanta, GA: AAOHN.

American Association of Occupational Health Nurses (AAOHN) Advisory. (2008). *Over the counter medications*. Retrieved from http://www.aaohn.org/advisories/over-the-counter-medications.html

American Association of Healthplans HIPAA information: Case Management Society of America (CMSA). (2002). *Standards of practice for case management*. Little Rock, AK: CMSA.

Centers for Disease Control and Prevention. (2006). *Clinical Laboratory Improvement Amendments (CLIA): How to obtain a CLIA certificate of waiver*. Retrieved from http://wwwn.cdc.gov/cliac/pdf/Addenda/cliac0210/Addendum%20F.pdf

Cham, E., Hall, L., Ernst, A. A., & Weiss, S. J. (2002). Awareness and use of over-the counter pain medications: A survey of emergency department patients. *Southern Medical Journal, 95*(5), 529–538.

Chenowith, D. H. and Garrett, J. (2006). Cost-effectiveness analysis of a worksite clinic: Is it worth the cost? *AAOHN Journal, 54*(2), 84–89.

Christiansen, J. R. (2003). HIPAA security compliance: It's all about risk management. *Health Lawyers News, 7*(5), 21–26.

Consumer Reports on Health. (2001). Over-the-counter drugs: How safe? *13*(8), 1–4.

D'Arruda, K. (2000). Confidentiality and disclosure of medical records under the Occupational Safety and Health Act. *AAOHN Journal, 48*, 458–460.

D'Arruda, K. (2001). HIPAA and USDHHS's Final Rule - First guidance from the Department of Health & Human Services. *AAOHN Journal, 49*, 542–544.

D'Arruda, K. (2002). HIPAA Update: Administrative simplification and national standards. *AAOHN Journal, 50*, 496–498.

DiBenedetto, D. V. (2002). Key HIPAA web sites and internet resources. *AAOHN Journal, 50*(9), 397–399.

DiBenedetto, D. V. (2003). HIPAA Privacy 101: Essentials for case management practice. *Lippincott's Case Management, 8*(1), 14–23.

Fitzmaurice, M. & Rose, J. (2000). What physician executives need to know about HIPAA. *The Physician Executive, 6*, 42–49.

Humphrey, H. L. & Gruber, C. R. (2008). Professional practice: Distribution of over-the-counter medications in the workplace. *AAOHN Journal, 56*(11), 445–446.

Integrated Benefits Institute. (2002). The impact of HIPAA privacy regulations on disability management. Retrieved from http://www.ibiweb.org

Kalina, C., Haag, A., & Wassel, M. L. (2001). How does the HIPAA privacy standards affect case management? *AAOHN Journal, 49*, 508–511.

Kibbe, D. (2001). HIPAA's here. *Nursing Management, 32*(4), 32–34.

Knoblauch, D., Childre, F., & Strasser, P. (1997). Legal and ethical issues. In M. K. Salazar (Ed.), *AAOHN core curriculum for occupational and environmental health nursing* (pp. 71–93). Philadelphia: W.B. Saunders.

Litchfield, S. M. (2010). Occupational health nursing currents: Medications in the workplace. *AAOHN Journal, 58(2)*.

The National Council on Patient Information and Education (NCPIE) & the Agency for Healthcare Research and Quality (AHRQ). (2003). Your medicine: Play it safe. Retrieved from ww.ahrq.gov/consumer/safemeds/safemeds.pdf

NIH Senior Health. (2004). Taking medicines—Medicines and your body. Retrieved from http://nihseniorhealth.gov/takingmedicines/medicinesandyourbody/01.html

Nurses Service Organization (NSO). (2003). Patient privacy and HIPAA hype. *NSO Risk Advisor, 12*(1), 4–5.

Oakley, Katie. 2008. *Occupational health nursing* (3rd ed.). Hoboken, NJ: Wiley.

OEM Press. (2003). HIPAA 2003: Medical privacy takes center stage. *The Occupational and Environmental Medicine Report, 17*(6), 37–44.

OEM Press. (2003). HIPAA 2003: Medical privacy takes center stage. *The Occupational and Environmental Medicine Report, 17*(7), 45–52.

OSHA. 29 CFR 1910.1020. Access to employee exposure & medical records. Retrieved from www.osha.gov

OSHA. (2011). Regulation 1910.10230, Occupational safety and health standards, toxic hazardous substances, access to employee exposure and medical records. Retrieved from http://www.osha.gov/pls/oshaweb

Rogers, B. (2003). *Occupational health nursing: Concepts and practice* (2nd ed.). Philadelphia: W.B. Saunders.

Rosati, K. & Shay, E. (2003). Your law firm signed that HIPAA business associate agreement. *Health Lawyers News*, 7(6), 9–13.

Shuren, A., & Livsey, K. (2001). Complying with the Health Insurance Portability and Accountability Act. *AAOHN Journal*, 49(11), 501–507.

Sitzman, K. (2003). Over the counter medications—Use caution! *AAOHN Journal*, 51(12).

U.S. Department of Health and Human Services (HHS). (2003a). Privacy rule preamble. Retrieved from http://www.hhs.gov

U.S. Department of Health and Human Services (HHS). (2003b). Summary of the HIPAA privacy rules & frequently asked questions & answers. Retrieved from http://www.hhs/gov/ocr/hipaa

U.S. Department of Health and Human Services. HIPAA administrative simplification. Regulation Text. 45 CFR Parts 160, 162, and 164 (Unofficial Version, as amended through February 16, 2006). Retrieved from http://www.hhs.gov/ocr/privacy/hipaa/administrative/privacyrule/adminsimpregtext.pdfwww.hipaaadvisory.com

U.S. Department of Health and Human Services. HIPAA privacy rule: Provisions relevant to public health practice. Retrieved from: www.cdc.gov

U.S. Food and Drug Administration. (2000). Use medicine safely. Retrieved from www.fda.gov/opacom/lowlit/medsafe.htm

U.S. Food and Drug Administration. (2005). Over-the-counter medicines: What's right for you? Retrieved from www.fda.gov/cder/consumerinfo/WhatsRightForYou.htm

U.S. Food and Drug Administration and the Consumer Healthcare Products Association. (2002). Over-the-counter medicines: What's right for you? Retrieved from www.fda.gov/cder/consumerinfo/whatsRightForYou.htm

Velez-McEvoy, M. (2006). What your employee needs to know about taking medication safely. *AAOHN Journal*, 54(2), 56–60.

WEB RESOURCES

www.aahp.org/Templage.cfm
American Association of Health Plans
www.aspe.hhs.gov/admnsimp/
US Department of Health and Human Services. Office of the Assistant Secretary of Planning and Evaluation
www.cms.hhs.gov/hipaa/
Centers for Medicare and Medicaid
www.sba.gov/advo/state_legislative03.pdf
Small Business Association

Workplace Regulatory Requirements

6

Health, safety and productivity.
A triad of priories for the workplace.

There are numerous regulatory concerns that must be taken into consideration that affect workers and workplaces. Occupational health nurses (OHN) should be keenly aware of the regulations that affect their specific workplace and strive to assist the employer in achieving compliance. This chapter provides a summary of some common workplace regulatory requirements; however this is in no means exhaustive.

OCCUPATIONAL SAFETY AND HEALTH ACT

The Occupational Safety and Health Act (OSH Act), established in 1970, is intended to "assure safe and healthful working conditions for working men and women" (OSHA, 2011). The primary intention was to develop and enforce standards that would lead to safe and healthful working conditions and to provide the mechanism for research, information, education, and training in the field of occupational health and safety. This Act led to the development of federal standards, but also allows states to develop and enforce their own standards as long as they are at least as stringent as the federal standards. The Act is administered by the Occupational Health and Safety Administration (OSHA), a division of the U.S. Department of Labor, with leadership from the assistant secretary of labor. The OSH Act addresses safety and health conditions in most industries, including some public sector employers. Any employer covered by the Act must comply with the regulations and standards. The prime principle of the Act is that employers have a "general duty" to provide workers with a workplace free from recognized hazards. The provisions of the Act are enforced by OSHA through inspections and investigations. OSHA, through a consultation service, also provides proactive assistance to employers to assist in the development of safety programs to ensure compliance. This consultation is

Essentials for Occupational Health Nursing, First Edition. Arlene Guzik.
© 2013 John Wiley & Sons, Inc. Published 2013 by John Wiley & Sons, Inc.

Table 6.1 OSHA information.

Who is Covered by Federal OSHA?
- Any employer with workers engaged in a business affecting commerce

Who is not Covered by Federal OSHA?*
- Self-employed business owners
- Farms at which only immediate members of the farmer's family are employed
- Persons who employ others in their own homes to perform domestic services such as housecleaning and child care
- Churches and nonsecular church activities
- Industries regulated by other federal agencies, such as mining, nuclear, or air transportation
- U.S., state, and local governments and political subdivisions

---

*Unless covered by State OSH regulations

confidential and provided at no cost to the employer. However, there is a caveat. If the employer does not heed the recommendations of the consultation and correct serious hazards within the timetable recommended, the consultation service will report the infractions to OSHA. The workplace may then be subject to formal inspection.

The OSH Act is a comprehensive law, and it covers most employers. Table 6.1 provides a list of common businesses that are covered and those typically not covered. Unless employers are sure their business is exempt, they should assume that the law is applicable to their operations. The OHS Act defines specific standards that apply to certain industries, and examples of standards for those specific industries are listed in Table 6.2. The laws, developed to ensure health and safety for the workforce, are a prudent guide for all employers, and it is in the best interest of employers to adopt the standards, even though their business may not be a covered entity.

OSHA's General Duty Clause states that "no employee will suffer impairment of health or functional capacity even if such employee has regular exposure to the hazard dealt with by such standard for the period of his working life." (OSHA, 2011). The expectation is that all workers have the right to work in a workplace that is free from recognized hazards that can cause or are likely to cause death or physical harm. It also requires that all workers are must be compliant with OSHA standards, along with other rules and regulations that are applicable to their work actions and job functions.

The OSH Act requires employers to notify workers, through awareness and training programs, of hazards that exist in the workplace, and the employer is required to maintain observant awareness of such hazards. Once aware of any hazards, the employer is required to determine the approach to protect workers (1) by eliminating the hazard, (2) by containing the hazard, or (3) by providing protection for workers. The employer is then responsible for measuring and monitoring the level of hazard exposure, as appropriate. The Act also requires

Table 6.2 Examples of standards for specific industries.

General Industry Standards
- Commercial diving
- Compressed gas/air equipment
- Electrical wiring and electronics
- Exit routes, emergency action plans and fire prevention plans
- Fire protection
- Handheld equipment
- Hazardous materials
- Machinery and machine guarding
- Material handling and storage
- Medical and first aid
- Personal protective equipment
- Radiation
- Sanitation
- Special industry standards
- Toxic and hazardous substances
- Ventilation
- Walking/working surfaces
- Welding, cutting and brazing
- Work platforms

Construction Industry Standards
- Concrete and masonry
- Cranes, derricks, hoists, elevators, conveyors
- Demolition and blasting
- Diving
- Electrical
- Excavations
- Fall protection
- Fire protection
- Hand/power tools, welding, cutting
- Material handling, storage, use, disposal
- Motor vehicles
- Overhead protection
- Personal protective and emergency response equipment
- Scaffolds
- Signs, signals, barricades
- Stairways, ladders
- Steel erections
- Hazardous substances

Maritime Industry Standards
- Cargo handling and equipment
- Electrical machinery
- Gangways
- Opening and closing hatches
- Personal protection
- Pressure vessels, drums, containers
- Rigging equipment and gear
- Scaffolds and ladders

(*Continued*)

Table 6.2 (*Continued*)

- Ship machinery and piping systems
- Surface preparation and preservation
- Terminal facilities
- Tools and equipment
- Toxic, hazardous substances
- Welding, cutting, heating

Agriculture Industry Standards
- Guarding of farm field equipment, farmstead equipment, and cotton gins
- Rollover protection structures
- Sanitation
- Use of cadmium

---

the employer to establish a mechanism for periodic health examinations and testing of workers who are exposed to specific hazards that could adversely affect their health. These examinations are to be made available by the employer at no cost to the worker.

To enforce the Act, provisions authorize an OSHA compliance officer to enter any workplace at any time to inspect and investigate the conditions and operations of the workplace and to validate adherence to the applicable standards. The visit from an OSHA compliance officer may be unannounced, meaning the officer may show up at the workplace unexpectedly. Visits may also be triggered by notice of or by frequency of accidents or even upon complaint from a worker. Should the employer attempt to refuse access to the workplace by the compliance officer, the officer has the right to obtain a legal warrant to inspect.

After the inspection tour, a closing conference is held between the compliance officer and the employer and/or the employer representative. This provides an opportunity for open discussion of findings and identification of any deficiencies, and it is a time for questions and answers. If the inspection leads to evidence that the employer has violated any section of the Act, the compliance officer is authorized to issue a citation to the employer. Each citation is issued in writing and includes a description of the nature of the violation, with reference to the standard, rule, regulation, or order that has allegedly been violated. The citation includes a proposed resolution and the reasonable timeframe for compliance. The officer also has the right to levy fines against the employer for violations. Table 6.3 provides a list of categories of fines. The employer is then required to post a copy of the issued citation in a prominent location on company premises, thus visible to all workers. The citation remains posted for 3 days or until the violation is abated, whichever is longer.

Employers have a right to appeal citations to Occupational Safety and Health Review Commission (OSHRC) and may request an informal meeting with

Table 6.3 Common OSHA penalties.

Level of Fine	Description	Impact on Employer
De minimus	The violation has no immediate relationship to safety and health	A documented violation without associated citation or fine
Other than serious	The violation has a direct relationship to safety and health; however, it would not likely cause serious harm or death	A penalty of up to $7,000 for each violation is *discretionary*. May be reduced based on good faith, history of prior violations, and size of business
Serious	The violation has the potential to cause serious injury or death and takes into consideration the fact that the employer should have recognized the hazard	A *mandatory* penalty of up to $7,000 for each violation is proposed. May be adjusted downward, based on the employer's good faith, history of previous violations, the gravity of the alleged violation, and size of business
Willful	Considers that the employer knowingly, deliberately, or intentionally committed the violation, with clear indifference to the law. The employer is aware that a hazardous condition exists and has made no reasonable effort to remove the hazard	Penalties of up to $70,000 may be proposed for each willful violation, with a minimum penalty of $5,000 for each violation. May be adjusted downward, depending on the size of the business and history of previous violations. Usually, no credit is given for good faith.
Criminal/willful	A willful violation that has resulted in the death of a worker	The offense is punishable either by a court-imposed fine, by imprisonment for up to six months, or both. A fine of up to $250,000 for an individual, or $500,000 for a corporation, may be imposed
Repeated violation	A recurrent violation of any standard, regulation, rule, or order. Is imposed when, upon reinspection, a substantially similar violation is found	Fine of up to $70,000 for each such violation
Failure to abate prior violation	Prior citation has been issued with failure to correct	May bring a civil penalty of up to $7,000 for each day the violation continues beyond the prescribed abatement date
Falsifying records, reports, or applications		Fine of $10,000, imprisonment for up to six months, or both
Violations of posting requirements	The employer fails to provide written postings required by OSHA standards	Civil penalty of up to $7,000
Assaulting a compliance officer	Includes resisting, opposing, intimidating, or interfering with a compliance officer	Fine of not more than $5,000 and imprisonment for not more than three years

Source: Created from information found at www.osha.gov.

Table 6.4 OSHA Citation and penalties, fiscal year 2010.

Top Ten Most Frequently Cited Standards	Top Ten Highest Penalties
1. Scaffolding, general requirements, construction	1. Fall protection, construction
2. Fall protection, construction	2. Electrical, general requirements, construction
3. Hazard communication standard, general	3. Safety training and education, construction
4. Ladders, construction	4. Control of hazardous energy (lockout/tagout), general industry
5. Respiratory protection, general	5. Machines, general requirements, general industry
6. Control of hazardous energy (lockout/tagout), general industry	6. General duty clause
7. Electrical, wiring methods, components and equipment, general industry	7. Excavations, requirements for protective systems, construction
8. Powered industrial trucks, general industry	8. Lead, general industry
9. Electrical systems design, general requirements, general industry	9. Grain handling facilities
10. Machines, general requirements, general industry	10. Ladders, construction

Source: Created from information found at www.OSHA.gov.

OSHA's area director to discuss the case. Workers also have the right to request an informal conference with OSHA to discuss findings of the inspection, the citation, and notice of proposed penalty.

The Act also requires employers to maintain accurate records connected to work-related deaths, injuries, and illnesses that involve medical treatment or for those that result in modification of the workers' duties as a result of a work incident. These reports are submitted to OSHA for the purposes of compiling the data for comparison to industry standards. OSHA is also authorized to use this data for research purposes and may publish the findings of any inspection or data from this record keeping. Specific information related to this record keeping will be discussed in Chapter 7. Table 6.4 lists a comparison of the top 10 cited standards and the top ten penalties for standards for 2010.

OSHA also sponsors a Voluntary Protection Program (VPP). This program serves to recognize the efforts of employers to provide worker protection by exceeding the minimum standards required by OSHA. There are three VPP categories: Star, Merit, and Demonstration. These VPP recognitions by OSHA serve to acknowledge outstanding achievement by workplaces that have incorporated a comprehensive health and safety approach their total management system through self-initiated efforts and cooperation, rather than just meeting minimum standards out of regulatory necessity. This means that the employers have voluntarily invited OSHA to conduct a comprehensive inspection of their workplace. This inspection consists of a rigorous, interactive methodology that includes active participation by not only management, but also by all workers. Workplaces that achieve VPP status are recognized at an OSHA award ceremony, receiving a certificate of approval and a VPP flag that can be proudly displayed at their worksite and on marketing material. VPP Star sites must apply for recertification every 3 years.

The OSHA Training Institute (OTI) Education Center Program provides support for OSHA's training and education mission through a variety of safety and health programs, including community outreach efforts. These programs are offered through community-based training and educational institutions and serve to conduct approved OSHA Training Institute courses. These institutions are selected through a national competitive process and support OSHA training based on their normal tuition and fee structures. This program serves as a valuable resource for employers for training management and workers in the basics of occupational safety and health. Common courses include training on occupational safety and health standards for general industry and construction, hazardous materials, machine guarding, ergonomics, confined space, excavation, electrical safety, and fall protection.

The OSH Act also served to create a National Institute of Occupational Safety and Health (NIOSH), part of The Department of Health and Human Services (DHHS), Centers for Disease Control and Prevention. NIOSH is the research body that serves to provide assistance to OSHA by conducting research on workplace risks and workplace health hazards. The findings of NIOSH research become the foundation for OSHA standards, supporting new or revised safety and health standards, and for the development of criteria for protection against toxic substances and physical agents. The research conducted by NIOSH is based on findings of investigations and information from worksites. Workers in certain industrial categories may also be summoned to participate in NIOSH research efforts through medical monitoring and physical examination for research purposes. The findings of such research serve to provide information related to the incidence of work-related illnesses among groups of workers.

NIOSH also provides competitive funding for 17 university-based Education and Research Centers (ERCs). These centers provide academic programs, continuing education, training, and research opportunities in the core areas of industrial hygiene, occupational health nursing, occupational medicine, and occupational safety. The ERCs serve to educate occupational safety and health professionals in order to provide an "adequate supply of qualified personnel to carry out the purposes of the Occupational Safety and Health Act" (NIOSH, 2011).

OSHA STANDARDS FOR GENERAL INDUSTRY

The following outlines some of the most common OSHA standards for general industry (29 CFR 1910). OSHA guidelines call for a systematic identification, evaluation, and prevention or control of general workplace hazards and the hazards involved in specific jobs and tasks.

Hazard Communication Program (29 CFR 1910.1200)
This program is designed to ensure that employers and workers are aware of the hazardous chemicals in the workplace and the protection that is necessary as a safeguard to avoid exposure to chemicals that may be harmful. The employer is required to establish and implement a written hazard communication program in order to comply with the requirements of the standard.

The basic concept of the standard is *the right to know,* that employees have both a need and a right to know the hazards and the identities of the chemicals they are exposed to when working. They also have the right to know what protective measures are recommended and available to prevent adverse health effects. The Hazard Communication Standard defines requirements for the evaluation of all chemicals imported into, produced, or used in U.S. workplaces. This information is to be made available to workers who may be affected by or exposed to these chemicals. Hazard information must be provided through labels on containers and through material safety data sheets (MSDSs). The employer is responsible for awareness and training efforts for workers to inform them about the hazards of specific chemicals used in their workplace.

Chemical Safety
Chemicals in sealed containers are required to have affixed labels that must remain intact. The employer must maintain on file and provide workers access to MSDSs. A written hazardous chemical program must detail the requirements for labels and other forms of warning, material safety data sheets, and the process for employee information and training. The employer's training for workers must include information on the use of the chemical and what actions to take in the event of a spill or leak.

The employer should ensure a standard approach to establishing compliance with the Hazard Communication standard by following these steps:

1. Obtain a copy of the rule
2. Determine if the standard applies to the workplace
3. Identify responsible staff
4. Establish policies and procedures to maintain and evaluate the effectiveness of the program
5. Identify hazardous substances in the workplace
6. Prepare and implement the program
7. Ensure that all containers are properly labeled
8. Obtain and make available to workers material safety data sheets for each chemical
9. Conduct employee awareness and training

All chemicals have the potential to cause health hazards. Exposures to chemicals may occur by absorption, commonly through contact with the skin, splashes to mucous membranes (such as the eye). Exposures may also occur through ingestion, or by inhalation. Exposures that cause or may lead to acute health issues should be referred to the OHN or to a healthcare facility immediately. When a worker has a significant exposure to a hazardous chemical, first aid intervention is critical and the employer is required to have supplies and equipment available for swift intervention. The second step is to retrieve a copy of the MSDS for that particular chemical to see what first aid interventions are warranted and to identify potential health hazards that may result from the exposure. If the worker is sent to an outside healthcare facility for further evaluation, the MSDS should accompany the worker as a resource for the healthcare provider.

Because of the focus on chemical safety within this standard, most exposures are now prevented by the use of protective clothing or apparatus; such as goggles, respirators, impervious gloves and aprons, etc. One must remember, however that exposure to chemicals may also have a cumulative effect and lead to chronic health conditions, such as cancers, birth defects, blood dyscrasias, liver and lung diseases. Therefore, the standard calls for routine health monitoring of workers exposed to specific chemicals.

Emergency Action Plan (EAP) Standard (CFR1910.38)

OSHA recommends that all employers have a plan that addresses emergencies that may reasonably occur in the workplace. There are also conditions in which an EAP is specifically mandatory when required by an OSHA standard. An EAP describes the actions workers should take to ensure their safety in the event of emergencies such as floods, hurricanes and tornados, fires, release of toxic gases or chemicals, irradiation accidents, or explosions. Workplaces are also required to have established emergency action plans in the event of workplace violence.

An EAP is a written document that addresses the procedures for reporting workplace emergencies. It includes evacuation procedures and emergency escape routes, assignment of employees who are critical to business operations during evacuation, procedures to account for all workers after an emergency evacuation, along with rescue and first aid duties for certain workers.

The emergency escape plan should define who is authorized to order an evacuation and under what conditions an evacuation would be necessary. The plan should also outline how workers will evacuate, and what routes they will take. Exit diagrams are typically used for this purpose. The plan should also define the workers who are critical to business operations during and after evacuation. Such workers would be required to operate fire extinguishers or shut down gas and/or electrical systems. They may also be responsible for operation of equipment that is critical to business functions or address operational issues that could create additional hazards during emergency response efforts.

The plan should also include procedures to account for workers after evacuation to ensure that all workers have safely evacuated. Workers who evacuate should be assigned to specific assembly areas, and the plan should identify a person responsible for conducting a roll call of workers. The plan may also outline specific rescue duties of certain workers, those well-trained in emergency response and first aid, to ensure appropriate triage for workers in need of further health evaluation.

Additional aspects of the standard require that an alarm system be in place to notify workers of such an emergency, and to ensure all workers know the actions to take should the alarm activate. The standard has provisions for training of all employees on initial hire and at times when revisions are made to the plan.

Although not specifically defined in the standard, it is prudent for the employer to ensure provisions are made for workers with impairments or disabilities. Examples would include evacuation alarm notices that have provisions for hearing-impaired workers; such alarms would not only be audible, but also visual. Evacuation plans should include providing support to sight-impaired workers and those who are physically incapacitated.

Walking/Working Surfaces Standard (29 CFR 1926.1050-1060)

The OSHA standards for walking and working surfaces applies to all permanent places of employment The only exceptions are those in which domestic, mining, or agricultural work is performed. The standard addressed requirements regarding breaks in elevation and single points of access/egress to allow for ample passage by workers.

The standard also addresses requirements for fall protection for elevated work surfaces, stairways, and ladders. A requirement for floor guarding for openings and holes in flooring or ground surfaces is also addressed. The standard also includes recommendations for the use of mobile ladders, scaffolds, man-lifts, and mounted and powered platforms.

Medical and First Aid Standard (29 CFR 1910.151)

OSHA requires employers to make provisions for first-aid interventions and health evaluations of workers. The specifics of a workplace health and first-aid program are dependent on the unique operations of each workplace, the hazards involved, and its resources. The aim is to provide prompt attention to workplace incidents and injuries in order to minimize these events. The employer is required to provide first aid supplies and equipment that are readily accessible to workers and to first aid providers. Table 6.5 outlines the minimum standards for first aid supplies required in the workplace.

The employer is also expected to establish a relationship with community emergency medical services (EMS) and local fire rescue. For industries with high-risk operations, it is also prudent to establish relationships with local healthcare providers and emergency departments. The OSHA First Aid standard

Table 6.5 Minimum standard first aid supplies.

Item and Minimum Size or Volume	Minimum Quantity
Absorbent bandage 4×4 in.	1
Adhesive bandages, 1×3 in.	16
Adhesive tape, 3/8 in.	1
Antiseptic, 0.14 fl oz.	10
Burn treatment, 1/32 oz	6
Exam gloves	2 pair
Sterile pad, 3×3 in.	4
Triangular bandage, 40×40×56 in.	1

Source: Created from information found in ANSI Z308.1-2003 Section 5.1.

also requires "trained first-aid providers at all workplaces of any size if there is no infirmary, clinic, or hospital in near proximity to the workplace which is used for the treatment of all injured employees" (OSHA, 2011). In workplaces where there is risk of extreme exertion, asphyxiation, electrocution, or other such danger, the OSHA standard requires training of workers in cardiopulmonary resuscitation (CPR). This requirement specifically applies to workplaces with confined spaces, logging operations, electric power generation, and dive operations.

The American National Standards Institute (ANSI, 2011) defines standards for workplace first aid kits (ANSI standard, Z308.1-2003). Kits sold to and purchased by employers for use in the workplace must meet the performance standards set forth by ANSI. There are specific classifications for kits used in the workplace:

Type I: This kit is intended for indoor use only. It is appropriate for office or service industries, as well as for light manufacturing settings. The kit is not intended to be portable and should be place in a fixed location, most likely mounted to the wall.

Type II: This kit, intended also for indoor use, is usually equipped with carrying handles, thus making it portable and valuable for response to remote locations. This type is suitable for use in services, light manufacturing, or light-industrial settings.

Type III: The kit is appropriate for use in heavy manufacturing, construction, transportation, and other heavy industrial settings because it is moisture resistant, has little potential for damage, and is portable.

Recent advances in technology have provided the availability of automated external defibrillators (AEDs) that can be placed in workplaces. These AEDs are appropriate for work settings with high potential for sudden cardiac arrest. The presence of an AED in the work setting is not only a benefit for workers, it is also a benefit for the general public who frequent that setting. Common settings for AEDs aside from high-risk industry include shopping malls, public libraries, government or municipal buildings, theaters, and event locations.

Each workplace should assess its own requirements for an AED program as part of establishing a first aid response protocol. Issues that should be considered when implementing a workplace AED program include physician oversight to write the prescription for the AED and provide medical direction; compliance with local, state, and federal regulations; location of the AED in the work or public setting; coordination with local EMSs; a quality assurance program; and medical director review of events requiring use of the AED.

Additional information and guidance for developing an AED program for the worksite can be found at the following websites:

- OSHA at www.osha.gov
- American College of Occupational and Environmental Medicine at www.acoem.org
- American Heart Association at www.americanheart.org
- American Red Cross at www.redcross.org
- Federal Occupational Health at www.foh.dhhs.gov
- National Center for Early Defibrillation at www.early-defib.org

Machine Guarding Standard (29 CFR 1910 Subpart O)
Employers with workers who operate machinery (e.g., saws, power presses, moving conveyors, etc.) are required to comply with the machine-guarding requirements.

Many hazards can be created by moving machine parts, leading to crushed hands and arms, lacerated fingers, extremity amputations, and other serious injuries. The OSHA standard for machine guarding requires that "any machine part, function, or process which many cause injury must be safeguarded. When the operation of a machine or accidental contact with it can injure the operator or others in the vicinity, the hazards must be either controlled or eliminated." (OSHA, 2011)

There are four strategies to machine guarding:

1. Prevent contact: Protection of hands, arms, and any other part of a worker's body eliminates the possibility of the worker or other workers placing parts of their bodies near hazardous moving parts.
2. Secure: The machine guard should not be able to easily remove or tamper with and must be firmly secured to the machine.
3. Protect from falling objects: Care must be taken to avoid falling objects that can land on moving parts of the machinery.
4. Create no new hazards: A safeguard should not create a hazard in and of itself.

5. Create no interference: The safeguard should not impede a worker from performing the job efficiently. If so, it may provoke the workers to override or disregard the machine guarding.
6. Allow for safe lubrication of the machine: Maintenance workers should be able to lubricate the machine without removing the safeguards.

Machine operator training should involve instruction or hands-on training that includes identification of hazards and their specific safeguards; the purpose of and reasons for the safeguards; how and for what reasons machine guards can be removed; and steps to take when a machine guard is missing or when it malfunctions.

Lockout/Tagout Standard (29 CFR 1910.147)

Employers are required to establish measures for controlling hazardous energy (electrical, mechanical, hydraulic, pneumatic, chemical, thermal, and other energy sources) as a safeguard for workers. This requires that those servicing machinery or equipment provide the necessary safeguards against the unexpected startup of the machinery or equipment. This is done by affixing appropriate lockout or tagout notices to the device. This standard was established to avoid physical harm as a result of the discharge of hazardous energy while the machinery or equipment is being serviced. It also serves as a safeguard to prevent the machine or equipment being turned on by another worker while it is being serviced. The standard requires that machines or equipment be de-energized (lockout) or tagged with appropriate notice (tagout) to provide a level of safety by providing adequate notice to workers. Lockout prevents use of the machine or equipment by disabling its operations so workers cannot turn on the machine/equipment. Tagout prevents use by providing appropriate written notice on the machine that it should not be used. This tag would be located at the area where the machine could be powered on.

The standard also requires that workers receive training regarding the control of hazardous energy and avoiding serious physical harm to or death of workers. Workers must receive training on procedures related to the unexpected energy discharge or unexpected start-up of the machinery or equipment should it occur. Workers must also receive training on how to apply the appropriate lockout or tagout devices. Training is intended to ensure that workers understand and follow the appropriate provisions for the lockout/tagout out program.

Electrical Hazards Standard (29 CFR 1910 Subpart S)

Electrical and wiring deficiencies are among the most common violations that receive OSHA citations. OSHA's Electrical Hazards Standard includes recommendations for design of electrical systems and safety-related work practices. The standard applies to engineers, electricians, and other professionals who work with electricity directly, including those working on overhead lines, cable harnesses, and circuit assemblies. The standard establishes electrical safety requirements necessary for the practical safeguarding of employees in their workplaces (OSHA, 2011).

The standard addresses four components for electrical safety: (1) design safety standards for electrical systems; (2) safety-related work practices; (3) safety-related maintenance requirements; and (4) safety requirements for special equipment.

Personal Protective Equipment (PPE) Standard (29 CFR 1910 Subpart I)
The first line of defence in protecting workers from hazards involves engineering controls—physically changing a machine or work environment by removing or controlling the hazard. The second line of defense, if the hazard cannot be eliminated or controlled, involves implementing and training workers on ways to perform the job to reduce their exposure to workplace hazards. OSHA generally considers PPE to be the third and last option for controlling worker exposure. If the employer determines that it is necessary for workers to use PPE, the employer must select the appropriate PPE for the hazard and require its use.

Examples of PPE include, but are not limited to, face shields, safety glasses/goggles, hard hats, safety shoes, coveralls, gloves, vests, aprons, earplugs, and respirators. Employers are required to communicate the requirement for and availability of PPE for workers; however, this is not enough. The burden is on the employer to routinely monitor workers' compliance with the use of PPE and reinforce the standard.

Respiratory Protection Standard (29 CFR 1910.134)
OSHA's respiratory protection program applies to workers who are exposed to airborne contaminants at a hazardous level (dust, grains, lead, pesticides, airborne bacteria, etc.) and for work conditions where the air is oxygen-deficient (mines, confined spaces, fires, etc.). The standard clearly states that the use of a respirator for protection should be considered only after exhausting all engineering control efforts, or while these controls are being instituted. Several other OSHA regulations specifically require the use of respirators for health hazard protection when workers are exposed to certain health-compromising contaminants.

The required components of a respiratory protection program include provisions for selection of the respirator, medical clearance for respirator users, procedures for proper use, respirator fit testing, and respirator maintenance procedures. In other words, the worker must be medically fit to wear the respirator and must wear the appropriate respirator for the associated work conditions. In order to do so, the worker must undergo health evaluation and testing to ensure that the respirator is the appropriate fit for protection. The cost of these evaluations must be covered by the employer. The employer must also ensure that the worker receives adequate training on the proper use and maintenance of the respirator.

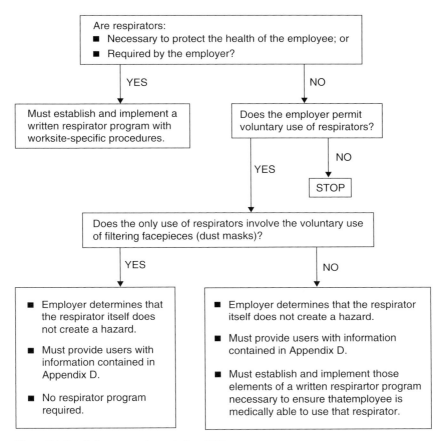

Figure 6.1 Respirator use requirements flow chart.
Source: Courtesy of the Occupational Safety & Health Administration. www.osha.gov

Employers with respiratory protection programs must assign a program administrator whose duty it is to ensure compliance with the standard. The program administrator must ensure that the respirators selected are certified by the National Institute for Occupational Safety and Health (NIOSH). Selection of the appropriate respirator for the associated work conditions is of critical importance. For example, only an air-supplied respirator will provide appropriate protection of the worker in an oxygen-deficient environment. The use of a non-air-supplied respirator in this type of environment will not provide adequate protection and the user will be exposed to death. Figure 6.1 displays OSHA's flow chart, which is useful for employers in determining the need for a respiratory protection program.

Types of Respirators
There are different types of respirators used in the workplace. The first type is the air-purifying respirator.

- Particulate respirators capture particles in the air, such as dusts, mists, and fumes. Typically called face-filtering respirators, they do not protect against gases and vapors.
- Gas/vapor respirators are used when there are hazardous gases and vapors in the air. They contain chemical filters (cartridges or canisters) and are made to protect against specific gases or vapors.
- Combination respirators have both particulate filters and gas/vapor filters.

Another type of respirator used in the workplace is the atmosphere-supply respirator.

- Air-supplied respirators provide a supply of clean air for long periods of time. They are lightweight and use a hose to deliver clean air from a fixed source of compressed air. Use of this type of respirator limits the mobility of the wearer.
- Self-contained breathing apparatus (SCBA) consists of a wearable supply pack of clean air, and as a result kit does not restrict movement of the wearer. Common use of SCBA is in fire fighting. For work performed underwater, a self-contained underwater breathing apparatus (SCUBA) should be used.

Combination respirators have an auxiliary wearable supply pack of clean air that can be used if the primary fixed supply fails. It is typically used for work in confined spaces.

Occupational Noise Standard (29 CFR 1910.95)
Since there are no visible effects of hearing loss, it often goes undetected until it has an effect on communication and responsiveness on the part of the worker. OHSA's Occupational Noise Standard is designed to protect the hearing of workers who are exposed to significant noise as a part of their work duties.

This standard is based on the principle that the health effects of noise exposure are dependent on the intensity and duration of the exposure. The health effect is primarily a loss of or reduction in the worker's hearing. These effects may be temporary, usually as a result of short-term exposure, after which normal hearing returns. Or, the effect can be permanent, usually related to exposure to high-pitched noise over a prolonged period of time. OSHA requires employers to determine if workers are exposed to excessive noise in the workplace. If so, the employer may be required to implement a hearing conservation program.

The standard requires employers to monitor noise exposure in areas of the workplace to determine if workers are exposed to noise at or above 85 decibels (dB) over an 8-hour work shift (8-hour time-weighted average [TWA]).

These work areas are usually in places where noise is generated by machinery, power tools, or other operational causes. If the noise level exceeds the permissible exposure limit (PEL), the employer must first consider engineering or administrative controls to reduce the noise level. If the noise cannot be eliminated or controlled, the employer must implement a hearing conservation program.

A hearing conservation program consists of worker training, the use of hearing protection, and periodic audiometric (hearing) evaluations of the workers. The employer must provide hearing protectors to all workers exposed to an 8-hour TWA noise level of 85 dB or higher. The protectors must be effective in reducing the workers' exposure to the noise to 90 dB or lower. The employer must then establish and maintain an audiometric testing program. The testing program is intended to test all workers at the time they begin work in the noise-induced area in order to provide a baseline of the worker's current hearing. Annual audiograms are performed thereafter, as long as the worker remains in the noise-induced work area. A comparison of the annual audiogram to the baseline test is conducted to determine if the worker has incurred hearing loss, defined as a standard threshold shift (STS), as a result of working in the noise-induced area. An STS is determined by calculating the results of the audiometric tests at 2,000, 3,000, and 4,000 hertz. If an average shift in either ear of 10 dB or more is identified, and no other causes of hearing loss can be identified by the occupational healthcare provider, the worker must receive additional training and counseling on hearing protection or be removed from the noise-induced area. Workers who terminate employment or transfer to a non-noise area of the workplace participate in an exit audiogram to memorialize the hearing of the worker at that time they exit the hearing conservation program.

The standard requires training, at least annually, of workers who are in the hearing conservation program. The training includes information on the effects of noise exposure, the purpose of the use of hearing protectors, the proper selection, fit, and care of the hearing protectors, and the purpose of audiometric testing. The standard also requires employers to maintain record keeping of the workplace noise exposure measurement results for 2 years and must also maintain records of the worker's audiometric test results for the duration of the worker's employment. The employer is also required to make these records available to current workers, former workers, representatives of the workers, and to OSHA.

Confined Spaces Standard (29 CFR 1910.146)
Many workplaces contain spaces that are considered "confined" because their configurations hinder the movement of the worker who must enter, work in, and exit from them. Examples of confined work spaces would include work in vessels, sewer lines, mines, containers, crawl spaces, etc. A general principle of a confined space is that the worker must enter and exit through narrow openings and/or perform work tasks while in a limited space, thus preventing free

movement. It also takes into consideration the type of work the worker is performing while in the confined space. Some work performed in a confined space can lead to the potential for the worker to be exposed to a variety of hazards, including toxic or flammable gases/vapors, oxygen-deficient air, and airborne contaminants. The potential for asphyxiation, incapacitation, the inability of self-rescue, injury, or even death are possible in confined spaces.

If the employer determines that a worker must perform work in a confined space, a confined space entry permit may be required. Some key principles in evaluating the workplace to determine if any spaces are permit-required confined spaces include:

1. Is the space large enough that a worker can bodily enter?
2. Is the space configured so that a worker can enter to perform work fully or partially inside?
3. Does the space in question have limited or restricted means for entry or exit?

If permit spaces are present and workers are required to enter such spaces, the employer must develop and implement a confined space program, which is an overall plan for protecting workers. An important element of the requirement is that entry of workers into confined spaces is allowed only by a written entry permit issued by the employer. The employer is required to identify confined spaces with signs, and entry must be limited to only authorized workers. The standard specifies strict procedures for evaluation and atmospheric testing of a confined space before and during entry by workers. When workers are performing work in a confined space, the standard requires that the confined space entry be attended outside the space by an attendant who is trained and equipped to respond to emergencies that may occur with the worker in the confined space. Provisions must also be made for rescue of the worker in the event of an emergency. The standard specifies training requirements and specific duties for authorized entrants, attendants, and supervisors. Rescue service provisions are required, and where feasible, rescue must be facilitated by a nonentry retrieval system, such as a harness and cable attached to a mechanical hoist.

Bloodborne Pathogens (BBP) Standard (29 CFR 1910.1030)

Recognizing that exposure to bloodborne pathogens present risk of serious and sometimes life-threatening illnesses, the BBP standard requires the use of engineering and work practice controls to eliminate or minimize exposure to bloodborne pathogens. This standard is applicable to all healthcare and emergency response workers. It is not only applicable in healthcare-related workplaces, but also applies when workers are assigned as emergency or first aid responders in the general workplace. In addition, the standard applies to workers who are not direct caregivers, those who handle potentially infectious waste (janitors, maintenance workers, medical devise handlers), and those who may be exposed to risk as a part of other job duties (housekeeping, linen facilities).

The standard requires that such employers establish an exposure control plan, a written plan intended to eliminate or minimize the risk of be BPP exposures. The written plan identifies workers in job classifications that would be at risk and a list of job duties performed by those workers that might result in exposure. The employer is required to update the plan annually.

A hallmark of the standard is the use of universal precautions. The key principle of universal precautions is that all human blood and other potentially infected material is considered to be infectious and puts the worker at risk for a bloodborne pathogen exposure. As a result, specific procedures must be in place for handling and disposing of contaminated sharps and medical instruments, handling of specimens, disposing of contaminated waste, and handling of soiled laundry. The standard has led to the development of many improvements, such as impervious sharps disposal containers, safer medical devices and procedures, and self-retracting or self-sheathing needles. Sharps containers and containers of contaminated waste must be labeled and identified as communicable hazards. Regulations for the storage, transport, and shipment of potentially infected material were also established as part of this standard.

The employer must provide personal protective equipment (PPE) to all workers at risk of exposure. This includes gloves, gowns, eye protection, and masks. The standard also requires employers to provide training regarding the potential for exposure and the use of PPE, and to make available hepatitis B vaccinations to all workers with the potential for bloodborne pathogen exposure. This training and the offer of vaccination must take place within the first 10 days of initial assignment to a job with potential exposure. Should the worker decline vaccination for hepatitis B, a signed notice of declination should be placed in the workers file. Training must also include information on the possible mechanisms of exposure to blood or other potentially infectious material, including incidents in which the worker incurs exposures by penetration of the skin and through splashes onto the skin or into mucous membranes. Workers must receive training on the appropriate methods of reporting such exposures, and the employer is required to provide medical evaluation regarding the exposure at no cost to the worker. The standard requires healthcare employers to maintain a sharps injury log as part of their record keeping and reporting of occupational injuries and illnesses.

Powered Industrial Trucks Standard (29 CFR 1910.178)
This standard defines powered industrial trucks as anything used to carry, push, pull, lift, stack, or tier materials. This standard was developed in an attempt to reduce injuries and illnesses as result of careless use of mobile equipment as part of the worker's job duties. Injuries occur not only to the mobile equipment operator, but incidents involving mobile equipment can also lead to considerable damage to company property and injury to others. Examples of such incidents and injuries include mobile equipment accidents, pedestrian

incidents as a result of being struck by mobile equipment, material that falls while being stacked at elevated levels, driving mobile equipment off an elevated platform or dock, and damage to overhead structures by lift equipment. It is acknowledged that most incidents and injuries are a result of unsafe use and operation of the equipment because workers have received insufficient or inadequate training on mobile equipment safety (OSHA, 2011).

The standard requires the employer to provide training to mobile equipment operators on a variety of topics. Among these topics are vehicle inspection and maintenance that the operator will be required to perform.

The standard requires that all mobile equipment be examined at least daily before being placed in service. Forklifts used on a round-the-clock basis must be examined after each shift.

- **Preoperation**—workers must be trained on preoperation inspection of the equipment. This includes knowing when equipment should be removed from service and when maintenance is indicated.
- **Traveling and maneuvering**—workers must receive training on mounting and dismounting the equipment. Instructions must be given on starting and stopping, appropriate operating speeds, audible notice to pedestrians, changes in direction, and parking. Practices for safe travel, including travel on inclines and on even surfaces must be covered. Procedures for pedestrian safety and procedures in the event of tip-over must also be covered.
- **Load handling**—mobile equipment is most often used to handle product. Training must include procedures for appropriately positioning the mobile equipment, lifting and lowering the load, and entry into other vehicles, such as truck trailers and railroad cars.

The employer is required to certify that each mobile equipment operator has received the appropriate training and has been evaluated and determined competent to operate the equipment. Although testing is not required, it is prudent for the employer to ensure the worker has a firm knowledge about the operation of the equipment. A written training certificate should include the date of the training, the date of the evaluation and the evaluator's signature. Annual recertification is not required; however, retraining is indicated whenever the worker has been observed operating the equipment in an unsafe manner, when the worker incurs a near-miss incident, or when the worker is involved in an accident. The worker must also receive training if they are assigned to operate a different type of equipment or when the workplace conditions change significantly.

Although not required by regulatory statute, it is prudent that the employer establish that the worker is physically fit and capable of performing the essential functions of operating mobile equipment on the job. Key aspects of medical evaluation should include review of a comprehensive medical history to identify any medical conditions of concern, such as uncontrolled high blood pressure, vision disorders, cardiac arrhythmias, and neurological disorders. The examination should include evaluation of the blood pressure and vision, at a minimum. A sample evaluation form for mobile equipment operator fitness for duty is provided in Appendix 9.

In addition to the preceding Standards for General Industry, OSHA also publishes a set of standards specific to the construction, maritime, and agriculture industries. Although these industries must also comply with the general industry standards, the industry-specific standards supersede the rules intended for general industry (Rogers, 2004).

Federal Mine Safety and Health Act

The Federal Mine Safety and Health Act (Mine Act), passed in 1977, is similar to the OHS Act; however, it covers aspects of health and safety specific to workers who work on mine property. The Act is administered by the Mine Safety and Health Administration (MSHA), a division of the U.S. Department of Labor, and applies to 2,100 coal mines and 12,500 metal and nonmetal mines nationwide (MSHA, 2011).

The efforts of the MSH Act are based on three aspects, referred to as the "triangle of success": education and training, technical assistance, and compliance enforcement (MSHA, 2011). Compliance officers assist mine operators with compliance with the Act and are available for technical and training assistance. Through the years, MSHA has established a culture of accident and injury prevention by establishing core standards for safety and health specific to mining operations. Mine operators are responsible for providing mandatory miner training, which must include basic health and safety training for workers, before employees begin work in underground and or surface mining. Workers must also receive specific job training, not only when they begin work, but also when they are assigned to new tasks. And each worker is required to participate in an annual training update.

Similar to OSHA compliance officers, MSHA inspectors maintain a presence in the workplace with the purpose of compiling information on health and safety issues. As a result of their observation or data collection, the industry continues to develop strategies to enhance mine-engineering techniques, to develop new engineering controls for worker protection, and to reduce health and safety hazards.

In addition to the Safety and Health Acts, there are other regulatory requirements that are of importance in most workplaces. A few of these will be discussed in the next section, however it is important for the OHN to identify other regulatory requirements that may be applicable to specific work operations and environments.

COMMUNICABLE DISEASE REPORTING

The Centers for Disease Control and Prevention (CDC), established in 1946, is the premier agency and global leader in public health. With the focus on health promotion, prevention, and preparedness, the CDC strives to "prevent and control infectious and chronic diseases, injuries, workplace hazards, disabilities, and environmental health threats" (CDC, 2010). The strategic areas of concentration for the CDC also support health and safety in the workplace. In addition to supporting state and county health departments, the CDC strives to improve global health. This becomes valuable for workers who travel for global business purposes. The CDC also supports efforts to conduct health surveillance and gather data used for epidemiological research. This strategy leads to the development of regulations and recommendations for protection of workers in the workplace. The epidemiological data also serve to strengthen initiatives in healthcare and can be helpful in the workplace when there is a focus on health risk reduction and wellness efforts.

A significant area of emphasis with the CDC is in relation to the collection and publication of data on notifiable diseases. A notifiable disease is "one for which regular, frequent, and timely information regarding individual cases is considered necessary for the prevention and control of the disease" (CDC, 2010). This regulation establishes guidelines for healthcare providers to report certain diseases and conditions. The public health departments, under the direction of the CDC, ensure appropriate evaluation, treatment, and follow-up of the cases. There is a focus on public safety, including the workplace, for communicable diseases that have the potential to spread amongst populations. Public health workers then follow up with contacts in need of further evaluation, treatment, or education. This is often helpful in the workplace among worker populations who may be at risk from an exposure.

The CDC is also responsible for surveillance of notifiable diseases, monitoring trends, identifying populations at risk, and making recommendations for preventive measures or further intervention. This public health initiative provides the ability to monitor changes in disease recurrence, identify changes and patterns related to infectious agents, and monitor the effects of healthcare interventions. Reportable conditions are determined at the state and county levels. The list of notifiable communicable diseases is published by the CDC at intervals and is posted on the CDC website (www.dc.gov). The 2008 list of notifiable diseases can be found in Appendix 10. For additional information and resources on communicable diseases, contact your local health department.

The CDC website hosts some valuable resources and information that is useful in the workplace. There is information and training material available on workplace hazards, such as asbestos, carbon monoxide, hazardous drug exposures, heat stress, and lead. Specific information for workplaces can be found related to specific industries, such as agriculture, healthcare, construction, and mining. The CDC also provides safety and prevention tools for the workplace related to chemicals, electrical hazards, eye safety, travel safety, motor vehicle safety, and workplace violence. The OHN will find that the CDC website is a valuable resource for a variety of aspects related to workplace health and safety.

HEALTH INFORMATION PORTABILITY AND ACCOUNTABILITY ACT—PUBLIC LAW 104-191 (HIPPA)

The Federal Health Insurance Portability and Accountability Act (HIPAA), enacted in 1996 under the U.S. Department of Labor, limits the ability of any employer to deny health insurance coverage to employees with preexisting health conditions. The law also directed the development of two specific rules under the U.S. Department of Health and Human Services related to the privacy of health information. Since the development of federal HIPAA law, several states have also enacted state laws specific to HIPAA.

There are two defined rules under HIPAA. The security rule protects the security of health information that is maintained or transmitted electronically, including health information that is maintained in an electronic medical record (EMR). The rule defines standards for EMRs and also defines provisions related to the transmission of health records and claims information, requiring safeguards for protecting disclosure of protected health information. The rule also provides the right for individuals to view their own health information and allows the individual to know who has previously accessed their health information and who has current access to their personal health information.

This rule defines specific "covered entities" that must comply with the provisions of the rule. These include healthcare providers, health clinics and healthcare institutions, and pharmacies, only if health information is transmitted in an electronic form. It also includes health plans and healthcare clearinghouses, such as healthcare insurance companies, government-sponsored insurance plans, and employer-sponsored healthcare plans.

The second aspect of HIPAA is the privacy rule, which prohibits covered entities (defined above) from releasing personal health information without the permission of the individual. The rule defines the conditions under which health information can be accessed, who has the right to access the information, and who can receive protected health information. The rule is intended to provide privacy protection for individuals while maintaining protection for public health, as well. The privacy rule permits covered entities to disclose protected health information without the individual's permission only for the purposes of treatment, payment, or for certain public policy purposes. Otherwise, the rule requires that the individual provide written consent for the release of protected health information. Healthcare providers must obtain signed authorization for the disclosure of information to employers or their representatives. This includes information related to employment physical examinations, wellness screenings, and health or disability insurance. Once the signed authorization is obtained, the information can be released to the employer, and the employer has the right to access this information. The privacy law applies also to information obtained by the OHN in an on-site occupational health service. The OHN must obtain a written consent from the worker before information obtained is shared outside the occupational health service. Exceptions to this rule would include information related to health and safety regulations, including workers' compensation.

In addition to maintaining compliance with federal HIPAA, employers must know which state and local regulations apply to their workplace and ensure that company-based policies and procedures are written in compliance with laws related to maintaining and releasing protected health information. The employer should have written policies that define who has access to a worker's health information, how this information is stored, and procedures on access to and release of protected health information. The employer is responsible for maintaining the integrity and security of the health information of the workers.

Before releasing protected health information, the employer must verify the reason for disclosure, the extent of the information required for that purpose, and who is requesting access to the information. If the release of this information falls under the provision of protection, the employer must ensure that a signed authorization for disclosure is obtained from the worker. The authorization should define the specific health information that will be disclosed, the reason for its disclosure, and to whom it will be disclosed. These rules for disclosure of protected health information apply to release of this information from human resources professionals and occupational health professionals (whomever are custodians of this information) to other entities within the company. Protected health information about workers should not be released to other entities within the company, including company attorneys, owners, or executives without written authorization from the worker.

Custodians of protected health information in the workplace must ensure that these records are secured, typically in a locked file. If this is not possible, a business associate's agreement may be required with those who may gain access to privacy information. This would include contracted medical, services, or housekeeping personnel.

The employer has legal, ethical, moral, and professional obligations to ensure compliance with HIPPA law (ACOEM, 2000) and must maintain current knowledge of changes in laws or regulations specific to their operations.

ENVIRONMENTAL PROTECTION AGENCY (EPA)
Created in 1970, the EPA provides standards for the protection and quality of water, air, and soil. This federal agency has the authority to inspect workplaces to ensure compliance with any law administered under the EPA. Since these laws are mandatory, EPA officials have the ability to impose sanctions and fines upon an employer for failure to comply with the laws administered by EPA. Many workplaces conduct operations that are regulated by the EPA. Examples include environmental emissions and pollutants, discharge of hazardous waste, and other operations that have potential to cause contamination of ground, water, or air.

FEDERAL TRANSPORTATION REGULATIONS

There are several laws with provisions regulating the transportation industry. Employers of workers in these safety-sensitive transportation roles must strive to ensure not only the safety of their workers, but also to ensure public safety. Fitness for duty for these safety-sensitive workers is of critical importance. Several regulations define the specific physical qualifications and physical abilities required for workers in these positions. A few of the laws governing transportation are covered; however, this is not an exhaustive list.

Department of Transportation (DOT)

The DOT was established in 1966 and functions under the leadership of the secretary of transportation. The DOT is responsible for the development and enforcement of policy related to all forms of national transportation. The DOT consists of several subdepartments, some of which are discussed here.

The **Federal Motor Carrier Safety Administration (FMCSA)** was established within the Department of Transportation in 2000 with the intention of preventing commercial vehicle fatalities and injuries. The FMCSA regulates both commercial transport and passenger vehicles. The FMCSA establishes standards for the qualification and certification for commercial vehicle drivers and also regulates the transportation of hazardous materials.

The **Federal Aviation Administration (FAA)** oversees the safety of air travel and transport. The functions of the FAA serve to develop and enforce regulations and standards for both commercial and passenger air transportation. The FAA also establishes standards related to the manufacturing, operation, certification, and maintenance of air vehicles.

The **Federal Railroad Administration (FRA)** supports the safety of both commercial and passenger rail transport. FRA officials enforce safety regulations, conduct research and development in support of improved rail safety, and support railroad worker training programs.

The **Federal Transit Administration (FTA)** assists in developing improved mass transportation systems for communities, including public transportation. The FTA develops regulations for and oversees transportation provided by bus, commuter ferryboats, trolleys, inclined railways, subways, and people movers.

The **Maritime Administration (MARAD)** promotes development and maintenance of waterborne commerce. The maritime safety standards not only apply to U.S. workplaces, but also are focused on the development and enforcement of laws and regulations that are globally enforced. The regulations address commercial and passenger transport as well as shipbuilding and repair service, ports, and the interrelationship between water and land transportation systems.

SUMMARY

The OHN plays a key role in developing health and safety policies and procedures for the workplace. In order to be most effective in this role, the OHN must know which specific regulations apply to company operations.

The regulations discussed in this chapter all fall under the realm of the OHN in efforts to establish and maintain mechanisms for regulatory compliance. Management commitment to maintaining a safe and healthful workplace is crucial, and the OHN must ensure that management understands their responsibility for protection of workers through compliance with appropriate regulations. Workplace hazards are identified through comprehensive hazard assessments and periodic monitoring and plans to eliminate or control hazards and protect workers should be a priority. Safety and health training for all workers, including management will not only ensure compliance with certain regulatory standards, but will also serve to create awareness of the potential impact of workplace hazards on the health and well-being of workers.

Several other laws and regulations come into play in the occupational health arena (see Table 6.6). The OHN must strive to stay abreast of any additions or revisions to these laws. In most cases, these changes will not be published directly to the employer. It is the professional obligation of those involved in health and safety to proactively stay abreast of changes through research and professional networking.

Table 6.6 U.S. Department of Labor (DOL) laws and regulations.

- Contract Work Hours and Safety Standards Act (CWHSSA)
- Copeland "Anti-Kickback" Act
- Employee Polygraph Protection Act (EPPA)
- Employee Retirement Income Security Act (ERISA)
- Energy Employees Occupational Illness Compensation Program Act (EEOICPA)
- Fair Labor Standards Act (FLSA)
- Family and Medical Leave Act (FMLA)
- Federal Employees' Compensation Act (FECA)
- Federal Mine Safety and Health Act (Mine Act)
- Immigration and Nationality Act (INA)
- Labor-Management Reporting and Disclosure Act (LMRDA)
- Longshore and Harbor Workers' Compensation Act (LHWCA)
- Mass Transit Employee Protections
- Migrant and Seasonal Agricultural Worker Protection Act (MSPA)
- Occupational Safety and Health (OSH) Act
- Rehabilitation Act of 1973, Section 503
- Uniformed Services Employment and Reemployment Rights Act (USERRA)
- Vietnam Era Veterans' Readjustment Assistance Act (VEVRAA)
- Walsh-Healey Public Contracts Act (PCA)
- Worker Adjustment and Retraining Notification Act (WARN)
- Whistleblower Protections

REFERENCES

American Association of Healthplans. *HIPAA information.* Retrieved from http://www.aahp.org/Templage.cfm

American Association of Occupational Health Nurses (AAOHN). (2006). *Role of OHNs and NCMs in protecting confidentiality of health information.* (Position Statement). Retrieved from http://www.aaohn.org

American Association of Occupational Health Nurses (AAOHN). (2006). Advisory. Confidentiality of Employee Health Information. Pensacola, FL: AAOHN.

American College of Occupational and Environmental Medicine (ACOEM). (2000). *Confidentiality of medical information in the workplace.* (Position Statement). Retrieved from http://www.acoem.org

American Heart Association. (2002). Respiratory Protection eTool. Publication 70-2562. Retrieved from http://www.osha.gov/SLTC/etools/respiratory/scope.html

American Nurses Association (ANA). (2001). ANA workplace health and safety guide for nurses: OSHA and NIOSH resources. Washington, DC: ANA Publishing.

American Red Cross. (2001). First Aid: Responding to Emergencies. (3rd ed.). Yardley, PA: American Red Cross.

Americans with Disabilities Act. (2004). *Delivery of occupational and environmental health services.* (Position Statement). AAOHN 42 USC §12112(D)(3)(B) (1990).

Center for Democracy and Technology. Health Privacy.: Retrieved from http://www.healthprivacy.org

Centers for Disease Control and Prevention. HIPAA Privacy Rule. Provisions Relevant to Public Health Practice Retrieved from http://www.cdc.gov

Centers for Disease Control and Prevention. (2008). Summary of notifiable diseases. *Morbidity and Mortality Weekly Report, 57*(54). Retrieved from http://www.cdc.gov/mmwr/mmwr_nd/

Centers for Disease Control and Prevention. (2010). Our History—Our Story. Retrieved from http://www.cdc.gov/about/history/ourstory.htm

Chalupka, S. (2011). Lockout and tagout procedures to prevent occupational injury and fatality. *AAOHN Journal, 59*(7), 324.

Federal Register. 29 CFR 1910.1020. *Access to employee exposure & medical records.* Retrieved from http://www.osha.govealth

Haag, A. B., Kalina, C. M., & Tourigian, R. (2003). Clinical rounds: Case management update: Short term disability, long term disability, Social Security Disability Insurance, and Family Medical Leave Act—Relationship to case management practice. *AAOHN Journal, 51*(10), 414–417.

Liaison Committee on Resuscitation. (2000). Guidelines 2000 for Cardiopulmonary Resuscitation and Emergency Cardiovascular Care: International Consensus on Science, Part 3: Adult Basic Life Support. *Circulation.*102, (suppl I), 22–59.

Litchfield, S. M. (2009). HIPAA and the Occupational Health Nurse. *AAOHN Journal*, *57*(10), 399.

Medicare and Medicaid HIPAA information: Retrieved from http://www.cms.gov/Regulations-and-Guidance/HIPAA.../HIPAA101-1.pdf

Occupational Safety and Health Administration (OSHA). (1998). *Respiratory protection standard. 29 CFR 1910.134*. Retrieved from http://www.osha.gov/pls/oshaweb/owadisp.show_document?p_table=STANDARDS&p_id=12716

Occupational Safety and Health Administration. (2011). The Occupational Safety and Health (OSH) Act. Retrieved from http://www.dol.gov/compliance/laws/comp-osha.htm

Rogers, B. (2004). Occupational health nursing, concepts and practice (2nd ed.). Philadelphia: W.B. Saunders.

Rogers, B., Meyer, D., Summey, C., Scheessele, D., Atwell, T., Ostendorf, J., Randolph, S. A., Buckheit, K. (2009). What makes a successful hearing conservation program? *AAOHN Journal*, *57*(8), 321–335.

Schuren, W. S., & Livsey, K. (2001). Complying with the health insurance portability and accountability act privacy standards. *AAOHN Journal*, *49*(11), 501–507.

Sickbert-Bennett, E. E., Weber, D. J., Poole, C., MacDonald, P., & Maillard, J-M. (2011). Completeness of communicable disease reporting, North Carolina, USA, 1995–1997 and 2000–2006. *Emerging Infectious Diseases*, *17*(1). Retrieved from http://www.cdc.gov/eid

Thompson, M. R. (2003). The three Rs of fire safety, emergency action, and fire prevention planning: Promoting safety at the worksite. *AAOHN Journal*, *51*(4), 169–179.

Thompson, M. C. (2006). Legislation affecting occupational health nursing: Identifying relevant laws and regulations. *AAOHN Journal*, *54*(1), 38–45.

U. S. Environmental Protection Agency. 40 CFR. *Protection of the Environment*. Retrieved from http://www.epa.gov/lawsregs/index.html

U.S. Department of Health and Human Services, Office of the Assistant Secretary for Planning and Evaluation. Administrative Simplification in the Health Care Industry. Retrieved from http://www.aspe.hhs.gov/admnsimp/

U.S. Department of Health and Human Services. *The HIPAA Standards for privacy of individually identifiable health information*. Retrieved from http://hhs.gov/ocr/hippa/

U.S. Department of Health and Human Services (USDHHS). (2003). *Privacy rule preamble*. Retrieved from http://www.hhs.gov

U.S. Department of Health and Human Services (USDHHS). (2003). *Summary of the HIPAA privacy rules & frequently asked questions & answers*. Retrieved from http://www.hhs/gov/ocr/hipaa

Mine Safety and Health Administration (MSHA), U.S. Department of Labor. (2011). Mine Safety and Health Act (MSHA). Retrieved from http://www.msha.gov/

RESOURCES

HIPAA Advisory.
http://www.hipaaadvisory.com
National Institute for Occupational Safety and Health (NIOSH). Education and
    Research Centers for Occupational Safety and Health.
http://niosh-erc.org/
National Safety Council.
http://www.nsc.org
OSHA Compliance Assistance.
http://www.osha.gov/dcsp/compliance_assistance/
SBA Toolkit Media Group. *Business owners tool kit.*
http://www.toolkit.com/small_business_guide/sbg
Small Business Association, Office of Advocacy.
http://www.sba.gov/advo/state_legislative03.pdf

Promoting and Maintaining a Safe Workplace

7

INTRODUCTION

With the advent of the Occupational Safety and Health Administration (OSHA) and the initiation of the Occupational Safety and Health Act (OSH Act) of 1970, all workers have the right to a safe workplace, and it is the employer's responsibility to help assure a safe and healthful workplace for all workers. OSHA was created within the U.S. Department of Labor to promote and to ensure workplace safety and health. The initial mission of OSHA was based on specific defined purposes and to reduce workplace fatalities, injuries, and illnesses that are still applicable today (Figure 7.1). Many years later, we have learned a lot about safety and how to get workers to buy into the commitment of a safe workplace.

A report from the Bureau of Labor Statistics (BLS, 2011a) estimates approximately 3.1 million serious work-related injuries and about 4,690 fatalities occurred in 2010, having a profound financial impact on businesses. Addressing safety and health issues in the workplace saves the employer money and adds value to the business. The total cost of preventable workplace injuries and deaths is difficult to measure since it includes not only direct costs of the workers' compensation claims and damage to facilities or equipment, but also includes indirect costs associated with worker replacement and lost productivity. Therefore, there are financial benefits, both direct and indirect, associated with having a safe and healthy workplace (see Figure 7.2). According to the 2011 Liberty Mutual Workplace Safety Index (2011), the direct cost of workplace injuries and illnesses in 2009 amounted to $50.1 billion in U.S. workers' compensation costs.

Recent studies show that injury and illness rates are trending in a favorable direction. Key findings from the 2010 Survey of Occupational Injuries and Illnesses Nonfatal (BLS, 2011a) reported that workplace injuries and illnesses in 2010 among private industry employers declined for all case types to a rate of 3.5 cases per 100 equivalent full-time workers. The manufacturing industry reported the largest decline, decreasing by 23%, and the construction industry reported a 22% decline, both lowering their incidence rates to 4.3 cases per 100 workers. The manufacturing and construction industries combined represent

Essentials for Occupational Health Nursing, First Edition. Arlene Guzik.
© 2013 John Wiley & Sons, Inc. Published 2013 by John Wiley & Sons, Inc.

Under the Act, the Occupational Safety and Health Administration (OSHA) was created within the Department of Labor to do the following:

- Encourage employers and employees to reduce workplace hazards and to implement new or improve existing safety and health programs
- Provide for research in occupational safety and health to develop innovative ways of dealing with occupational safety and health problems
- Establish "separate but dependent responsibilities and rights" for employers and employees for the achievement of better safety and health conditions
- Maintain a reporting and record-keeping system to monitor job-related injuries and illnesses
- Establish training programs to increase the number and competence of occupational safety and health personnel
- Develop mandatory job safety and health standards and enforce them effectively
- Provide for the development, analysis, evaluation, and approval of state occupational safety and health programs

Figure 7.1 OSHA's purposes.
Source: Courtesy of the Occupational Safety & Health Administration. http://www.osha.gov/doc/outreachtraining/htmlfiles/introsha.html

Direct Cost Savings

- Lower workers' compensation insurance costs
- Reduced medical expenditures
- Smaller expenditures for return-to-work programs
- Fewer faulty products
- Lower costs for job accommodations for injured workers
- Less money spent for overtime benefits

Indirect Cost Savings

- Increased productivity;
- Higher quality products
- Increased morale
- Better labor/management relations
- Reduced turnover
- Better use of human resources

Figure 7.2 Financial benefits of a safe workplace.
Source: Courtesy of the Occupational Safety & Health Administration. http://www.osha.gov/Publications/smallbusiness/small-business.html#appb

more than half of the total private industry decline in injuries and illnesses. The report indicates that public entity (local, state, county, government) workers had much higher rates of injuries and illnesses requiring days away from work than did workers in private industry.

Despite this favorable trend, billions of dollars are still spent each year for treatment of work-related injuries and illnesses. The top five injury causes (overexertion, fall on same level, bodily reaction, struck by object, and fall to lower level) accounted for 71.7% of the total cost burden. Overexertion (musculoskeletal injuries related to lifting, pushing, pulling, holding, carrying, or throwing) has for years been the number one category, costing businesses $13.40 billion in direct costs and accounting for nearly 25% of the overall burden (Liberty Mutual, 2011). Injuries in the categories of fall on same level, struck by object, bodily reaction, fall to lower level, caught in/compressed by, and assaults/violent Acts are on the increase. Costs related to overexertion injuries, repetitive motion, highway incidents, and struck against object have shown declines. Despite declines in incident and injury rates, the overall direct financial impact to business is still quite great. OSHA officials encourage all employers, both private and government, to use the data released from these annual surveys to focus on areas with high incidence rates and to identify and eliminate hazards to prevent future occurrences.

To achieve this expectation, two things must change and must become a consistent part of the business philosophy: attitudes and behaviors. The owners or boards of directors of any business must understand that their attitude toward job safety will be reflected by management and workers. If there is little interest in preventing incidents, injury, and illness at the top of the organization, the workers will probably not care about safety. It is therefore essential that an attitude for safety is demonstrated at all times and at all levels, and it must become a prime priority in the workplace. Safety must receive as much attention as operations and production. It must receive as much attention as customer service. It must receive as much attention as business success and profitability. And it must be a part of everyone's agenda.

OSHA does not require employers to have a comprehensive safety program; however, employers have certain responsibilities under the OSH Act (Figure 7.3). Yet, experience shows that the development and implementation of a solid safety program is an effective way to comply with OSHA standards and prevent workplace injuries and illnesses. The following steps form OSHA's Program Evaluation Profile provide a solid foundation for developing a comprehensive safety and health program (OSHA, 1996). Figure 7.4 outlines OSHA's four basic elements for safety and health programs.

MANAGEMENT COMMITMENT AND EMPLOYEE INVOLVEMENT

"We've been doing it like this for years. What we are doing works and we don't need to change." This mantra is often heard at all levels of the organization. If business is successful and profitable, leaders will use this excuse to avoid change, even if it compromises safety of workers. Some highly successful businesses have managed to ignore attention to safety because they produce a great product or service, and have been doing so for years. So why change now? Managers can be heard using this excuse in order to avoid investments in safety initiatives or to avoid additional expense, resources, and effort. As for the

- Provide a workplace free from serious recognized hazards and comply with standards, rules, and regulations issued under the OSHA Act.
- Examine workplace conditions to make sure they conform to applicable OSHA standards.
- Make sure employees have and use safe tools and equipment and properly maintain this equipment.
- Use color codes, posters, labels, or signs to warn employees of potential hazards.
- Establish or update operating procedures and communicate them so that employees follow safety and health requirements.
- Provide medical examinations and training when required by OSHA standards.
- Post, at a prominent location within the workplace, the OSHA poster (or the state plan equivalent) informing employees of their rights and responsibilities.
- Report to the nearest OSHA office within 8 hours any fatal accident or one that results in the hospitalization of three or more employees.
- Keep records of work-related injuries and illnesses. (Note: Employers with 10 or fewer employees and employers in certain low-hazard industries are exempt from this requirement.)
- Provide employees, former employees, and their representatives access to the Log of Work-Related Injuries and Illnesses (OSHA Form 300).
- Provide access to employee medical records and exposure records to employees or their authorized representatives.
- Provide to the OSHA compliance officer the names of authorized employee representatives who may be asked to accompany the compliance officer during an inspection.
- Do not discriminate against employees who exercise their rights under the act.
- Post OSHA citations at or near the work area involved. Each citation must remain posted until the violation has been corrected, or for 3 working days, whichever is longer. Post abatement verification documents or tags.
- Correct cited violations by the deadline set in the OSHA citation and submit required abatement verification documentation.

Figure 7.3 OSHA—employer responsibilities under the Occupational Safety and Health Act of 1970. *Source*: Courtesy of the Occupational Safety & Health Administration. http://www.osha.gov/as/opa/worker/employer-responsibility.html

workers, although there are some workers who have an inherent attention to safety, most will take the lead of management. And there are those who, despite a strong management commitment to safety, will choose to ignore safety when focused on other goals or outcomes. If workers are expected to meet certain production standards, they may develop a work-around to meet quota by ignoring safety. Or, they may choose to ignore safety because it gets in their way, such as the use of personal protective equipment (PPE).

Although safety must be a both a top-down and bottom-up commitment, the company's leadership provides the motivating force and ultimate support. Safety must become one of the highest priorities of the business, and management must show active participation in all aspects of the safety program, including

1. Management Commitment and Employee Involvement

   • Management's commitment provides the motivating force and the resources for organizing and controlling activities.
   • Employee involvement provides the means by which workers develop and/or express their own commitment to safety and health protection for themselves and for their fellow workers.

2. Worksite Analysis

   • Analysis involves a variety of worksite examinations to identify existing hazards and conditions and operations in which changes might occur to create new hazards.

3. Hazard Prevention and Control

   • Hazards must be eliminated or controlled to prevent unsafe and unhealthful exposure.

4. Safety and Health Training

   • Training helps communicate the safety and health responsibilities of both management and employees at the site.

Figure 7.4 OSHA's four basic elements of a health & safety program.
Source: Courtesy of the Occupational Safety & Health Administration. http://www.osha.gov/Publications/Const_Res_Man/1926_C_SH_guide.html

worksite inspections, incident reviews, and safety audits. Safety should be included as agenda items on all management and operations meetings, and visible management leadership must clearly demonstrate involvement and support for the importance of safety of every worker and of every worksite.

Management must clearly state the goals and objectives of the company's safety program. OSHA (2005a) provides several sample policy statements (examples provided in Figure 7.5). There should also be a written policy and procedure that clearly defines management's commitment to safety, along with the expectation for active involvement of management and workers. The written safety policy (see sample in Appendix 11) should be posted where it is visible to all workers, and it should be covered in orientation for all new workers. When initiating or revising a safety program, management should hold a meeting with all workers to communicate the aspects of the policy and to discuss objectives and expectations related to safety. The policy must clearly outline specific assigned responsibilities, and accountability at all levels must follow. Appendix 12 outlines OSHA's Strategic Map for Change and Continuous Improvement for Safety and Health, which can serve as a guide to the development and implementation process. A focus upstream requires a commitment to root causes analysis and grass roots involvement by workers.

There must be an expectation for everyone to follow all applicable safety requirements, including senior management. For example, if an area of the

"Safety and health in our business must be a part of every operation. Without question it is every employee's responsibility at all levels."

"Our objective is a safety and health program that will reduce the number of injuries and illnesses to an absolute minimum, not merely in keeping with, but surpassing, the best experience of operations similar to ours. Our goal is zero accidents and injuries."

"The personal safety and health of each employee of this company is of primary importance. The prevention of occupationally induced injuries and illnesses is of such consequence that it will be given precedence over operating productivity whenever necessary. To the greatest degree possible, management will provide all mechanical and physical facilities required for personal safety and health in keeping with the highest standards."

Figure 7.5 Sample policy statements.
Source: Courtesy of the Occupational Safety & Health Administration. http://www.osha.gov/Publications/smallbusiness/small-business.html#appb

workplace requires the use of PPE (such as a hard hat, safety glasses, or hearing protection); it must be worn by anyone entering the area, including senior management and visitors, even if they are in the area for a brief period of time. This simple gesture displays to all a sincere commitment to safety. Management must also provide support by committing enough people, time, training, and financial resources to support the safety mission. In return for this commitment by management, all workers must know that they will be held accountable for not adhering to safety policies and procedures designed to promote a safe workplace. And at least once a year, management should review what has been accomplished in meeting the objectives of the health and safety program, redefine their commitment, and determine needed revisions to the plan.

Every workplace should have an assigned safety officer. Large workplaces usually have the resources to support hiring a safety manager who has the prime responsibility for executing and managing the safety program. Often hired as the safety professional, this individual holds specialized knowledge and skills in the area of safety or risk management and may also hold an educational degree or specialty certification in safety or risk management. Additional areas of responsibility for a safety officer may include training, industrial and environmental hygiene, security, and fire protection (Balge & Krieger, 2000). Ideally, this position would report directly to top management or actually hold a top management position and have responsibility for both administrative and execution elements of the safety program. Administrative responsibilities include development of safety policies and procedures, safety training, and leading the safety committee. The execution elements of the safety officer's role would include conducting safety inspections and audits, hazard prevention and risk mitigation, loss control, job analysis, ergonomics, and incident investigation. Smaller workplaces may assign the key responsibility for safety to a supervisor or manager who holds other responsibilities as well, and oftentimes this responsibility is assigned to the occupational health nurse (OHN). This safety officer would serve as an advocate between management and workers to ensure the elements of the safety program are executed using a variety of resources. In this situation, the administrative and execution elements of the safety program are shared among others in the organization.

To fully execute an upstream approach to health and safety, each manager and supervisor must clearly understand their role and responsibilities and must also be given the adequate resources and support for execution. Typically, these tasks are the responsibility of the supervisor with the assigned authority and for which they are held accountable. They should also agree that these tasks are of key importance to safety and health of workers and the workplace. OSHA describes the need for the supervisor to have the responsibility, authority, and accountability for execution: "The essential tools are the assignment of responsibility for a function or activity, the authority to do the job, and account-ability to senior management to see that it is done." (OSHA, 2002b) OSHA's Responsibility, Authority, and Accountability Checklist (see Appendix 13) pro-vides a tool to assist the supervisor in determining if they have the responsi-bility and authority to execute the health and safety plan in order to assure accountability to workers and to senior management.

Worker involvement in supporting safety initiatives is critical, and if workers are expected to be accountable for safety, they must be invited to participate in the establishment and evolution of the safety program. This is often accom-plished by the establishment of a safety committee, representative of workers in all departments. The composition of the safety committee varies on the type and size of business. The committee should include at least one representative from each major department or business unit, and include representatives from line workers, senior and middle management, supervisors, and union repre-sentatives (if applicable). Along with representative of workers and management, the safety committee may also include OHNs, safety specialists, physicians, and human resources specialists. To support a true upstream approach, grassroots involvement is essential, and the committee should be more representative of line workers than of management.

Members of the safety committee should participate in the development of the safety and health program including hazard and job analysis strategies, as well as training and education initiatives. The safety committee should also review safety audits, have access to program reviews conducted by management or consultants, and review all incident and injury reports. In doing so, strat-egies for eliminating hazards and reducing injuries and illnesses becomes a core responsibility of the committee. Committee members then relay information back to their respective departments and ask for input from workers at all levels of the organization. The expectation that all workers have a role in identifying and resolving safety and health problems creates an atmosphere where workers will apply their unique perspectives and initiatives to achieving the goals and objectives of the program. Management must therefore authorize both workers and committee members to identify and cease activities that present potential safety and health hazards (OSHA, 1996).

Safety incentive programs often become a focus of the safety committee, yet they have long been controversial. Although OSHA neither approves nor disapproves the design or the effectiveness of safety-incentive programs, those that encourage underreporting of workplace injuries are discouraged. OSHA addresses two incentive models: The "traditional" model and the "nontraditional" model. The traditional safety-incentive program is one that offers rewards for reduced injury rates, such as when the workers, departments, or business reach certain milestones without a lost time due to accident (time away from work). In this approach, the number of accidents, incidents, and near misses are tallied. If the numbers fall below a certain level, workers would be rewarded. If they were above the designated levels, they would not be rewarded. Some companies tie the rewards to individual performance, while others tie rewards to team, departmental, or even company performance. Some even establish programs that are designed to have departments compete against one another for having the best safety record. A common theme that is heralded includes celebrations for achieving "a million man-hours without a lost-time injury." These types of incentive programs encourage workers to avoid reporting injuries and may also encourage supervisors and managers to pressure workers not to report incidents and injuries. And besides, what worker wants to be the one who incurs the injury and wrecks the chances of winning the award?

The nontraditional incentive program is one that rewards workers based on positive behaviors, often referred to as "behavior-based" safety incentives. Workers under this program are rewarded for positive behaviors, such as attending safety meetings; for their ability to articulate and demonstrate safety awareness; or for making safety suggestions that will lead to process improvements or risk reduction. Companies that adopt a nontraditional incentive program are implementing "leading indicator" safety incentive programs. Management defines certain positive behaviors or indicators, and the program is then designed to reward workers for safety-related behaviors and activities, rather than for results. Examples of leading indicators include reporting safety violations, identifying potential or actual risks, making safety suggestions, taking steps to remedy unsafe situations, positive work practices, and volunteering for safety committee activities (Atkinson, 2004).

A significant aspect of behavior-based safety is to establish an expectation for reporting incidents and near misses, rather than just reporting injuries and illnesses. Heralding an upstream approach, this encourages workers to report situations that could have led to a more serious outcome. This then creates an opportunity for an incident analysis, looking for root causes that can be eliminated to prevent future occurrence. Strategies for improvements may include such efforts as facilities improvements, equipment maintenance, and worker training.

Under a behavior-based approach, employers should strive to implement incentive programs that reward workers for positive performance rather than those that discourage reporting of accidents, symptoms, injuries, or hazards. The program should offer rewards that are linked to support for safety-related activities, that encourage safe work practices, and that are based on the strategy of prevention, recognizing those workers who work safely. The focus is on long-term behavior change as a result of workers having a greater sense of awareness and on establishing rewards for positive behavior. A focus on three guiding principles will help achieve an upstream approach to safety.

Attitudes

It is very difficult to change a worker's attitude or perceptions because these factors are typically a consequence of one's life experience. As a result, the workplace will host a variety of attitudes that influence safety, so it becomes important to assess the attitudes and awareness of workers in order to enhance their commitment and motivation in attaining a safe workplace. Maslow (1943) proposed that each person has an inner nature unique to himself or herself, with basic needs, one of which is safety and security, and it is best to bring out or encourage this need rather than suppress it. Maslow goes on to state that this inner nature is weak and delicate and can easily be overcome by habit, cultural pressures, or a bad attitude. Although Maslow defined safety as a fundamental human need, we often find workers with indifferent attitudes toward safety and security in the workplace. Rather than blame the worker for their frustration, procrastination, denial, and complacency, we might stop and think that their attitude may be a result of management's lack of focus on safety.

It becomes important then to increase awareness and to make safety a habit for all workers. Once a person learns the correct way to do something, emphasis on reinforcing the practice becomes important so that the behavior becomes part of a natural work routine. We all have learned that we must look both ways before crossing a street. This behavior was reinforced by our elders to keep us safe. Once we mastered this habit, we could be trusted to cross the street alone without supervision. This same leadership initiative must take place with workers.

When a worker is unaware that certain steps or practices are necessary to prevent accidents and injuries, external motivation is necessary to influence a behavior change. However, dictating and mandating safety will not be effective. Education of the workers is critical and continued motivation is needed to maintain awareness and support positive behavior. A workplace culture must be created that enables or facilitates personal responsibility and personal accountability for working safely, one that encourages personal involvement and commitment for safety.

Attitudes can be influenced by management's commitment to walk and talk safety, and managers must be committed to abide by all safety standards as an example to the workers. Safety must be addressed at all department meetings by addressing any safety issues and new processes and by asking input from workers regarding safety improvements. An emphasis on safety can be displayed through posting slogans throughout the workplace; such as "Think Safety,"

"Safety is our #1 Priority," and "Safety Prevents Injuries." In some of the best workplaces, you can find safety posters displayed at every turn in the facilities, so every time workers round a corner, they come face-to-face with a safety slogan. This encourages a positive reinforcement for everyone to be safety-minded.

Behavior

The behavior-based approach focuses on observing what people do, analyzes why they do it, and targets specific behaviors in order to effect change. When we analyze behavior and implement interventions to improve behavior, improvements in attitude, commitment, and motivation follow (Laws, 2005).

Williamsen (2003) defines four steps to addressing safety behaviors. First, identify and address all behaviors that must be implemented in order to eliminate unsafe Acts and prevent injuries. This would include adherence to all OSHA regulations such as use of PPE, fall prevention, and machine guarding. Other strategies might include implementing a safe lifting program or simply maintaining a clean workplace to avoid slips and falls. Next, train workers on the expected behaviors. Use a variety of training techniques, such as videos, demonstrations, or handouts. Make safety training a mandatory part of the workers' annual performance evaluations. Third, monitor and enforce safe work behaviors, such as the use of protective equipment. Promote the reporting of all injuries, incidents, and near misses, along with property damage. Check the cleanliness of the work environment. Perhaps initiate a peer review system whereby workers are encouraged to maintain alertness for unsafe conditions or behaviors and stop it by bringing it to the attention of the worker or the supervisor. And lastly, reward positive, safe behaviors, clearly supporting an upstream approach.

Consequences

Practice makes perfect, and reinforcement of positive behavior supports habitual practice. Workers must know there are consequences for behaviors in the workplace, both negative and positive. Oftentimes, a focus is placed on identifying and addressing negative behavior in the workplace, such as absenteeism or poor performance. Workers may receive disciplinary action for not adhering to certain expectations, receive verbal or written warnings, and may even face termination of employment. But with behavior-based safety, reinforcement of positive behavior often leads to a more desirable outcome, thus reinforces habitual positive behavior. Recognition, rewards, and celebrations help to support and reinforce these positive behaviors. In keeping with Maslow's (1943) theory, if workers' behavior does not gain the support and approval of others, they will be "ruled by the laws of their own character," rather than by that which is expected in the workplace. Through the promotion of behavior-based safety, the worker's thoughts, feelings, and behaviors become consistent with rewards, incentives, and recognitions.

When incidents and injuries occur, conduct investigations, including assessments of the environment, the processes, and behaviors that may have been contributing factors. Hold workers accountable for behaviors they can control and have a system in place to evaluate the behavioral aspects contributing to the incident or injury. The accountability to evaluate the safety performance of individual workers, departments, and the entire workforce influences whether workers feel empowered and responsible for improving safety. Strive toward establishing a more synergistic atmosphere in which what is good for the individual is also good for the workplace and contributes to both the personal fulfillment of the worker and the prosperity of the organization (Maslow, 1943). Behavior-based safety then focuses on environmental conditions, processes, and behaviors that can be changed upstream to prevent potential injury.

JOB HAZARD ANALYSIS

OSHA (2002) defines "hazard" as the potential for harm, often associated with a condition or activity that, if left in place or uncontrolled, could result in an injury or illness. Appendix 14 lists common hazards and descriptions as defined by OSHA. Job hazard analysis is intended to eliminate and prevent risk in the workplace by identifying hazards in order to eliminate or control them as early as possible to prevent injuries and illnesses. The analysis looks at work tasks and identifies what could possibly go wrong and the associated consequences. The analysis then looks for contributing factors and proposes changes that would eliminate or control the hazard. The intended outcomes include safer work practices, fewer injuries and illnesses, reduced workers' compensation costs, and increased productivity of the workforce.

Management's commitment to safety should be demonstrated by looking at hazards from a multidimensional perspective, taking into consideration the environment in which the work is taking place, the potential exposure, precipitating factors, and consequences (OSHA, 2002). In conducting the analysis, it is often helpful to establish a team of workers who will evaluate the job tasks, including workers who routinely perform the job tasks and those who do not, both management and nonmanagement workers. Various perspectives will be helpful in the analysis since workers who routinely perform the tasks may not perceive inherent components of the job as risks. Remember the quote earlier stated: "We've been doing it like this for years. What we are doing works and we don't need to change." The analysis involves observing a worker perform the job task while listing each step of the process. The workers who routinely perform the work can be helpful in defining and labeling the tasks. Photographs or videotapes of the work are often catalogued, along with the analysis, to provide a visual reference for further analysis and comparison.

OSHA (2002) provides the following suggestions for prioritizing the jobs selected for hazard analysis:

- Jobs with the highest injury or illness rates
- Jobs with the potential to cause severe or disabling injuries or illness, even if there is no history of previous accidents

- Jobs in which one simple human error could lead to a severe accident or injury
- Jobs that are new to the operations or have undergone changes in processes and procedures
- Jobs complex enough to require written instructions.

Once the analysis is completed and documented, workers should be involved in reviewing the results and making recommendations for eliminating or controlling hazards that exist. This serves to demonstrate management's commitment to making changes that will improve the safety of the workers. Hazards that pose immediate danger must receive immediate attention and intervention.

There are many agents that may pose risk to workers, including physical, chemical, and biological hazards. Physical agents that may pose risk include a variety of external factors that may cause injury or illness. Workers who are exposed to extremes in weather, both heat and cold, can be affected by heat exhaustion or stress, heat rash, sunburn, frostbite, and hypothermia. Associated hazard prevention includes protective clothing, job rotation, time limits, and hydration. Energy sources such as electricity, lightening, laser, and radiation also pose risk. Physical hazards can also include vehicles, mobile equipment, machinery, or structures; things that can cause workers to slip, trip, fall, get struck by, or get caught between things that would cause injury.

Chemical hazards can be found in many industrial workplaces and can be present in many forms. Common forms include gases, liquids, and particulates that can be inhaled, ingested, injected, or that come in contact with the skin, eyes, and mucous membranes. Chemicals may be systemic toxins, carcinogens, reproductive toxicants, neurological toxicants, sensitizers, immunological agents, dermatopathic agents, pneumoconiotic agents, or asthmagens (NIOSH, 2010). Workers exposed to hazardous chemicals, such as benzene, chromium, hazardous or toxic waste, latex, lead, mercury, and many others may be prone to acute injury or illness that sometimes result in chronic health conditions. Since the result of a chemical exposure is dependent upon the dose, route of entry, and exposure time, regulatory and professional agencies (such as OSHA, National Institute for Occupational Safety and Health [NIOSH], and American Conference of Governmental Industrial Hygienists [ACGIH]) have established statutory threshold level values (TLVs), recommended exposure limits (RELs), and permissible exposure limits (PELs) for most chemicals used in the workplace. Workplaces that pose hazards as a result of chemicals must conduct assessment methods to determine the risk to workers. This is accomplished through area monitoring to determine the level of chemical hazard over a time-weighted average (TWA). Action levels are defined determining the need to implement a hazard control program usually when the area monitoring is measured at or above 50% of the TLV/REL/PEL; however, some OSHA standards define a mandatory action level with use of certain hazards, such as the Lead Standard and the Noise Standard. OSHA's Hazard Communication Program was discussed in Chapter 6.

Biological hazards include naturally occurring substances known to cause illness and include agents, viruses, and bacteria. Examples include asbestos, bloodborne pathogens, botulism, mold, and tuberculosis. Outdoor work also poses hazards from vector-borne diseases from insects or animals, venomous wildlife and insects, and poisonous plants.

Once a list of the jobs is documented, establish a ranked priority for intervention, obviously intervening on tasks that present the most risk. For all tasks that pose unacceptable risk, immediately evaluate the options for removing or controlling the hazard and minimizing risk of illness or injury. For instance, work that poses danger to the worker for eye injury should result in the implementation of the use of mandatory eye protection and the installation of eye-wash stations near the areas of potential exposure. Work that poses risk of slips and trips should result in addressing housekeeping, floor safety, and footwear. Work that poses risk of bloodborne pathogen exposure should result in the implementation of universal precautions.

HAZARD PREVENTION AND CONTROL

There are three primary interventions for hazard control (see Figure 7.6): engineering controls, administrative controls, and the use of PPE. Of highest priority is to evaluate whether the hazard can be removed or eliminated through the use of engineering controls. If this can be done, it reduces the risk to zero. In many types of work, however, hazards are a natural part of the job, especially in manufacturing, plant and distribution operations, and use of certain machinery. In these settings, despite what seems to be inherent risk, it is sometimes possible to remove or eliminate the hazard. In some cases it can be "engineered out," meaning the machinery can be redesigned, retooled, or a change in processes may be implemented. Consideration can also be given to isolating the risk through the use of shields or barriers for machines, equipment, or for the workers themselves.

If the risk cannot be eliminated or isolated, administrative controls will assist to establish guidelines and procedures that serve to reduce that risk, such as controlling the time a worker is exposed to the risk, monitoring an area or biological risk, and improving housekeeping procedures. Improvements in ergonomic conditions, job rotation, and mandatory stretching routines, have proven effective in reducing overuse and repetitive use syndromes. Limiting time of worker exposure is also effective in reducing heat exhaustion. Alarm systems that are triggered to go off when exposure limits reach a concerning level are effective in monitoring the atmospheric levels of dangerous chemicals. Other jobs such as healthcare carry inherent risks that cannot be eliminated, for example, the risk of bloodborne pathogen exposure. It is impossible to eliminate the healthcare worker's need to work with human blood and waste products. As a result, procedures for universal precautions and the use of PPE have become mandatory in the healthcare environment. Other jobs that pose risk that cannot be eliminated or controlled require the use of personal protective

The order of precedence and effectiveness of hazard control:

1. Engineering Controls

   - Elimination/minimization of the hazard—Designing the facility, equipment, or process to remove the hazard, or substituting processes, equipment, materials, or other factors to lessen the hazard
   - Enclosure of the hazard using enclosed cabs, enclosures for noisy equipment, or other means
   - Isolation of the hazard with interlocks, machine guards, blast shields, welding curtains, or other means
   - Removal or redirection of the hazard such as with local and exhaust ventilation.

2. Administrative Controls

   - Written operating procedures, work permits, and safe work practices
   - Exposure time limitations (used most commonly to control temperature extremes and ergonomic hazards)
   - Monitoring the use of highly hazardous materials
   - Alarms, signs, and warnings
   - Buddy system
   - Training.

Personal Protective Equipment

   - The use of respirators, hearing protection, protective clothing, safety glasses, and hardhats is acceptable as a control method in the following circumstances:
     ○ When engineering controls are not feasible or do not totally eliminate the hazard
     ○ While engineering controls are being developed
     ○ When safe work practices do not provide sufficient additional protection
     ○ During emergencies when engineering controls may not be feasible

Figure 7.6 Hazard control measures.
Source: Courtesy of the Occupational Safety & Health Administration. http://www.osha.gov/Publications/osha3071.html

equipment such as safety eyewear to prevent foreign bodies in the eye from grinding; respirators as protection from airborne gases, particulates, or biological hazards; the use of chaps or aprons to prevent splashes of hazardous chemicals on the worker's clothes; ear plugs to prevent exposure to loud noise. Ensure that PPE is used and that workers understand the principles and rationale for its use, how and when to use it, and how to maintain it.

Medical Surveillance
The goal for any workers exposed to hazard is to prevent illness and injury from ever occurring, and workers should know their possible exposure risk and the adverse health effects that could result from the exposure. Medical surveillance is a concept of conducting biological and medical monitoring, and it is

designed to identify signs or symptoms of exposure in its early stages. Medical surveillance consists of two components: biological monitoring and health monitoring. Biological monitoring calculates the dose of the exposure through laboratory or diagnostic studies that measure chemical markers related to the exposure by looking for the chemical agent itself and/or one of its metabolites using samples of the worker's blood, breath, hair, nails, urine, and/or stool. Reference values for certain chemicals, published by the American Conference of Governmental Industrial Hygienists' (ACGIH's) Biological Exposure Committee, are referred to as biological exposure indices (BEIs) (ACGIH, 2012).

Medical monitoring, thorough health assessment, evaluates the worker to determine any health effect from the exposure in addition to the measured BEI. The health assessment should be conducted by a health professional with specialized knowledge in the areas of epidemiology, toxicology, and industrial hygiene. Since several personal factors may come into play when assessing workers for effects from workplace exposures, these must be considered as part of the medical surveillance process. Therefore, knowledge in these specialty areas proves valuable in making the determination based on all contributing causes of the exposure. Age, gender, physiology, and metabolism of the worker can have an influence on the results. In addition, diet, smoking, drug intake, and exposures outside the workplace may also be contributing factors. For this reason, when biological markers show indication of possible exposure, it is vital to conduct medical monitoring to fully evaluate all contributing causes that may explain the result. For example, mercury is present in seafood. When a worker's BEI is elevated, a review of the worker's dietary intake and patterns is quite important. If the worker admits to eating a diet high in seafood, advise the worker to abstain from eating seafood for a period of a few weeks and repeat the laboratory test. If the lab result declines, despite the worker continuing work with mercury, the worker's diet may be determined to be the major contributing cause to the elevated lab result. Many OSHA standards define specific intervals for medical surveillance and/or health monitoring. Workers exposed to respiratory hazards with requirements to wear respiratory protection must undergo initial and annual medical review to establish their medical qualification to wear a respirator. Workers exposed to chemicals, such as lead, mercury, and cadmium, are required to have biological monitoring at specific intervals during the course of the work with these hazards. And workers exposed to noise must undergo baseline, annual, and exit hearing exams as part of the hearing conservation program. Knowing the hazards that exist in the workplace and assuring adherence to specified standards and requirements will assist in maintaining the health and safety of the workers.

If the hazard cannot be prevented entirely, control measures must be put in place considering a combination of all three hazard control strategies. A routine review of each job, at least annually, to analyze the steps of the work process will identify any new or prior undiscovered hazards in the equipment or processes. Institute safe work practices and written procedures based on an analysis of the hazards and ensure that management and workers are fully aware of the hazards and the hazard control strategies. Involving workers in the analysis and development of procedures will usually result in better compliance. Since all hazards cannot be eliminated, be sure to plan for emergencies, including fire, chemical spills, explosions, entrapment, and natural disasters. Have written emergency plans in place and conduct routine emergency drills to ensure that management and workers know what to do under emergency conditions. (See Chapter 6 for a summary of OSHA's emergency action plan [EAP] standard). Post emergency numbers, including poison control, in conspicuous places and at all telephones. Develop written emergency medical procedures to handle ill or injured workers and establish a plan with local medical facilities for triage and treatment.

Practice makes perfect, and routine inspections serve to evaluate compliance and immediately address any noncompliance with workers and supervisors. The inspection should, not only look at hazards already identified, but serve to identify any new or additional hazards. Enforcement of the rules related to safe work practices is critical, therefore coordination with Human Resources is essential in establishing a disciplinary system that will be firm, fair, and consistently applied. This comprehensive process of hazards analysis and hazard prevention and control is extremely effective in training workers on the hazards that pose risk in the workplace.

Case in Point

Excessive noise is the best example of an OSHA standard designed to protect workers from physical hazard. Noise is a physical agent that may cause a temporary or permanent impairment of a worker's hearing. OSHA requires noise level monitoring for any workplace that poses a risk to worker's hearing. Noise level testing must be conducted in various locations throughout the worksite to identify noise levels above OSHA's defined permissible noise level exposure limit (when noise exposures for workers equals or exceeds an 8-hour time-weighted average sound level [TWA] of 85 decibels) and monitoring must be repeated whenever a change in production, process, equipment or controls increase noise exposures. Efforts to reduce noise levels must be initiated and may include isolating, limiting, or dampening the noise using engineering and administrative controls. If noise levels cannot be controlled below the permissible level using engineering and administrative controls, the employer must implement a hearing conservation program. This includes notification to workers through a hearing conservation training program, audiometric testing at baseline and annually, testing at other specified intervals and when the workers exit the noisy area, and issuance of appropriate hearing protection devices for workers. Annual audiograms are then conducted and results compared to those from the baseline test to detect a significant change in the workers' hearing. This is defined as a standard threshold shift: a change in hearing threshold relative to the baseline audiogram of an average of 10 dB or more at 2,000, 3,000, and 4,000 Hz in either ear. Training must be repeated annually, and there are standards for types of hearing protectors and guidelines for notice of results to the workers (OSHA, 2012).

SAFETY AND HEALTH TRAINING

Safety and health training has proven most effective when incorporated into other mandatory training related to human resources, job performance requirements, and job practices. The training should become an expected competency that is required as an aspect of performance. The training should be conducted within 30 days of initial employment or job transfer to a safety sensitive position and should include all components necessary to address the hazards of the job, potential consequences, and hazard control measures (OSHA, 2002). The training should also be required as an annual update and be addressed on annual performance appraisals for hourly workers, supervisors, managers, contractors, and temporary workers.

As part of mandatory training, OSHA mandates that employers are required to display the OSHA "Job Safety and Health: It's the Law" poster, unless the employer's workplace is located in a state that operates an OSHA-approved state plan, and display it in a conspicuous place where workers and applicants for employment can see it (OSHA, 2005a).

INCIDENT INVESTIGATION

Despite what is sometimes thought, workers are the most valuable asset of most companies: not buildings, not machines, not tools. But there is no way to incident-proof the workplace, since incidents are generally unforeseen and are a result of an unplanned event. While incidents can and do happen, the same type of incidents should not happen repeatedly. Effective and thorough investigations lead to prevention of future occurrences and also send a message to workers that the company is concerned for their safety and well-being. Additional rationales for incident investigations include the following:

- Identifying root cause of the incident/injury (people or processes)
- Identifying and eliminating hazards
- Correcting unsafe Acts and unsafe conditions
- Making recommendations in structures or processes that will prevent future incidents

Investigations and interviews must be fact-finding, and not fault-finding. Prompt establishment of an incident investigation team is of great importance, and the team should be organized before an incident occurs and trained in incident investigation procedures. Issues to consider are: Who is in charge of the incident investigation? Who will gather the evidence (statements, photographs, faulty equipment, etc.)? Who will interview witnesses and victims? Who will prepare the final report?

When conducting incident investigation, the following six questions must be answered:

1. *Who.* Gathers information on what workers or other people were involved in the incident. For example: Who was involved in the incident? Who was

injured? Who witnessed the incident? Who was responsible for the cause of the incident? Who failed to follow safety procedures? Who installed the equipment?

2. *What*. Addresses the actions, events, and physical objects were involved in the incident. For example, What happened to cause the incident? What were the workers doing? What equipment or facilities were involved?

3. *Where*. Ties the incident to a specific location. For example, Where was each worker located? Where was the equipment? Where was the personal protective equipment?

4. *When*. Elicits information on relationships between the incident and associated activities or events. For example, When did the incident occur in relation to the worker's injury or illness? When was the incident reported in relation to its occurrence? When was training last completed? When was the equipment last checked?

5. *How*. Provides information on the relationship among activities and events. For example, How did the incident occur? How did the worker get injured?

6. *Why* Looks at root cause analysis, focusing on unsafe Acts or hazardous conditions. For example, Why wasn't the worker wearing personal protective equipment? Why wasn't the machine locked out? Why was the floor wet?

The investigation and resultant findings provide valuable information for identifying root cause and preventing future occurrence. It is also valuable in defining a relationship between the injured worker's symptoms and the mechanism of injury. Figure 7.7 provides a stepwise approach to incident investigation.

SAFETY AND HEALTH RECORD KEEPING

Employers are encouraged to document all interventions and maintain record keeping that is required for workers' compensation, insurance audits, and government inspections, according to their respective standards. Records of policies and procedures, training sessions, safety and health committee meetings, educational information provided for workers, and arrangements for emergency response and medical treatment should all be maintained for reference purposes. Certain OSHA standards also define requirements for maintenance of records related to exposures to toxic substances and hazardous exposures, along with biological and health-monitoring records. The following records must be maintained in accordance with OSHA requirements:

- Records of workplace hazard monitoring (noise, lead, etc.)
- Records reporting results of biological monitoring (lead, mercury, etc.)
- Chemical inventories and material safety data sheets specific to hazardous chemicals used in the workplace
- Health records of workers covered under specific OSHA standards for biological and health monitoring, or for those who have incurred workplace exposures requiring medical treatment. These must be maintained on file for the duration of the worker's employment, plus 30 years.

a. Workers report all accidents/incidents to their supervisor or manager immediately at the time of occurrence.
b. Render first aid and/or appropriate referral for medical evaluation.
c. Secure the scene of the incident and confine or remove the hazard in order to prevent additional risk.
d. The injured worker(s) and his/her supervisor complete a written incident report.
e. Obtain written statements from witnesses.
f. Report the incident to the safety officer.
g. Further investigation is based on the severity or potential severity of the incident.

Step 1: Incident Reporting

Reported Incident → Render First Aid or Refer for Medical Care → Secure the Scene → Abate the Hazard → Submit Incident Report to Safety Officer

---

h. The incident investigation process is conducted to identify the root cause and contributing factors and to establish appropriate corrective actions to prevent future occurrences.

Step 2: Incident Investigation

Review Incident Report → Conduct Incident Scene Investigation → Interview Witnesses to the Incident → Determine Root Cause → Establish and Implement Corrective Action → Notify Workers and Management → Retrain Workers, If Indicated → Review Incident and Investigation at Monthly Safety Committee Meeting → Update Written Procedures as Needed

---

i. Implement corrective actions in a timely manner, with defined dates and responsible parties for intervention and follow up.
j. Communicate results of the incident investigation to workers and management.
k. The safety committee reviews all incidents, actions, and recommendations and addresses issues to prevent future occurrence.
l. Update written procedures, as appropriate.

Figure 7.7 Incident reporting and investigation process.

OSHA's (2005) 29 Code of Federal Regulations (CFR) 1904 requires record keeping related to all accidents, injuries, illnesses, and property losses with the primary purpose of retaining information to help determine contributing causes, identify trends, and develop procedures to prevent a recurrence. OSHA compliance officers find this data valuable in identifying patterns and trends of injuries and illness, not only within a specific workplace, but also within certain industries and hazard-specific workplaces. The agency, in collating data recorded by employers, finds this information useful in evaluating industry-specific strategies for developing new or improving existing regulatory standards. The Bureau of Labor Statistics (BLS) also uses this data to compile the Annual Survey of Occupational Injuries and Illnesses, citing national industry-specific trends in health and safety. The BLS Injuries, Illnesses, and Fatalities (IIF) program "provides annual information on the rate and number of work related injuries, illnesses, and fatal injuries, and how these statistics vary by incident, industry, geography, occupation, and other characteristics" (BLS, 2011b).

This process is consistent with the upstream approach to maintaining a safe and healthy workplace. Employers can review this data to benchmark how their company compares to industry average overall and by type of injury/illness. All workplaces are required to participate in OSHA record keeping with the exception of businesses with 10 or fewer workers, or specific industries considered low risk, such as retail, service, finance, insurance, and real estate. A complete list of exempt industries can be found at: http://www.osha.gov/recordkeeping/pub3169text.html.

The OSHA record-keeping standard requires employers to "report" and/or "record" specific incidents, illnesses, and injuries. Employers are required to "report" or notify OSHA by telephone within 8 hours all work-related fatalities or hospitalizations involving three or more workers. They must also report to OSHA cases where the death occurs within 30 days of the work-related incident. Employers must also report to OSHA all fatal heart attacks occurring in the work environment.

The employer's obligation also requires that a record of certain incidents, illnesses, and injuries be recorded on an OSHA-specific log. These conditions are considered "recordable" in that they must be logged according to specific standards set by OSHA (see Appendix 15). The OSHA record-keeping system includes five aspects related to recordable data (OSHA, 2005b):

1. Employers must obtain a written report on every work-related injury or illness requiring medical treatment (other than basic first aid).
2. The employer must record each work-related injury or illness on the OSHA Form 300 (Log of Work-Related Injuries and Illnesses).
3. The employer must complete a supplementary record of occupational injuries and illnesses for each recordable case on OSHA Form 301 (Injury and Illness Incident Report).
4. The employer must prepare an annual summary using OSHA Form 300A (Summary of Work-Related Injuries and Illnesses). Since workers, former workers, and their representatives have the right to review the OSHA Form 300 Log, the report must be posted for review by workers no later than February 1 of each year, and remain posted through April 30.
5. The employer is required to retain these records for at least 5 years.

Medical treatment is defined as "the management and care of a patient to combat disease or disorder" (OSHA, 2005b). However, it is sometimes easier to define what does not constitute medical treatment and use this as a guide to determine if the case must be recorded. OSHA specifies the following scenarios that do not constitute medical treatment (OSHA, 2005b):

146

- First aid treatment; including the administration of over-the-counter medications
- Visits to a healthcare professional solely for evaluation, observation, or counseling
- Diagnostic procedures (radiology and laboratory testing) or evaluations that require use of prescription medication for diagnostic purposes.

OSHA (2005) has defined specific interventions that constitute "first aid" in order to guide the employer's decisions related to recordability of the event. The following is a list of interventions that constitute "first aid only" for cases that are not required to be recorded:

- Use of nonprescription medication at nonprescription strength
- Tetanus immunizations; other immunizations administered strictly for prevention not in relation to an exposure incident
- Cleaning, flushing, or soaking wounds and using wound bandages for wounds on the surface of the skin
- Use of butterfly bandages or adhesive wound-closing devices
- Using heat or cold therapy
- Use of any nonrigid means of support, such as elastic bandages, wraps, nonrigid back belts, etc.
- Use of temporary immobilization devices while transporting an accident victim (e.g., splints, slings, neck collars, back boards, etc.)
- Drilling of a fingernail or toenail to relieve pressure, or draining fluid from a blister
- Use of eye patches
- Removing foreign bodies from the eye using only irrigation or a cotton swab
- Removing splinters or foreign material from areas other than the eye by irrigation, tweezers, cotton swabs, or other simple means
- Use of finger protectors
- Use of massage
- Administration of oral fluids for relief of heat stress.

See Appendix 16 for an OSHA Recordable Reference Chart.

As part of OSHA record keeping, the employer is obligated to track and log the number of calendar days each worker is unable to work as a result of the injury or illness, regardless of whether or not the worker was scheduled to work on those day(s). Weekend days, holidays, vacation days, or other days off are included in the total number of days recorded. If the worker incurs 1 or more days away from work (DAFW), these days are entered onto the OSHA log. Restricted work days must also be entered in the OSHA log. These are days when workers are unable to perform one or more of the essential, routine functions of their usual job or when a licensed healthcare professional renders opinion that workers not perform one or more of the usual job functions. If a worker cannot work a full shift or is transferred to another job, this must also be logged. Essentially, these scenarios are referred to as DART days (days away, restricted, transfer). OSHA also requires that certain serious health conditions be entered onto the OSHA log, even if the injury did not incur DART days. Complete information on OSHA record guidelines may be found at www.OSHA.gov.

SUMMARY
The upstream approach to safety involves involvement at all levels and identification or root causes of hazards and risks. A company's safety program should provide adequate authority and resources, while holding managers, supervisors, and workers accountable for their responsibilities. The safety program should be reviewed annually and specifically include a review of the OSHA log. The purpose of the review is to identify opportunities for program improvement and revision that will lead to further reductions in workplace incidents, injuries, and illnesses.

Several key principles are necessary for a successful safety program. The first and foremost principle is management buy-in and support for the health and safety of the workers. This commitment will then exude through the workplace, building trust and developing allegiance from the workers as the program evolves. A roadmap of success is only evident if management tracks the success of the program. This requires data collection and benchmarking strategies, which are not only valuable to compare against industry standards, but also vital in order to track changes and effectiveness of strategies and initiatives. Measures of success can be achieved through statistical reports and risk analysis. Periodic assessment of the opinions of workers and management is also valuable to assure satisfaction, and sporadic, unannounced workplace inspections to validate and assure compliance will validate success of the program.

The safety committee, composed of management and workers, is intended to provide the overall guidance and direction that will align the organization with the shared vision for health and safety in the workplace. The committee will drive the upstream approach by encouraging positive change, open communication, and accountability. The initiatives of the committee are intended to strive to combine operational standards with safety and health standards through support from management. Through this bottom-up approach, with input from workers at all levels, workers will begin to talk the talk and walk the walk in their everyday work performance.

The return on investment is significant through direct cost saving as a result of fewer workplace incidents and injuries that lead to lower insurance costs. Indirect cost savings are also reaped through decreased lost work time, increased productivity, and enhanced morale of the workforce. A continual process for measuring safety performance will result in a process for communicating results and celebrating successes that lead to a safe and healthy workplace for all.

REFERENCES

ACGIH. *Biological Exposure Indices (BEI®) Introduction*. (2012). Retrieved from http://www.acgih.org/tlv/

American Conference of Governmental Industrial Hygienists (ACGIH). (2012). Retrieved from http://www.acgih.org/home.htm

Atkinson, W. (2004). Safety incentive programs: What works? *EHS Today*. Retrieved from http://ehstoday.com/safety/incentives/ehs_imp_37145/

Balge, M. Z. & Krieger, G. R. (Eds.). (2000). *Occupational health & safety* (3rd ed.). Chicago: National Safety Council.

Burton, B. C. & Halprin, L. P. (2003). *Training for first aid teams or first aid responders: Part I. Occupational health & safety*. Retrieved from http://www.ohsonline.com

Burton, B. C. & Halprin, L. P. (2003). *Training for first aid teams or first aid responders: Part II. Occupational health & safety*. Retrieved from http://www.ohsonline.com

Eckenfelder, D. J. (2003). Getting the safety culture right. *EHS Today*. Retrieved from http://ehstoday.com/mag/ehs_imp_36651/

Geller, S. (2006). The human dynamics of injury prevention (Part 1): From behavior-based to people-based safety. *EHS Today*. Retrieved from http://ehstoday.com/safety/ehs_imp_39434/

Geller, S. E. (2005). Behavior-based safety and occupational risk management. *Behavior Modification, 29*(3), 539–561.

Geller, S. E. (2010). *Cultivating a self-motivated workforce: The choice, community and competence of an injury-free culture*. Retrieved from http://ehstoday.com/safety/management/cultivating-selfmotivated-workforce-0510/index1.html

Laws, J. (2005). Taking an upstream approach. *Occupational Health & Safety*. Retrieved from http://www.oshonline.com

Laws, J. (2012). Getting to zero. *Occupational Health & Safety*. Retrieved from http://www.ohsonline.com

Liberty Mutual Insurance Research Institute. (2011). *Liberty Mutual workplace safety index*. Retrieved from http://www.libertymutualgroup.com/omapps/ContentServer?pagename=LMGroup/Views/LMG&ft=2&fid=1138356633468&ln=en

Maslow, A. H. (1943). A theory of human motivation. *Psychological Review, 50*(4), 370–396.

National Institute for Occupational Safety and Health (NIOSH). (2004). *How to evaluate safety and health change in the workplace*. DHHS (NIOSH) Publication No. 2004-135. Retrieved from http://www.cdc.gov/niosh/docs/2004-135/pdfs/2004-135.pdf

National Institute for Occupational Safety and Health (NIOSH). (2010). *Workplace safety and health topics. Chemical safety*. Retrieve from http://www.cdc.gov/niosh/topics/chemical-safety/

National Institute for Occupational Safety and Health (NIOSH), Education and Information Division. (2011). *The emergency response safety and health database*. Retrieved from http://www.cdc.gov/niosh/ershdb/glossary.html

National Institute for Occupational Safety and Health (NIOSH). (2012). *Small business resources guide: Regulations.* Retrieved from http://www.cdc.gov/niosh/topics/smbus/guide/guide-4.html

National Institutes for Health (NIH). The National Institute of Environmental Services. (2012). Occupational Health. Retrieved from http://www.niehs.nih.gov/health/topics/population/occupational/index.cfm

Occupational Safety and Health Administration (OSHA). (1996). *Program evaluation profile.* Retrieved from http://www.osha.gov/dsg/topics/safetyhealth/pep.html

Occupational Safety and Health Administration (OSHA). (2002). *Responsibility, authority, and accountability checklist.* Retrieved from http://www.osha.gov/SLTC/etools/safetyhealth/mod4_tools_checklist.html

Occupational Safety and Health Administration (OSHA). (2005a). *Model policy statements.* Retrieved from http://www.osha.gov/Publications/smallbusiness/small-business.html#appb

Occupational Safety and Health Administration (OSHA). (2005b). *Small business handbook: Small business safety and health management series.* OSHA 2209-02R. Retrieved from http://www.osha.gov/Publications/smallbusiness/small-business.html

Occupational Safety and Health Administration (OSHA). *Injury and illness prevention programs.* Retrieved from http://www.osha.gov/dsg/topics/safetyhealth/index.html

Occupational Safety and Health Administration (OSHA). *Occupational noise exposure.* Retrieved from http://www.osha.gov/SLTC/noisehearingconservation/

Occupational Safety and Health Administration (OSHA). *Occupational safety and health guidelines.* Retrieved from http://www.osha.gov/SLTC/healthguidelines/index.html

Perce, K. H. (2007). Disaster preparedness. *AAOHN Journal.* 55(5), 197–207.

Rogers, B. (2003). Occupational and environmental health nursing: Concepts and practice. (2nd ed.) Philadelphia: W. B. Saunders.

Roy, D. R. (2003). Safety is everyone's responsibility. *AAOHN Journal, 51*(4), 158–159.

Salazar, M. K. (Ed.). *Core curriculum for occupational and environmental health nursing* (2nd ed., pp. 3–32). Philadelphia: W.B. Saunders.

Schultz, D. (2004). Employee attitudes—A must have. *Occupational Health and Safety.* Retrieved from http://ohsonline.com/articles/2004/06/employee-attitudesa-must-have.aspx

Stroschein, J. (2010). Incentives: Is behavior the key to an effective program? *EHS Today.* Retrieved from http://ehstoday.com/safety/news/incentives-behavior-key-effective-program-1113/index.html

Thatcher, J. J. (2009). Core practices: Culture or behavior: Which comes first? *EHS Today.* Retrieved from http://ehstoday.com/safety/ehs_imp_36298/index.html

U.S. Department of Labor, Bureau of Labor Statistics (BLS). (2011a). *Injuries, illnesses, and fatalities*. Retrieved from http://www.bls.gov/iif/

U.S. Department of Labor, Bureau of Labor Statistics (BLS). (2011b). Workplace injury and illness summary. *News Release: Workplace injuries and illnesses—2010*. Retrieved from http://www.bls.gov/news.release/osh.nr0.htm/

Williamsen, M. (2003). Getting results from safety meetings. *Occupational Health and Safety*. Retrieved from http://www.ohsonline.com

RESOURCES

OSHA Technical Manual (OTM). (1999). OSHA Directive TED 01-00-015 [TED 1-0.15A].

Small Business Handbook. (2005). OSHA Publication 2209-02R.

Informational Booklet on Industrial Hygiene. (1998). OSHA Publication 3143.

OSHA Regulations (Standards-29 CFR).

Safety and Health Information. Mine Safety and Health Administration (MSHA). http://www.msha.gov/safeinfo.HTM

National Institute for Occupational Safety and Health (NIOSH) http://www.cdc.gov/niosh/

Fitness for Duty

8

A key aspect in assuring health and safety in the workplace is to determine if the worker is fit for duty, therefore capable of performing the essential functions of the job.

Why can't just anyone do the job? This is a question that must always be asked related to worker fitness. This chapter covers the rationale for determining fitness for duty and defines the components of the evaluations used to determine the fitness of a worker. Certain regulatory requirements regarding work fitness will also be addressed.

A RATIONALE FOR OCCUPATIONAL HEALTH SERVICES

A significant role that is specific to occupational healthcare professionals is that of ensuring an employer's workforce is medically qualified, fit, and available for work. The occupational health nurse (OHN) should strive to assure that workers are of the highest calibre and are able to perform the essential functions of their assigned jobs. Knowing the job and what it entails is the first step in the process of determining fitness. This is accomplished through the development of job descriptions that provide details related to essential functions. The second step is evaluation of the worker, through health assessments and physical-demand testing. Health assessments may include review of the worker's health history, health testing, and physical examination. In addition, the use of substance testing is considered a significant aspect of fitness for duty.

The healthcare provider conducting the fitness for duty assessment holds a critical role in making the determination of whether or not an individual is medically qualified for the job. Diligence and consistency in the standard of care as to how fitness is determined is crucial, especially with those individuals who have preexisting health conditions that may pose a liability risk for the employer. The healthcare provider must use critical decision making in reviewing the candidate's medical history, reviewing prior medical records, and making the fitness determination.

Essentials for Occupational Health Nursing, First Edition. Arlene Guzik.
© 2013 John Wiley & Sons, Inc. Published 2013 by John Wiley & Sons, Inc.

Many entities have regulated fitness standards, such as the Federal Aviation Administration, Department of Transportation, and U.S. Merchant Marine. Otherwise, employers reserve the right to determine the standards related to fitness for duty in regard to the essential functions of the job. The standards are specified in job descriptions that outline the essential functions and the physical demands the job entails.

In addition, there are many unwritten standards that surround a fitness for duty determination that may present a concern for the employer. How do you address the actual or potential effect of medications on a person's ability to perform the essential functions of the job? What about certain health conditions that may pose a risk to climbing, operating hazardous equipment, or work with dangerous chemicals? Oftentimes, the healthcare provider is faced with making a judgment based on the "potential" risk that may be posed by certain health conditions and the use of certain medications. This judgment is often based on a reasonable degree of probability, the knowledge of job risks, and the underpinnings of healthcare science. The primary principles of occupational health also serve to support and further justify these decisions.

ISSUES AFFECTING FITNESS FOR DUTY

There are a number of issues that can interfere with the ability of a worker to perform essential job functions that can then place the worker at risk for injury or illness. This interference can also create a liability for the employer, especially if it creates a hazard for other workers or has an impact on public safety. Medical conditions, impairments, and the use of certain medications may affect a worker's ability to perform in certain safety-sensitive jobs and may also affect a worker's ability to perform at the potential expected by the employer. Drug use, both legal and illegal, can present certain challenges for workers and impede their ability to perform their jobs in a safe and effective manner.

The primary purpose of determining a worker's fitness for duty is to put the right person in the right job, determining the ability of the worker to meet certain physical demands and to perform the essential functions of the job, with or without accommodation. A secondary purpose is to identify serious health conditions that may qualify for protection under the Americans with Disabilities Act and to determine if reasonable accommodation is warranted. Employers also face increasing responsibility under the Occupational Safety and Health Act to assure that certain workers are fit, ensuring the safety and health of the worker and the workplace. To determine fitness for duty, two aspects must be considered: (1) knowing the job and (2) knowing if the worker is fit to do the job.

Know the Job

The ability to determine a worker's ability to perform the job safely requires knowledge of what the job entails. This is typically provided in a job description, provided by human resources. Traditional job descriptions only gave a "description" of the job, including the knowledge and skills required of the worker. Today's job descriptions contain additional information that details specific essential job functions and the physical, mental, or psychological demands required to carry out these functions. According to the Job Accommodation Network (Loy, 2008) a job description should consist of the following components: (1) essential job functions, (2) knowledge and skills, (3) physical demands, (4) environmental factors, and (5) regulatory requirements.

Essential job functions can be determined by conducting a job analysis. This job analysis, accomplished by observing workers while performing the job and by interviewing workers who have done the job, serves as a foundation for the job description. The job analysis also takes into consideration the environment and structure of the job setting, equipment and supplies used to perform the job, and the activities performed while completing the job tasks.

The Americans with Disabilities Act (1990) defines essential functions as the "fundamental job duties of the employment position the individual holds or desires. The term *essential function* does not include the marginal functions of the position." The essential functions exist so that the work will be accomplished. In some cases, the worker must hold certain skills and abilities in order to perform the essentials of the job. The function, in order to be essential, must entail a significant portion of the job tasks that are critical to completing the work. Should these tasks not be completed, the outcome would not be desirable or meet the needs and expectations of the business. In some cases, the essential functions of a job are defined by regulatory requirement or by collective bargaining agreements. The employer holds the right to determine what is essential in regard to specific jobs and should detail these functions in the written job description.

Once the essential job functions are determined, the next step is to determine the physical, mental, and sometimes psychological demands that are required in order for the worker to accomplish the job. The demands of the job are based on skills, knowledge, and abilities the worker must possess in order to qualify for the job. These factors provide guidance for completing the job tasks. (KSA Writing, 2011).

Knowledge
To have the appropriate knowledge, the worker would need to possess intellectual information or procedural competence regarding how the job is performed or what the job process entails. The job demands for an administrative assistant would include knowledge on how to use a computer and specified applications, how to answer the phone, how to plan a meeting, how to make travel arrangements, and how to file documents. In contrast, a construction worker may need knowledge related to building codes, plumbing, laying tile, or even OSHA regulations. Knowledge, as a job demand, may have been gained by the worker through formal education or through prior experience in a similar job.

Skills

The worker may be required to hold certain physical, verbal, or mental skills. The physical skills required to meet the demands of a job may include standing, walking, sitting, kneeling, bending, twisting, crawling, stooping, squatting, lifting, carrying, pushing, pulling, reaching, and climbing stairs or ladders. The worker may also need to be capable of using a computer, driving a vehicle, operating a fork lift, taking a blood pressure, or using a drill. Verbal skills may include singing, answering the phone, or speaking a particular language. Mental skills may include being able to compare and contrast, analyze, judge, negotiate, solve problems, and to learn and comprehend.

The job demands for an administrative assistant would include the ability to sit for long periods of time, lift up to 20 pounds occasionally, and type; the mental skills for the administrative assistant would include the ability to multitask, calculate an expense report, handle customer complaints, and work under short deadlines. In contrast, the construction worker would need to meet the different job demands of standing for long periods of time, frequently lifting up to 75 pounds, climbing, and working at heights; the mental demands may involve the ability to deal with difficult clients, work under deadlines, process information, make decisions, and supervise work of others.

Abilities

The workers hold certain talents required of the job duties, which are referred to as abilities. These would include physical abilities specific to the job demands or being capable of performing certain procedures. Beyond the physical abilities, mental abilities may also be required, such as the ability to supervise, coordinate, communicate, teach, concentrate, or the ability to remain calm. For workers in high-pressure jobs, such as law enforcement, fire fighting, and emergency response, they may be required to have the ability to work under stressful conditions and perhaps be required to complete psychological testing as part of the fitness for duty evaluation.

Using the example of these same job categories, you can now see how the job demands build on one another by populating the specific knowledge, skills, and abilities required of the worker.

The job demands required for an administrative assistant would include the following:

- Use a computer and specified applications
- Answer the phone
- Plan a meeting
- Make travel arrangements
- File documents
- Sit for long periods of time
- Lift up to 20 pounds occasionally
- Multitask

- Calculate an expense report
- Handle customer complaints
- Work under short deadlines

The job demands required for a construction worker would include:

- Knowledge of building codes and OSHA regulations
- Install and repair plumbing
- Install tile
- Lift up to 75 pounds frequently
- Use hand and power tools
- Kneel, crawl, and climb
- Work at heights
- Operate a backhoe
- Work in confined spaces
- Work in hazardous and changing environmental conditions

It is important to also know if the job falls under any specific regulatory requirements. Often, regulatory requirements define the skills, knowledge, and the abilities that are essential for the job. Therefore, one job does not fit all workers, and one worker does not fit all jobs.

Know the Worker

The employer, having the right to determine job categories that require fitness for duty evaluation, must be consistent regarding which employees are evaluated, for what jobs they are evaluated, and how they are evaluated. This consistency is important to assure fairness and uniformity in the workplace in compliance with the regulations set forth by the Equal Employment Opportunity Commission (EEOC).

A determination of fitness for duty may be required or requested by the employer and for a variety of situations. A fitness for duty evaluation may be conducted to measure a person's ability to do the job. This may be performed prior to placing the individual in the job or may also be performed as a regulatory requirement on a periodic basis. Employers also have the right to conduct fitness for duty evaluations to address the ability of the worker when performance or safety issues have raised question in regard to the worker's ability to perform the essential functions of the job in a safe and effective manner.

The fitness for duty evaluation is a procedure conducted by a health professional that seeks information about the individual's physical or mental health status. It is usually conducted in a healthcare setting, and it involves the use of medical equipment or testing. The fitness for duty evaluation may also involve tests to measure the worker's performance of specific tasks or to measure physiological or psychological responses in relation to job demands (EEOC, 2007).

The employer must be consistent in its requirements for fitness for duty evaluations. The requirements must in accordance with civil rights statutes and must be specific to the work environment and job requirements. The employer is precluded from denying an individual a job based on any physical or mental disability. The employer is able, however, to extend a job offer contingent upon passing a fitness for duty evaluation that verifies the candidate would be able to perform the essential functions of the job in a safe manner. The candidate can only be disqualified if the fitness of the individual is not compatible with the physical demands of the job, and reasonable accommodation is not an option.

The fitness for duty evaluation must be specific to the essential functions of the job; however, it can consist of a variety of procedures. Substance testing is considered an aspect of fitness for duty in relation to an employer's drug-free workplace program and regulatory mandates. Further evaluations can be conducted by reviewing an individual's health history using a health history form that has been completed by the worker or job candidate. More extensive evaluations would be conducted through physical examinations or through physical testing. Common tests used for fitness for duty determination include laboratory tests; vision, hearing and pulmonary function tests; physical ability or agility tests; and psychological testing.

SUBSTANCE TESTING

Substance testing, as a measure of fitness for duty, should be used in compliance with an employer's drug-free workplace program (DFWP). Realizing that DFWP statutes are state specific, the employer must ensure testing is in compliance with all applicable regulatory statutes. The rationale for this testing is to ensure a drug-free workforce in attempt to increase safety and to enhance the quality of the workplace and worker productivity.

According to a survey of members conducted by the Society for Human Resource Management, 84% of employers conduct some form of substance testing as a measure of fitness for duty. The survey results revealed that 39% conducted random screening, 73% conduct for-cause testing, and 58% require drug tests associated with work-related incidents and accidents. The report indicates that 55% of the employers reported that this substance testing applied to all workers, 17% indicated the testing applied to only select workers (such as safety-sensitive positions), and 7% tested for regulatory purposes only (SHRM, 2010).

The use of preemployment and random testing of workers for illicit drugs such as heroin, cocaine, amphetamines, and marijuana is most common. However, today the use of legally prescribed drugs raises new issues in regard to fitness for duty for workers and their employers. Drug use, both legal and illegal, can have an effect on safety and productivity of the worker.

Because there are common panels for drug screens that identify specific drugs, the worker can be under the effects of drugs despite a negative substance test. Therefore, a "negative" result from a substance test does not mean the worker is not under the influence of drugs. Street drugs now include prescription narcotic drugs that are abused, such as hydrocodone, OxyContin, Soma, and fentanyl. These drugs would not be found on standard drug screen panels commonly used by employers.

Laboratory reports for drug screens indicate results only for drugs that have been requested on the Custody and Control Form. Depending on what panel of drugs is requested, the laboratory performs testing only for those drugs. If any of the specified drugs are found through the confirmed laboratory analysis, the drug screen report must be reviewed by a medical review officer (MRO). The MRO then has the obligation to notify the donor of the specimen to discuss the substances found in the drug screen. If the donor can provide, and the MRO can verify, a legal prescription for the identified substance, the drug screen result is reported to the employer as "negative." Therefore, a negative drug screen report may reflect the fact that the individual has a legal prescription for the drug. It does not mean that he or she is not taking drugs that may affect his or her ability to perform the job safely.

The MRO, however, has an ethical and moral obligation to notify the employer of safety-sensitive concerns, especially if the drug screen was conducted for regulatory purposes or for the purposes of reasonable suspicion. If the MRO has knowledge that the donor is or will be involved in safety-sensitive work or presents a risk to himself/herself or others through the performance of his or her job duties, the MRO should report the fact that the findings on the drug screen, despite being reported as negative, have safety-sensitive implications. The MRO is precluded from identifying the drugs in question; therefore, this report should prompt the employer to move to a higher level of fitness for duty evaluation.

HEALTH EVALUATIONS
Preplacement
The employer reserves the right to make inquiries into the ability of an individual to perform the functions of the job and/or to ask the individual to describe or to demonstrate how they will be able to perform job-related functions (EEOC). The term *preplacement* in lieu of *preemployment* is used since it further generalizes the purposes of the fitness for duty evaluation to apply not only to individuals being hired for jobs, but also to current workers who apply for job transfers and to those workers who have had a change in health status.

Preplacement fitness for duty evaluations are conducted for three specific reasons:

1. New hire: As an evaluation of fitness for a new-hire job candidate.
2. Job transfer: Before transfer into a new position within the same company.
3. Change in health status: Change in the worker's health condition while on the job or after absence from the job for health reasons.

Table 8.1 Essential job function defined.

What Is an Essential Job Function?

• The primary reason for the job position is to perform that function
• There are a limited number of workers available to perform that job function
• The function requires highly specialized expertise or ability to perform the particular function

What Determines If a Job Function Is Essential?

• The employer's judgment
• Written job descriptions
• The amount of time spent on the job performing that particular function
• The consequences of not requiring performance of the function
• Collective bargaining agreement
• Work experience of former workers requiring the function
• Current work experience of workers in similar jobs

Source: Adapted from 29 CFR Part 1630 Regulations to Implement the Equal Employment Provisions of the Americans With Disabilities Act.

The fitness for duty evaluation serves several purposes. One purpose is to identify substance use, health conditions, or disabilities that may interfere with the ability of the individual to perform the essential functions of the job in a safe manner. The fitness for duty evaluation also serves to establish a baseline of the individual's health status for comparison purposes during the course of employment. This becomes important in regard to compliance with specific regulatory statutes, such as hearing conservation, work with hazardous substances, or the worker's risk of exposure to communicable diseases. This baseline data also proves valuable in the process of establishing preexisting history in the event of a work-related injury or illness. Most importantly, this evaluation will serve to ensure that an individual is physically and mentally capable of performing the essential functions and demands of a particular job. The definitions related to essential job functions are outlined in Table 8.1.

For new hires and job transfers, the employer must conduct any preplacement fitness for duty evaluations, including substance testing, after providing the individual a conditional offer for the job. This means the job candidate must first be found otherwise qualified (by knowledge, skills, or abilities) and offered the position. The Americans with Disabilities Act (1995) states: "After the employer extends an offer for the new position, it may ask the individual disability-related questions or require a medical examination as long as it does so for all entering employees in the same job category. If an employer withdraws the offer based on medical information, it must show that the reason for doing so was job-related and consistent with business necessity." Therefore, the job offer is made dependent upon successful completion of the fitness for duty evaluation to determine if the individual is physically qualified to perform the essential functions of the job.

Although preplacement fitness for duty evaluations are not regulatory mandated for most jobs, it is prudent for the employer to conduct the evaluations for job categories requiring specific physical demands or for job categories that are safety sensitive in nature. Components of the fitness for duty evaluation must be consistent with job requirements. As a result, the employers, along with the healthcare provider conducting the evaluations, have the right to define specific components of the fitness for duty evaluation. Fitness for duty evaluation commonly consists of one or more of the following:

- Review of a completed health history form
- Physical examination
- Physical capacity tests to evaluate certain capabilities such as lifting, pushing, pulling a predetermined amount of weight, climbing, or kneeling
- Physical agility tests consisting of an aerobic component such as running, walking, stair stepping, or other exercise endurance testing
- Respirator clearance, including chest x-ray and pulmonary function testing
- Hearing evaluations
- TB testing for healthcare workers
- Baseline laboratory testing for positions involving work with hazardous materials
- Psychological evaluations

Change in Heath Status
Fitness for duty evaluations may also be conducted when a worker has had a change in health status during the course of employment. For certain jobs that are safety sensitive or have regulatory requirements related to worker fitness, the employer has the right to require the worker to provide notice to the employer of any significant change in health status that may interfere with their ability to perform the essential functions of the job in a safe manner. This includes the use of certain safety-sensitive medications. The employer should have a written policy that advises workers of this responsibility.

For workers whose jobs require the specific essential physical demands, the company's fitness for duty policy should define the fact that workers are required to notify the employer of any changes in health status that would interfere with their ability to meet the physical qualifications specified in the job description. For example, there are many safety-sensitive jobs that require workers to be able to see and hear, such as school-crossing guards, mobile equipment operators, and security officers. These workers, who may experience a change in vision or hearing, would be required to notify the employer of this change. Certain jobs also have statutory requirements that address standards for seeing and hearing. Examples include Department of Transportation (DOT) medical qualifications for truck drivers, National Fire Protection Standards for fire fighters, and the Federal Aviation Administration medical qualifications for aviation pilots. These standards define specific physical requirements and also define how certain health conditions impact decision making in relation to the worker's fitness for duty. For example, the DOT defined physical qualifications for truck drivers using guidelines, established through evidence-based research, that address cardiovascular, neurological, musculoskeletal, and many other disorders. So if the driver incurs a heart attack or is diagnosed with multiple sclerosis, guidelines are available to assist with decision making on how soon after the diagnosis the worker can resume driving, what information is required to determine the stability of the condition, and how often the worker's health status should be reevaluated.

A change in the worker's health status may also occur as a result of a work-related injury. Depending on the extent and severity of the health condition, the worker may be left with certain permanent impairments or work restrictions as a result of the injury. Should this occur, it may be important to evaluate the worker's health status and ability to continue to return to his or her original job based on these impairments or restrictions. In the process of closing a workers' compensation claim, a fitness for duty evaluation may be requested by the treating healthcare provider to objectively define the permanent restrictions and level of impairment that will be assigned to the worker. In addition, a fitness for duty evaluation may be requested by the employer, claims administrator, workers' compensation attorney, or judge in order to gather objective information related to impairment and to establish the need for future care and the disability rating. The question to be answered in this situation is "can the worker, with the assigned impairment or restriction, return to his or her original job, and if not, what is the worker physically capable of doing.

Return to Work

An additional indication for a worker's fitness for duty evaluation would be when the worker has experienced a change in their health after absence from the job for health reasons. This not only applies to absences related to on-the-job injuries, but also to absences related to personal health reasons. Workers who take leaves of absence for medical reasons may or may not be able to return to work in the same physical capacity. The purpose of this evaluation then is to determine if the worker has recovered sufficiently to return to the workplace and to measure the worker's ability to meet the essential physical demands of the job. Once a worker is released back to work by the treating healthcare provider, the employer has the right to refer the individual to the company's occupational health provider for a fitness for duty evaluation. The rationale to support this approach is based on the fact that the individual's personal healthcare provider, despite providing the individual with a return-to-work note, may not be familiar with regulatory guidelines, safety implications, or the physical demands that are involved with the job position. Therefore, this evaluation uses the same principles as preplacement evaluation in conducting an objective measure of health status, including the use of medications and physical abilities, while considering all health and safety implications.

Benefits Eligibility or Regulatory Entitlement

A fitness for duty evaluation may also be indicated to determine worker's eligibility for benefits entitlement. Examples of requirements for benefits eligibility include social security disability benefits, short- or long-term disability benefits, and life insurance policy eligibility. Certain eligibility criteria, established by the insurance carrier, would be used to determine if the individual is qualified to obtain or retain certain benefits. Prior to the issuance of life insurance or disability insurance policies, the individual may be required to submit to a fitness for duty evaluation to establish a baseline of health status before issuance of insurance certificate.

Fitness for duty evaluations may also prove beneficial to validate a request for accommodation from a worker or their personal healthcare provider, especially when the disability or need for accommodation is not known or not obvious. For example, a worker may requests a change to day shift from the night shift because of diabetes. In this situation, the employer has the right to conduct an evaluation to determine the medical necessity of the request. The occupational health profession will, after interviewing and examining the worker, conduct a review of the personal health records to determine if the condition warrants the change. In some situations, the occupational health provider, acting as intermediary between the employer and the worker, will also have a conversation with the worker's treating healthcare provider to discuss the condition and options for accommodation. The occupational health provider will evaluate the stability of the condition and the current treatment modalities in order to validate the need for reasonable accommodation to further stabilize the condition. Options for accommodation would be explored with the employer as well.

Reasonable Suspicion

If the employer has reasonable belief, based on objective evidence, that a worker's performance is affected by a health condition or that the worker's health condition poses a direct threat to the worker, the workplace, or to public safety, a fitness for duty evaluation may be requested (EEOC, 2007). Objective evidence would include observed performance issues, such as the inability to follow direction, unexplained incidents or injuries, falling asleep on the job, or simply because a worker states he or she cannot perform certain functions of the job because of a health condition. Another reason for evaluation would exist when a worker is exhibiting risky or unacceptable behavior, verbal or physical violence, incoherence, or the suspicion of alcohol odor on the breath.

The objective evidence needed to make health-related inquiries must be reliable, either observed by the supervisor or learned from another credible source. An evaluation for reasonable suspicion should include a written report from the supervisor or other company official of the specific behavior in question describing the factors of concern and the aim of the evaluation. Factors to be considered that support the need for fitness for duty evaluation include the seriousness of the issue and its impact on the workplace environment. The employer reserves the right to conduct such inquiries and examinations, including substance testing, physical examinations, psychological tests, or tests of physical fitness or ability. When the individual is exhibiting unacceptable behavior, seems incoherent, or appears to be under the influence, the individual should be escorted by a company representative to the evaluation and should not be left unattended until it is determined safe to do so.

Periodic Health Monitoring

Periodic fitness for duty evaluations and other health status monitoring may be indicated under specific circumstances or for regulatory purposes. This includes periodic physical examinations and testing, such as firefighter physicals, audiograms, exams for respirator users, medical surveillance monitoring for those who work with hazardous chemicals and for other jobs where periodic health evaluations are required based on regulatory mandate. These evaluations must be job-related and consistent with business necessity.

PHYSICAL ABILITIES TESTING

Tests of physical ability are intended to measure the ability to perform specific tasks necessary to perform the essential functions of the job. The test may consist of measures of strength and flexibility of specific muscle groups, as well as physical endurance. The test could also include the performance of several tasks that mimic portions of the job. The intended purpose of physical abilities testing is to provide the employer with an analysis of the individual's ability to perform essential job functions that may be physically demanding.

Common uses of physical abilities testing are for jobs in firefighting, law enforcement, and security administration. However, employers with jobs that are physically demanding, such as material handling or construction, have found this a useful screening process to measure the physical capabilities required for the job. Typical components of a physical abilities test include measures of the following:

- Grip strength or manual dexterity
- The ability to lift, carry, push, and pull defined amounts of weight
- Trunk strength, including sit-ups
- Endurance, including running, step tests, or exercise treadmills
- Physical agility, including the ability to climb, jump, enter or exit a confined space

Despite the trend in the use of physical abilities testing in attempt to put the right person in the right job, the fact that an individual meets or exceeds the physical demand testing does not predict or ensure that the individual will perform the job in a safe and effective manner. Nor does it guarantee that the individual will not incur an injury during the course and scope of their work duties.

Table 8.2 Key elements of a fitness for duty evaluation.

1. Signed consent from the individual being tested, including permission to communicate finding with the employer
2. Review health history
3. Physical examination
4. Ancillary testing specific to the physical demands
5. Review of personal health records, when applicable
6. Discussion with the individual's healthcare provider, when appropriate
7. Decision making for fitness for duty:
   - Determine the presence or absence of a permanent impairment that substantially limits one or more major life activities.
   - Evaluate the patient's work capacity (mental and physical) and delineate workplace restrictions.
   - Assess workplace demands (mental and physical) and essential functions of the job.
   - Ascertain the patient's ability to perform the essential functions of the job with, or without, accommodations.

DETERMINING FITNESS FOR DUTY

The capture of a thorough health history is the foundation for the fitness for duty evaluation. A sample health history form is provided in Appendix 17. This evaluation is obtained not only through a health history completed by the worker, but also through interview and a review of the personal health records, if applicable. If the evaluation is triggered as a result of performance issues, it is most helpful to discuss with the worker and the employer the performance or health issues underpinning the fitness concern. The key components of the fitness for duty evaluation are listed in Table 8.2.

The determination of fitness can result in the following possible recommendations (AHRQ, 2005):

- **Fit for duty**—The individual is fit to perform the essential functions of the job without accommodation. This implies that the individual has met the physical, mental, and psychological requirements to perform a specific job.
- **Temporarily fit for duty**—The individual is fit for a defined period of time. This may be due to the need for reevaluation or periodic review of the worker's health condition.
- **Fit for duty with permanent restrictions**—The individual is not fit for the job because of a disability, one that substantially limits one or more life activity and that interferes with their ability to perform the essential functions of the job. The employer must now assess their obligation to provide reasonable accommodation through job modification, use of adaptive equipment, or by reallocating marginal job functions that the individual is unable to perform because of their disability.
- **Fit for duty with temporary restrictions**—The individual has a health condition that renders them incapable of performing certain functions of

the job for a temporary period of time. In this case, the restrictions may apply only to marginal functions and the individual may perform most functions of the job in a safe manner. It is expected that the health condition will improve, at which time the restrictions would be removed and the individual would be able to perform all essential functions of the job. The employer is not required to consider accommodation for temporary conditions.

- **Temporarily not fit for duty**—The individual has a health condition that may or may not improve with time, or there are uncertainties surrounding the determination of fitness. At the time of evaluation, it is determined that the individual's presence in the workplace would present a risk to the individual or others. This designation is often used when the determination of fitness is dependent on the need for additional testing or the gathering of additional information.
- **Permanently not fit for duty**—It is expected that the individual will never be capable of performing the essential functions of the job, with or without reasonable accommodation. This determination must be based on objective evidence that proves a direct risk or documents the inability of the individual to meet specific standards.

The results of a fitness for duty evaluation should be documented in the worker's medical file and considered protected health information. Use and disclosure of this information must be compliant with the regulations of the Americans with Disabilities Act (ADA) and the Health Information Portability and Accountability Act (HIPAA).

THE FITNESS FOR DUTY POLICY AND PROCEDURE

A written policy and procedure (Appendix 18) regarding fitness for duty should identify the rationale for evaluation and detail both the employer's and the individual's rights and responsibilities. For regulatory or safety-sensitive job positions, the policy and procedures should include the requirement for workers to self-report medical conditions, symptoms, diagnoses, or prescribed drugs between qualifying periods. The policy should also define the employer's right to conduct fitness for duty evaluations based on reasonable suspicion or based on performance concerns. The policy should define the rights of individuals protected under ADA and the employer's obligation to offer reasonable accommodation. This may include the individual's option to transfer or apply for another vacant, budgeted position for which they are qualified, or to take a leave of absence. Aspects of the policy must also address what right the individual has to a second opinion and the process for resolution of conflicts. This is of particular importance to evaluations conducted on individuals who are already employed. However, it must also take into consideration rights of candidates for positions who are disqualified, but may otherwise be reconsidered at a later time.

SUMMARY

Fitness for duty is a serious issue that directly influences not only the health and safety of the workplace, but also has an impact on workplace productivity. Of particular concern is the fact that the workforce is aging, and older workers, especially those with acute or chronic health conditions, present concern. These concerns include the declining physical ability of the worker and the use of prescription medications to treat certain health conditions.

Best practices for addressing fitness for duty are built on the foundation of a solid and practical policy and a process for evaluation of the workforce. A prudent employer will maintain a solid knowledge of regulations that require fitness for duty evaluations and that address the implications for both the individuals and the employer. The healthcare provider must conduct fitness for duty evaluations in a manner in which the individual's capabilities are compared to the essential functions and demands of the specified job and provide a report to the employer regarding the individual's capabilities, limitations, and any applicable restrictions.

The goal of attaining and maintaining a workforce that is fit for duty should be a shared strategy for both management and workers. The employer must strive to make fitness for duty a core component and expectation for the workforce and must communicate this expectation through written policies and continued education of management and workers.

REFERENCES

Agency for Healthcare Research and Quality (AHRQ) , National Guideline Clearinghouse. (2005). *Work loss data institute. Official disability guidelines fitness for duty*. Corpus Christi, TX: Work Loss Data Institute.

American College of Occupational and Environmental Medicine (ACOEM). (2006). *Preventing needless work disability by helping people stay employed*. Retrieved from http://www.acoem.org

American College of Occupational and Environmental Medicine (ACOEM). (2007). *Position statement transportation and public safety*. Retrieved from http://www.acoem.org

DePaul Brown, N. & Tourigian, R. (2006). What resources are available for creating documents describing essential job functions? *AAOHN Journal, 54*(12).

Equal Employment Opportunity Commission (EEOC), 56 Fed. Reg. 35,734 (July 26, 1991) (29 C.F.R. Chapter XIV [7/1/02 ed.] 1630.2 [n]). Retrieved from http://a257.g.akamaitech.net/7/257/2422/14mar20010800/edocket.access.gpo.gov/cfr_2002/julqtr/pdf/29cfr1630.2.pdf

Equal Employment Opportunity Commission (EEOC). (1992). *A technical assistance manual on the employment provisions (Title I) of the Americans with Disabilities Act*. EEOC-M-1A. Retrieved from http://askjan.org/links/ADAtam1.html

Equal Employment Opportunity Commission (EEOC). (1995). *Enforcement guidance: Preemployment disability-related questions and medical examinations.* Retrieved from http://www.eeoc.gov/docs/preemp.html

Equal Employment Opportunity Commission (EEOC). (1996). *Enforcement guidance: Workers' compensation and the ADA.* Retrieved from http://www.eeoc.gov/docs/workcomp.html

Equal Employment Opportunity Commission (EEOC), ADA Division, Office of Legal Counsel. (2000). *EEOC enforcement guidance on disability-related inquiries and medical examinations of employees under the Americans with Disabilities Act (ADA).* Retrieved from http://www.eeoc.gov/policy/docs/guidance-inquiries.html

Equal Employment Opportunity Commission. (2007). ADA: Pre-offer medical exams. Retrieved from http://www.eeoc.gov/eeoc/foia/letters/2003/ada_pre-offer_exams.htm

Goetzel, R. Z. (2003). The health and productivity cost burden of the "top 10" physical and mental health conditions affecting six large U.S. employers in 1999. *Journal of Occupational and Environmental Medicine*, 45(1), 5–14.

Job Accommodation Network. (2009). *Employers' practical guide to reasonable accommodation under the Americans with Disabilities Act (ADA).* Retrieved from http://askjan.org/Erguide/three.htm

KSA Writing. (2012). KSA writing. Retrieved from http://www.ksa-writing.com/

Loy, B. (2008). *Accommodation and compliance series: job descriptions.* Retrieved from http://askjan.org/media/JobDescriptions.htm

Mitchell, J. & Kessler, E. (2009). EHS today. Medical exams: A driver of workforce wellness. Retrieved from http://ehstoday.com/health/wellness/medical-exams-drive-wellness-0409/

National Guideline Clearinghouse. (2011). *Fitness for duty.* Retrieved from http://www.guideline.gov/content.aspx?id=25689

Russi, M., Buchta, W., Swift, M., Budnick, L., Hodgson, M., Berube, D., Kelafant, G. (2010). Guidance for occupational health services in medical centers. Retrieved from http://www.acoem.org/uploadedFiles/Public_Affairs/Policies_And_Position_Statements/Guidelines/Guidelines/MCOH%20Guidance.pdf

Society for Human Resources Management. (2010). *Background checking: Drug testing SHRM poll.* Retrieved from http://www.shrm.org/Research/SurveyFindings/Articles/Pages/BackgroundCheckDrugTesting.aspx

U.S. Department of Labor, Bureau of Labor Statistics. (2006). *Employment situation summary.* Retrieved from http://www.bls.gov/news.release/empsit.nr0.html

RESOURCES

The Job Accommodation Network (JAN) is a free consulting service that provides information about job accommodations, the Americans with Disabilities Act (ADA), and the employability of people with disabilities.

Office of Disability Employment Policy 200 Constitution Avenue, NW, Room S-1303 Washington, DC 20210 Toll Free: (866)633–7635.

WEB RESOURCES
American College of Occupational and Environmental Medicine
http://www.acoem.org
American Association of Occupational Health Nurses
http://www.aaohn.org
America's Career InfoNet.
http://www.acinet.org/acinet/
Career Onestop
http://www.careeronestop.org
Job Description Writer.
http://www.acinet.org/acinet/jobwriter/default.aspx
National Drug Free Workplace Alliance.
http://www.ndwa.org/Editor/assets/statistics.pdf
Office of Disability Employment Policy (ODEP). U.S. Department of Labor.
http://www.dol.gov/odep/
Substance Abuse and Mental Health Services Administration.
http://www.workplace.samhsa.gov

Drug-Free Workplace

9

How do you spot a drug user at work? Poor performance? Absenteeism?
Mood swings? Accidents? Arguments?
Any or all of these could be indicators of a worker with a substance abuse problem. But
don't be surprised if it's that loyal worker who never misses a day's work and always
does an outstanding job . . . identified through a random drug screen.

Despite initiatives since the early 1900s aimed at reducing, eliminating, or
controlling the use of drugs and alcohol, the problem of drug abuse continues
to affect America's communities and work places. In the 1960s the use of illegal
drugs became an increasing problem. Drugs such as marijuana, heroin, cocaine,
and other street drugs began to have an influence on America's youth. In
the late 1980s, as part of an effort called the "war on drugs," the Reagan
Administration developed the first drug-testing laws. Workplaces where
workers under the influence of an illegal substance could harm themselves or
others began testing for drugs. Employers were required to develop and circu-
late a written policy regarding drug use in the workplace and could then
administer drug tests to certain employees.

As part of this national initiative, random drug testing for workers in the
Department of Transportation was permitted. Subsequent modifications to the
law now require compliance with drug-testing laws by all organizations that
contract with any U.S. federal agency for work in the amount of $100,000 or more
that is performed entirely in the United States. Organizations receiving federal
grants and all individual contractors must now also comply with the law
(SAMHSA, 2010).

The Substance Abuse and Mental Health Services Administration (SAMHSA),
established in 1992, is the federal agency designed to target the need for and
establish substance abuse and mental health services. SAMHSA's goal is to
improve the quality of and access to preventive, treatment, and rehabilitative
services in order to reduce illness, death, and disability resulting from substance
abuse and mental illness.

Essentials for Occupational Health Nursing, First Edition. Arlene Guzik.
© 2013 John Wiley & Sons, Inc. Published 2013 by John Wiley & Sons, Inc.

STATISTICS
According to SAMHSA's National Survey on Drug Use and Health Statistics (2008), an estimated 19.9 million Americans were current illicit drug users, and 23.6 million (9.6%) persons aged 12 or older needed treatment for an illicit drug or alcohol abuse problem. Approximately 10.8% of those who needed treatment received it at a specialty facility. An estimated 22.3 million persons (9.0% of the population age 12 and over) were classified with substance dependence or abuse in the past year. Of these, 15.5 million abused or were dependent on alcohol, 3.7 million abused or were dependent on illicit drugs, and 3.2 million abused or were dependent on both alcohol and illicit drugs. These individuals are in our workplaces.

EFFECT ON THE WORKPLACE
Nearly 75% of all current illegal drug users and heavy alcohols users hold jobs. In a study on workplace drug use conducted in the year 2000, it was estimated that the overall cost to business for drug and alcohol abuse was nearly $160.7 billion. The study estimated that 69% of these costs were from losses in productivity due to drug-related illnesses and deaths. (SAMHSA, 2006).

Alcoholics and problem drinkers are absent from work 3.8–8.3 times more often than normal. Drug users are absent from work an average of 5 days per month due to drug use. Substance abusers are 33% less productive and cost their employers $7,000 in lost productivity annually (SAMHSA, 2006). In addition to the acute effects of alcohol and drug use on judgment and psychomotor skills, "substance use that occurs hours before a worker begins his or her shift can cause spillover effects, such as fatigue and hangovers, that may independently increase injury risk" (Ramchand, Pomeroy, & Arkes, 2009).

Nearly 40% of workplace fatalities can be linked to alcohol use, abuse, or alcoholism. Drug-using workers are 3.6 times more likely to be involved in workplace accidents and 5 times more likely to file a workers' compensation claim. Studies show that 38% to 50% of all workers' compensation claims are related to some form of substance abuse (National Council on Compensation Insurance, 2009). Hangovers can not only be a result of alcohol use, but also workers may experience hangover effects from drug use as well. Studies have demonstrated a variation in the correlation between substance use and occupational injuries that can be seen across different industries (Ramchand, Pomeroy, & Arkes, 2009).

Issues with drug use in the workplace are not limited to illicit drugs. The use of prescription drugs, for both medical and nonmedical use, is a serious concern. In the 2007 National Survey on Drug Use and Health, 6 million people were current users of psychotherapeutic drugs taken for nonmedical reasons. SAMHSA (2008) reported that 25% of drug-related emergency department visits were related to nonmedical use of prescription and over-the-counter drugs.

Drug and alcohol use invades the workplace in exactly the same way it invades the family. Nearly 80% of drug abusers steal from their workplaces to support their drug use. Drug use is most common in the following occupations (SAMHSA, 2008):

- Food preparation workers (19%)
- Waiters, and bartenders (15%)
- Construction (14%)
- Service and accommodation occupations (13%)
- Transportation and material moving (10%)

Common effects of substance abuse on the workplace include:

- Worker absenteeism
- Worker tardiness
- Workers who are less productive
- Work performance issues
- Work-related accidents, injuries, and fatalities
- Increased workers' compensation costs
- Higher medical costs
- Increased worker turnover
- Workplace theft
- Workplace violence

The most common reasons for having a drug- and alcohol-testing program are to avoid hiring workers who use illicit drugs, to provide a mechanism for deterring drug and alcohol use/abuse by workers, and to identify need and refer workers for treatment for drug- and alcohol-related problems. Support for the implementation of a drug-free workplace is driven by facts demonstrating that the cost of drug testing is offset by savings in productivity, accident prevention, absenteeism, illness, and crime. In addition, some states allow insurers to offer discounts on premiums for workers' compensation insurance for having a drug-free workplace program.

DRUG-FREE WORKPLACE REGULATIONS

The Division of Workplace Programs (DWP) is mandated by executive order and public law to provide oversight for the federal Drug-Free Workplace Program. Additionally, DWP addresses primary substance abuse prevention through comprehensive drug-free and health/wellness workplace programs. These programs are intended to promote a safe, healthy, and productive workplace. The components of these programs focus on promoting substance abuse awareness, health and wellness assessments, drug testing, early intervention efforts, treatment, and recovery. DWP is committed to helping workplaces meet the demands of healthcare reform while reducing healthcare costs (SAMHSA, 2010).

One of the most important pieces of federal legislation affecting safety-sensitive industries is the Omnibus Transportation Employee Testing Act of 1991, requiring drug and alcohol testing of all safety-sensitive transportation employees in aviation, trucking, railroads, mass transit, pipelines, and other transportation industries (SAMHSA, 2010).

When developing a drug-free workplace policy, certain federal laws and regulations come into play, specifically addressing substance abuse in the workplace, requiring workplaces to adopt policies and procedures for substance testing and administer drug tests to certain workers. Examples of these regulations include the Drug-Free Workplace Act of 1988, Omnibus Transportation Employee Testing Act of 1991, National Institute on Drug Abuse (1993), U.S. Department of Defense's Rules and Regulations for Defense Contractors, Department of Transportation, Department of Health and Human Services, and the Nuclear Regulatory Commission.

Although substance testing has become common in the workplace, the potential for legal challenges must be recognized. This includes challenges related to worker privacy, unreasonable search and seizure, due process violations, violations of collective bargaining agreements, and wrongful terminations (Balge & Krieger, 2000). Regulations that address the rights and benefits of workers also influence the implementation and management of a drug-free workplace policy. These include Civil Rights Act, Equal Employment Opportunity Act, National Labor Relations Act, Americans with Disabilities Act, and Family and Medical Leave Act. In addition, company-specific policies and benefits, as well as labor bargaining agreements, should be considered. Workplaces impacted by one or more Federal agencies that require drug testing should refer to the specific regulations to determine the scope of the requirements.

DETERMINING THE NEED

One of the first steps in evaluating the development of a drug-free workplace is to define the reason for substance testing and to analyze the business to determine the range and extent of the program.

Employers are responsible for providing workers with a safe workplace, and any worker whose behavior on the job presents a risk to self or others creates a liability for the employer (Balge & Krieger, 2000). Support for substance testing is gained by identifying certain factors within the workplace and developing a philosophical commitment for the company's rationale for the substance testing program. Implementation of a substance testing program may simply be done to deter drug use in the workplace. It may also be implemented as a need because of regulatory requirements. Or, companies with safety-sensitive work may find it valuable in support for a safer workplace. The philosophy of the substance testing program is typically based on whether testing is implemented because of regulatory or business need, or if it is established because of management's commitment to a safe workplace as a social responsibility to employees and to the community.

Businesses with essential functions that are not safety sensitive and pose little risk to workers can often have a basic drug-free workplace program. This type of program would include a written policy and an awareness program. It may or may not include a drug testing component, but probably would not include drug testing for workers, unless they are in a job that has a regulatory requirement for drug testing. Sometimes, the program would only include drug screening for new applicants. This is primarily intended to deter hiring drug users. The risk of this approach is that once hired, the employee may resume drug habits that were ceased before being hired in order to get the job.

Businesses with moderate-high risk may consider implementing a drug-free workplace program that not only includes a written policy and an awareness program, but one that also includes other aspects of testing. Workers in safety-sensitive jobs may be subject to not only preplacement testing, but also may be required to participate in random and/or postaccident testing. In this type of business, the company may provide a benefit where workers also have access to a community Substance Abuse Professional (SAP) or an Employee Assistance Program (EAP).

Large business with workers in a variety of roles may have a formal, comprehensive drug-free workplace program including all aspects of testing.

According to SAMHSA (2011), employers most commonly report the following reasons for having a substance testing program:

- To comply with federal regulations
- To comply with customer or contract requirements
- To comply with insurance carrier requirements
- To minimize the chance of hiring workers who may be users or abusers
- To reinforce the organization's "no drug use" position
- To identify current users and abusers and refer them for assistance
- To establish grounds for discipline or firing
- To improve safety
- To deter recreational drug use that could lead to addiction
- To reduce the costs associated with alcohol and other substance abuse in the workplace.

IDENTIFYING RESOURCES

ACOEM (2009) recommends that employers "obtain expert legal, medical and employee relations advice before making a decision to require screening of employees or applicants for drugs." A physician or clinic specializing in occupational health can serve as an exceptional resource, both in the development of a drug-free workplace program and in facilitation of the testing program.

The employer must assign a medical review officer (MRO), a licensed physician (MD/DO) with appropriate certifications, who will be designated to evaluate positive results prior to a report being made available to the employer. An

MRO is a physician holding specialized knowledge in the pharmacology of prescription drugs and holds knowledge related to the toxicology and effects of prescription, nonprescription, and illicit drugs. To qualify as an MRO, the physician must receive specialized training on regulatory aspects and specimen procedures, satisfactorily complete a certification examination through a nationally recognized board, and meet mandatory requirements for continuing education and recertification.

The MRO serves as a point of contact between an employer and the individual who has been tested by reviewing the laboratory report and validating results. The review process by the MRO certifies that the correct specimen was obtained and that the integrity of the specimen was maintained. The MRO also reviews the laboratory report for completeness and then uses a stepwise process to determine if there is a legitimate explanation for the nonnegative result. This includes an interview with the individual who provided the specimen. Prescription drug use must be validated through the pharmacy that issued the drug. If a legitimate reason for the drug found in the specimen is established, the MRO reports a "negative" result to the employer. If prescription drugs found in the specimen cannot be validated, the result is reported as "positive." The issue of illicit drug use must also be addressed. The individual who provided the specimen must be notified of the findings. In a drug-free workplace, illicit drug use is prohibited on or off the job; therefore, explanations as to where or when the substance was encountered are irrelevant.

After the MRO's review, a final report is provided to the employer.

A list of certified MROs can be found on the following websites:

- Substance Abuse and Mental Health Services Administration, www.samhsa. gov
- American Society of Addiction Medicine, www.asam.org
- American College of Occupational and Environmental Medicine, www. acoem.org
- American Association of Medical Review Officers, www.aamro.com
- Medical Review Officer Certification Council, www.mrocc.com

The MRO, company's medical director, or an occupational health specialist can assist with development of policies and procedures, defining specific needs for testing based on the business operations. These professionals may also assist in identifying collection sites, conducting worker education and supervisor training, and facilitating relationships with substance abuse professionals.

Since some states have regulations guiding the development and management of a drug-free workplace, it is important to research state regulations that are specific to the location of the business. State agencies may also provide support and resources that may prove helpful for the development of the drug-free workplace program.

The facility used for specimen collection should be a National Institute on Drug Abuse–approved (NIDA-approved) collection site for urine drug screenings and an approved collection site for any state-specific drug-free workplace programs. Both drug specimen collectors and breath alcohol technicians must be certified. Because there are legal implications related to the integrity of specimens and the collection process, the collector must be competent in the collection method, as well as understand the importance of the "chain of custody." The chain of custody accounts for the collection procedures and for the integrity of the specimen by tracking the handling, storage, and transportation of the specimen from the point of collection to its final disposition (SAMHSA, 2010). The laboratory used for analysis of drug screening specimens should be certified by The National Laboratory Certification Program.

DEVELOPING A DRUG-FREE WORKPLACE POLICY

Components of a drug free workplace policy are outlined in Table 9.1.

Because of the sensitive nature of substance testing and the associated regulatory statutes, ACOEM (2009) recommends that a company's drug-free workplace policy be reviewed by "a legal consultant, such as a labor/employment attorney, prior to distribution and implementation." This may provide protection for the company in the event the procedure is challenged from a liability or civil rights perspective. It also serves to ensure employee rights are protected and that the policy and procedure is written in a way that assures compliance with all applicable laws and regulations.

The U.S. Department of Labor provides an on-line Drug-Free Workplace Adviser. This valuable resource will assist in the development of a drug-free workplace policy by walking the user through a series of questions. The Drug-Free Workplace Adviser can be accessed at http://www.dol.gov/elaws/asp/drugfree/drugs/screen2.asp.

Table 9.1 Components of a drug-free workplace policy

1. What is the purpose/goal of the policy?
2. Who will be covered by the policy?
3. When will the policy apply?
4. What behavior will be prohibited?
5. Will workers be required to notify the employer of drug-related convictions?
6. Will the policy include searches?
7. Will the program include drug testing?
8. What will the consequences be if the policy is violated?
9. Will there be Return-to-Work Agreements?
10. What type of assistance will be available?
11. How will worker confidentiality be protected?
12. Who will be responsible for enforcing the policy?
13. How will the policy be communicated to workers?

The DOL strongly recommends that the policy be reviewed by a legal consultant, such as a labor/employment attorney, prior to distribution and implementation.

Consequences of violations of the drug-free workplace policy must be clearly defined. The company may choose to have a zero-tolerance policy. This means that any candidate for employment who tests positive for tested substances will not be hired and that any current worker who tests positive for tested substances will have their employment terminated. An alternative is to allow current workers a chance to enter a substance rehabilitation program. In this case, workers who test positive for tested substances must be removed from safety-sensitive work or placed on leave of absence. The worker is then subject to random, unannounced follow-up testing at the discretion of the employer. If subsequent testing is positive, most likely employment would be terminated.

A sample drug-free workplace policy can be found in Appendix 19.

WORKER EDUCATION AND AWARENESS

Having a plan for introducing and explaining the drug-free workplace program to employees is vital. The educational program serves to inform workers about substance abuse issues, the effect on the workplace, and resources that are available. Support for the program, not only from management but from all workers, is important to the program's overall success. In order to maintain documentation of awareness and training efforts, the employer should maintain signed acknowledgement that all new hires, workers, supervisors, and managers have received a copy of the company's drug-free workplace policy.

Components of worker education and training regarding the drug-free workplace policy include:

1. The purpose and rules of the drug-free workplace program
2. What resources are available: substance abuse professional, employee assistance program, etc.
3. When the policy will take effect
4. Details regarding the reasons for testing, procedures, and other elements of drug testing
5. What workers are subject to testing and under what circumstances
6. How will worker confidentiality be protected
7. Who will be responsible for enforcing of the policy
8. How will the policy be communicated to workers and candidates for employment

The educational program should target aspects of the drug-free workplace program for all workers. The introduction of a drug-free workplace program should be conducted in an open forum where workers have the opportunity to interact and ask questions. If the company uses the services of an employee assistance program or substance abuse professional, it may prove valuable to include them in the education process for workers. The company's medical director could also serve as a valuable resource for education for both workers and management. Education and awareness for the drug-free workplace program should be supported in an ongoing fashion through the use of posters and printed material. Entry doors to the company facilities should have notice that this is a drug-free workplace. Posters can also be placed in break rooms, in waiting areas, at time clocks, and in the occupational health clinic.

TYPES OF TESTING

The testing program must establish a procedure and protocol for testing, define the types of testing, and specifically outline the drugs that will be included in the testing.

Protocol for Testing

The employer can choose one or more of the following testing options:

- **Postoffer, preplacement testing**. All final job candidates to whom employment has been offered will be tested. This testing is conducted after a conditional offer of employment has been made, although candidates may begin work pending the results of the drug test. Postoffer testing is intended to prevent hiring of individuals with drug or alcohol problems. Preplacement testing is intended for current workers who apply for a different job within the same company. The candidate to whom job transfer is offered is subject to testing as a condition for transfer. The employer has the right to limit testing of applicants and job transfers to only certain positions based on specific job categories and essential functions. A most important consideration is that all workers in those specific job categories are equally subject to testing.
- **Post incident, injury testing**. When workers are involved in workplace incidents or accidents (especially workers in safety-sensitive positions) or when property damage occurs as a result of the incident, the involved workers will be subject to testing. The worker need not be injured as a result of the incident. The main purpose of testing post incident is to identify if drug or alcohol use was a contributing underlying cause of the incident. Additionally, workers who incur injuries on the job will also be tested. Some state workers' compensations regulations allow for denial of benefits if the accident or injury is proven to be a result of worker substance impairment or intoxication.
- **Random testing**. The employer has the right to conduct unannounced testing on a periodic basis. This type of testing is intended to identify workers who are under the influence of drugs and/or alcohol while on the job. This method sometimes proves to be a significant deterrent and may provide an opportunity for early intervention with current workers. Random testing is specifically indicated for workers in safety-sensitive positions or for those subject to random testing based on regulatory requirements. Workers are usually chosen through a random selection process conducted either by the employer or by the medical review office. Workers who receive notice of being selected for random testing must report for testing immediately.
- **Reasonable suspicion/for-cause testing**. This type of testing is used when the employer has suspicion that the worker is under the influence of drugs or

alcohol while working. It is most often triggered by an observed performance issue or a demonstration of unsafe work practices by the worker. This includes signs such as falling asleep on the job, incoherence, inability to comprehend or follow instructions, direct observation of the worker using drugs and/or alcohol while on work time or on company property, suspicions related to being "under the influence," or other suspicious behavior or communication. It is important that these behaviors and the effect on job performance or the workplace are properly documented by management. Additional triggers for reasonable suspicion testing include a report of worker's drug use by a reliable, credible source; evidence that the worker has tampered with a drug test; or evidence that a worker has possessed, sold, or solicited drugs while working or while on company property.

- **Return to work/follow-up testing**. When a worker tests positive for drugs or alcohol and participates in a rehabilitation program, the employer has the right to conduct unannounced periodic testing after the worker returns to work. If the employee voluntarily enters the program, the employer has the option to not require follow-up testing.
- **Routine fitness-for-duty testing**. Routine annual or periodic physical fitness-for-duty examinations may include substance testing.

SUBSTANCE TESTING—WHAT CAN BE TESTED?

When establishing a drug-free workplace, the employer must decide what process will be used for drug testing. Consideration must be given to the need for compliance with any regulatory mandated testing that outlines the specific mode of testing required. Otherwise, the employer can choose one or more of the following modes of testing. Importantly, the mode(s) of substance testing must be applied consistently according to the employer's drug-free workplace policy.

Urine

Urine specimen analysis is the most common method for substance testing. With urine testing, a urine sample is obtained and sent to a certified laboratory for analysis. Negative results are normally available within 24 hours. Nonnegative tests require the laboratory to run a secondary confirmation test. If the confirmation test results are positive, it requires review by a medical review officer and mandates retention of the sample for the availability of retesting at the donor's request. In this case, the *same* specimen can be sent to a different laboratory for repeat testing. Most employers require that the donor pay for the cost of repeat testing.

There are also instant urine test kits on the market. The procedures for these tests allow for immediate testing of a urine sample. These tests are considered quite accurate and provide an efficient means for the employer to obtain negative results at the time of testing. If the result is nonnegative, the urine sample must be sent to the laboratory for traditional testing, confirmation, and MRO review, if applicable.

Urine drug testing is sometimes criticized because of the opportunity for the donor of the specimen to adulterate the specimen either by dilution or the addition of substances to the urine sample. These challenges can be overcome by selecting a credible collection site that uses drug screen certified collectors. These sites are often audited by regulatory agencies, such as the Department of Transportation and the Federal Aviation Administration, to ensure compliance related to collection techniques, the use of certified laboratories, and document retention.

Dilution can occur by the donor adding liquid to the specimen or by the donor drinking large amounts of water to overhydrate themselves, which in turn dilutes the specimen. Common substances used to adulterate the urine sample include soap, bleach, acidic substances, or the use of commercial products intended specifically for this purpose. In addition, the opportunity exists for the donor to substitute urine from another individual. Specific collection techniques and procedures are recommended to overcome these attempts to cheat the system, and a quality-oriented substance testing facility will assure adherence to these standards. To assure quality results, certified laboratories are now employing technologies that are more precise in measuring specific gravity, pH, and creatinine levels in the urine specimen, and are able to determine "positive" or "negative" results in an extremely accurate and efficient manner. For postoffer testing, instant tests can give immediate results, which serves to expedite the hiring process.

Urine testing is the most common type of testing and meets requirements for all regulated drug testing (except for instant testing). A significant advantage of urine testing is that the employer can choose to screen for a variety of drugs through the use of specific drug panels. Various panels or lists of drugs can be included in the test at the discretion of the employer. The basic drug panel is a five-panel drug screen that tests for marijuana, cocaine, amphetamines, opiates, and phencyclidine (PCP). Additional panels also include barbiturates, benzodiazepines, synthetic opiods, methaqualone, propoxyphene, and others.

One disadvantage of urine testing is that collection errors can occur as a result of poor collection techniques. In addition, urine testing offers the greatest opportunity for adulteration or substitution of the specimen. Of particular note, specific substances have expected life spans in the urine and thus create an opportunity for the donor to abstain prior to testing. Most employers require that a worker or job candidate submit the urine sample within a specific time frame in order to capture that period or time when testing would be optimum. Examples of drug life spans in urine are as follows:

- Marijuana: 2–5 days (in a heavy user, 14–30 days)
- Cocaine: 1–2 days
- Amphetamines: 1–2 days
- Opiates: 1–3 days
- PCP: 1–8 days

Hair

A hair drug test is designed to detect drug use over a period of months. The rationale for using hair samples for drug testing is to "ensure that a drug user cannot evade the test by simply abstaining for a few days" (Psychemedics, 2011). Additional advantages to hair testing are that it does not require the collection of body fluids, which is sometimes considered intrusive, and it virtually eliminates the possibility for substitution and adulteration of the specimen. It is estimated that hair testing can detect as many as 5 to 10 times more drug users than urine testing (Psychemedics, 2011); however controversy exists as to the inability to determine if the drug use is current or in the past. The collection of a specimen for substance testing requires that a small sample of the donor's hair is cut from the back of the head just below the crown, packaged, and sent to a specialized laboratory for testing. The same procedure is followed for validation of positive results, requiring a medical review process. A significant advantage of hair testing is that it identifies substance use over a longer period of time than does other modes of testing. The disadvantage of using hair testing is that it only offers a five-panel test that is designed to detect the following drugs and their metabolites: cocaine, opiates, phencyclidine (PCP), amphetamines, and marijuana. Controversies exist over hair testing because it remains unclear how drugs enter hair and there is uncertainty in regard to limitations regarding dose (how much of the drug) and time (when it was used) relationships between drug use and testing (Cone, 1997). Collection challenges also exist when donors do not have enough hair to provide an adequate sample or when donors wear wigs and hairpieces. An additional disadvantage is that hair testing is often not recognized as an acceptable means of testing under federal or state regulations.

Saliva

Saliva tests are convenient for preemployment drug testing and allows for immediate results. A basic panel identifies the presence of the five substances (marijuana, cocaine, amphetamines, opiates, and phencyclidine); however, a seven-panel is available that includes barbiturates and benzodiazepines.

Saliva testing is cost effective and efficient, providing results within minutes. This allows fast interpretation and decision making. It is a nonintrusive collection method of drug testing, can be conducted virtually anywhere, and can also be conducted under direct observation. Adulteration of a saliva sample is nearly impossible. A disadvantage is that most drugs do not remain present in saliva more than 12–24 hours from use of the drug; therefore, a short window of opportunity exists for drug detection. The reliability of saliva drug testing is also limited because of the possibility of contamination of saliva from other substances, including some over-the-counter medications. Drugs smoked or used through intranasal routes of inhalation may also go undetected (Cone, 1997).

Sweat

Research on sweat testing for drugs has been limited mostly because of the difficulty in collecting sweat samples. The sample is collected by applying a patch to the donor's skin. Over a period of several days, sweat should saturate the pad, and the drug should slowly concentrate. The patch is then removed, and the absorbent pad is detached from the device and analyzed for drug content. Although this also provides a nonintrusive process for substance testing, variations of sweat production in individuals contribute to its unreliability. Collection of a sweat sample may prove challenging in colder climates or in less humid environments. Disadvantages of the sweat patch include this high inter-subject variability, the possibility of environmental contamination of the patch before application or after removal, and risk of accidental removal during a monitoring period (Cone, 1997).

SUBSTANCES COMMONLY TESTED

Employers have the right to choose the number of drugs tested, unless this is mandated under certain federal regulations. This decision is based on the type of risk related to certain jobs or may be decided based on workers' access to controlled substances as part of the job duties. For example, healthcare workers have higher rates of abuse with benzodiazepines and opiates, most prevalent in the specialties of anesthesia, emergency medicine, and psychiatry (Baldisseri, 2007). Abuse of certain drugs may also be specific to regions of the country, such as the abuse of methamphetamines. A list of commonly abused drugs can be found in Table 9.2.

A basic drug screen includes a standard 5-panel test of common drugs consisting of marijuana, cocaine, amphetamines (including methamphetamine), opiates (codeine and morphine), and PCP. Additional options include 8-panel, 9-panel, or 10-panel tests, which also test for controlled drugs (barbiturates, benzodiazepines, methadone, propoxyphene, methaqualone) that are legal to possess and use, but have high abuse potential. Tests for alcohol and nicotine may also be included.

A basic drug-free workplace is well supported by the use of a five-panel drug test. The trend for use of higher panel tests typically involves testing workers involved in safety-sensitive job functions, such as driving, climbing, use of hazardous materials, power tools/equipment, etc. Larger "professional" or "medical" panels are sometimes employed by healthcare organizations whose workers have access to highly controlled substances on a regular basis. These panels are sometimes employed as part of a fitness-for-duty evaluation regarding suspected impairment or to evaluate suspected theft of pharmaceutical drugs from the premises.

Tests for alcohol are often used, specifically when required by federal regulatory mandates. Alcohol can be tested through the breath or by blood analysis. Impairment related to alcohol use was originally defined by blood

Table 9.2 Commonly abused drugs.

Cannaboids

- Hashish
- Marijuana

Opioids

- Heroin
- Opium

Hallucinogens

- LSD

Depressants

- Barbiturates
- Benzodiazepines

Opioids

- Codeine
- Fentanyl
- Morphine
- Opium
- Hydromorphone, oxycodone, propoxyphene, meperidine

Stimulants

- Amphetamines
- Methamphetamine
- Cocaine

Others

- Anabolic steroids
- Nicotine
- Alcohol
- Inhalants

From: The National Institute of Drug Abuse
For a more comprehensive list, visit http://www.nida.nih.
gov/DrugPages/DrugsofAbuse.html

alcohol levels; however, breath alcohol analysis has now evolved to a process that is low cost, highly accurate, and efficient. The process is simple and non-intrusive; a sample is collected by having breath blown into the breath alcohol machine. The machine calculates an immediate result. Drug testing done in accordance with federal regulations requires that breath testing be done with analyzers approved by the National Highway Traffic Safety Administration. Alcohol testing can also be achieved through the analysis of saliva. The degree to which the central nervous system function is impaired is directly proportional to the concentration of alcohol in the blood (NIDA, 2010). The body uses several different metabolic pathways for the oxidation of alcohol, including the liver; however, two significant pathways for elimination of alcohol from the body are through the breath and through saliva. Some federal regulations mandate that the safety sensitive job functions of a worker are prohibited under the following circumstances: if breath alcohol results are 0.04 or more, while using alcohol, within 4 hours of alcohol use, or when refusing to be tested (Salazar, 2001).

Workplaces focused on health and wellness strategies have also started to test for nicotine as part of the substance awareness program and as part of a wellness strategy to control healthcare costs. Nicotine testing is typically done by blood analysis.

HOW A DRUG TEST IS CONDUCTED
Although substance testing can take place through various modes of specimen collection, only the collection process for urine drug screening will be discussed in this section. Although the testing procedures will vary, the process for maintaining specimen integrity, chain of custody, and the medical review process are the same. Refer to the test kit instructions for procedures for other modes of testing.

Urine Collection Process
For urine drug screen collection, the restroom facility must be in compliance with certain regulatory requirements. Specific rules are published in the current version of the *Federal Register* (DOT, 2010), which often changes; therefore, the reader is encouraged to check the updated version of the rules when implementing testing procedures.

Soaps and other possible adulterants must be removed from the restroom. The water to the restroom can also be controlled from a location outside the restroom, thus preventing the donor from running water inside the restroom while providing the specimen. The toilet water is tinted blue, so if it is used in an attempt to dilute a specimen, it will discolor the specimen. The restroom should be free of cabinetry, trashcans, towel holders, removable ceiling tiles, or other containers that could pose an opportunity to hide paraphernalia or adulterants. There should be a specific location for processing the specimen with enough space for both the collector and donor.

- The donor must provide photo identification when the process begins, and the collector must assure the photo identification matches the donor. This starts the chain of custody.
- A Custody and Control Form (CCF) is initiated that includes information regarding the employer, the collector, the medical review officer, and the donor.
- The donor is asked to remove coats, purses, hats, bags, or other objects that may be used to conceal an adulterant. They must remove all items from pockets, except for money or wallets, and these items should be placed in a lock box for security purposes.
- The donor is instructed to choose a lab-certified drug collection kit from a group of kits appropriate for the specific test being conducted. This kit is

packaged in a sealed wrapper that protects its integrity before use. The collector then opens the kit in the presence of the donor.

- The donor is instructed to wash his or her entire hands with soap and water and then dry them or to sanitize both hands using a hand sanitizer, completely covering the hands to the wrists.
- The donor is instructed to enter the restroom to provide a specimen and instructed not to flush the toilet.
- Once the specimen is provided to the collector, the collector makes note of an unusual color or odor of the specimen, checks the temperature of the specimen noted by a temperature strip that is imbedded in the specimen cup, and notes these on the CCF. The specimen must meet certain temperature requirements to be considered a valid specimen.
- The specimen must remain in the presence of the collector and donor until it is completely sealed. The specimen is poured into the appropriate containers and sealed in the presence of the donor. Both the collector and the donor initial the seal.
- The collector completes the CCF and both the collector and the donor sign the CCF. There are five carbon pages of the CCF, individual copies for the donor, the collection facility, the employer, the laboratory, and the MRO.
- The collector then inspects the restroom and the toilet for anything unusual that may have been done to tamper with or adulterate the specimen.
- Urine drug screen specimens are typically shipped to the laboratory. The specimens are picked up by a designated courier and sent to the laboratory via overnight express. The courier must also sign a log indicating that the specimen was taken from the collection facility, thus maintaining documentation of the chain of custody of the specimen.

For quality control and auditing purposes, a Urine Drug Screen Collection Checklist is provided in Appendix 20.

SUMMARY

Advances in the technology of substance testing continues to evolve providing the employer with cost-effective and efficient means of testing. Studies continue to demonstrate the harmful effects of substance use and abuse in the workplace. Specifically, studies continue to support that workers who engage in harmful, substance-using behaviors may be more likely to take risks at work (Ramchand, Pomeroy, & Arkes, 2009).

The burden of proof is on the individual who is tested for drugs, to prove or disprove the findings of a substance test. One must remember that all drug use is not illegal. Beware of the prevalence of legal prescription drugs at work. Many controlled substances that are legally prescribed lead to dependence and tolerance, producing a risk of overuse and a false veil of safety. Prescription drug abuse is the intentional use of a medication without a prescription, in a way other than as prescribed, or for the experience or feeling it causes (NIDA,

2010). Factors contributing to abuse of prescription drugs include misperceptions about their safety—thinking that if they are prescribed by a healthcare provider, they must be safe.

Popular abused drugs include central nervous system depressants, stimulants, and narcotics, such as hydrocodone and oxycodone, that carry a high "street value" and that are sold and obtained illegally. These drugs can present great risk. The use of herbal supplements, teas, medicinal bath salts, and other "natural" drugs can also have an effect on workers and the workplace. A new chemical product on the market is a synthetic marijuana, known as K2, Spice, Blaze, or Red Dawn, which people have been using recreationally for the past few years to imitate the feeling they would get from smoking marijuana. It is reported to produce a mellow "high" similar to smoking marijuana. However, there are also reports of frequent adverse side effects: disorientation, anxiety, convulsions, increased heart rate and blood pressure, vomiting, and other unpleasant symptoms. These products are relatively new, and the scientific community has not yet performed much human testing on their effects. Currently, these products do *not* show up in the standard test panels used for workplace drug testing.

A formal industry now exists to advise donors and provide devices and techniques that assist individuals in cheating on a drug test, resulting in invalid tests or hindering positive results. An employer must be astute to the fact that a negative drug test report does not mean the individual is not taking drugs. It only means they have a valid, legal prescription for the drug, or that the drug was not detected due to the donor's success in influencing the results.

Important considerations that must be addressed in the design and implementation of a drug screening program include biological factors concerning rates of absorption and elimination of drugs, technical factors relating to specificity and accuracy of testing, legal ramifications, regulatory requirements, and employee relations concerns. Employers that include an aspect of due diligence in planning and managing a drug-free workplace are likely to have carefully designed and managed programs for the screening of workers and applicants for drugs and alcohol. These programs then serve to protect and improve the health and safety of workers in an ethical manner (ACOEM, 2009).

REFERENCES

American College of Occupational and Environmental Medicine (ACOEM). (2009). *Position statement: Ethical aspects of drug testing*. Retrieved from http://www.ACOEM.org

Baldisseri, M. R. (2007). Impaired healthcare professional. *Critical Care Medicine* 35(2), S106–116.

Balge, M. A. & Krieger, G. R. (2000). Occupational health and safety (3rd ed., pp. 409–430). Chicago: National Safety Council.

Cone, E. J. (1997). *New developments in biological measures of drug prevalence.* Retrieved from http://archives.drugabuse.gov/pdf/monographs/monograph167/108-129_Cone.pdf

Golden-McAndrew, K. (2005). Pagliaros' comprehensive guide to drugs and substances of abuse. *AAOHN Journal, 53*(2).

Kuntz, D. J. (2008*). Laboratory perspective on additional drug testing and associated costs.* Retrieved from http://nac.samhsa.gov/DTAB/Presentations/Aug08/DavidKuntzDTAB0808.pdf

Lipton, B., Laws, C., & Li, L. (2009). *Narcotics in workers compensation.* National Council on Compensation Insurance Research Brief. Retrieved from https://www.ncci.com/documents/Narcotics_in_WC_1209.pdf

Substance Abuse and Mental Health Services Administration (SAMSHA), Office of Applied Studies (OAS), Department of Health and Human Services (DHHS). (2008). *Misuse of Prescription Drugs.* Retrieved from http://www.oas.samhsa.gov/prescription/TOC.htm

National Council on Compensation Insurance. (2009). Retrieved from https://www.ncci.com/nccimain/DataReporting/Reports/

National Drug-Free Workplace Assistance. (2005). *Drug-free workplace statistics.* Retrieved from http://www.drugfreeworkplace.gov/

National Institute on Drug Abuse (NIDA). The science of drug abuse and addiction. Retrieved from http://www.NIDA.com

National Institute on Drug Abuse (NIDA). (2010). *A research update from the National Institute on Drug Abuse.* Retrieved from http://www.nida.nih.gov/tib/prescription.html

National Institute on Drug Abuse (NIDA). (2011). *Research report: Prescription drugs: Abuse and addiction.* Retrieved from http://www.nida.nih.gov/ResearchReports/Prescription/prescription.html

OHS Health & Safety Services, Inc. (2004). *What every employer should know about drug-abuse in the workplace!* Retrieved from http://www.ohsinc.com

Psychemedics Corporation. (2011). *Advantages over urinalysis.* Retrieved from http://www.psychemedics.com

Ramchand, R., Pomeroy, A., & Arkes, J. (2009). *The effects of substance use on workplace injuries.* (Santa Monica, CA: Center for Health and Safety in the Workplace, The RAND Corporation).

Salazar, M. (2001). *Core curriculum for occupational and environmental health nursing* (2nd ed.). Philadelphia: W.B. Saunders.

Substance Abuse and Mental Health Services Administration (SAMSHA), Office of Applied Studies (OAS), Department of Health and Human Services (DHHS). (2006). *Substance abuse and mental health statistics.* Retrieved from http://www.samhsa.gov.

Substance Abuse and Mental Health Services Administration (SAMSHA). Office of Applied Studies, Department of Health and Human Services (DHHS). (2008). Results from the 2007 national survey on drug use and health: National findings. NSDUH Series H-34, DHHS Publication No. SMA 08-4343. (Rockville, MD: SAMSHA Office of Applied Studies).

Substance Abuse and Mental Health Services Administration (SAMHSA), Center for Substance Abuse Prevention, Department of Health and Human

Services (DHHS). (2010). *Urine specimen collection handbook for federal agency workplace drug testing programs.* Retrieved from http://www.workplace.samhsa.gov/DrugTesting/pdf/specimen_collection_handbook_2010_100908.pdf

Substance Abuse and Mental Health Services Administration (SAMHSA), Center for Substance Abuse Prevention, Department of Health and Human Services (DHHS). (N.D.). *Coping with work and family stress.* Retrieved from http://www.modelprograms.samhsa.gov/pdfs/model/Coping.pdf/

Substance Abuse and Mental Health Services Administration (SAMHSA), Center for Substance Abuse Prevention, Department of Health and Human Services (DHHS). (N.D.). *Team awareness.* Retrieved from http://www.modelprograms.samhsa.gov/pdfs/model/TeamAwareness.pdf/.

Substance Abuse and Mental Health Services Administration (SAMHSA), Center for Substance Abuse Prevention, Department of Health and Human Services (DHHS). (N.D.). *The healthy workplace.* Retrieved from http://www.modelprograms.samhsa.gov/pdfs/model/Healthy.pdf/

Substance Abuse and Mental Health Services Administration (SAMHSA), Center for Substance Abuse Prevention, Department of Health and Human Services (DHHS). (N.D.). *Wellness outreach program.* Retrieved from http://www.modelprograms.samhsa.gov/pdfs/model/Wellness.pdf/

U. S. Department of Defense, Office of the Under Secretary, Defense Procurement and Acquisition Policy. (2005). *Defense Federal Acquisition Regulation Supplement. Subpart 223.5: Drug-free workplace.* Retrieved from http://www.acq.osd.mil/dpap/dars/dfars/html/r20070212/223_5.htm/

U. S. Department of Health and Human Services (DHHS), Substance Abuse and Mental Health Services Administration (SAMSHA). http://www.workplace.samhsa.gov/

U. S. Department of Labor. *Working partners for an alcohol and drug free workplace.* Retrieved from http://www.dol.gov/workingpartners/welcome.html

U. S. Department of Labor (DOL). elaws—Drug-Free Workplace Adviser. *Drug-free workplace policy builder. Developing a policy statement.* Retrieved from http://www.dol.gov/elaws/asp/drugfree/drugs/screen2.asp

U. S. Department of Transportation (DOT), Office of Drug and Alcohol Policy and Compliance. (1988). *Drug Free Workplace Act.* See U.S.C. 701–707, 105–584. Retrieved from http://www.dot.gov/ost/dapc/NEW_DOCS/part40.html?proc/

U. S. Department of Transportation (DOT), Office of Drug and Alcohol Policy and Compliance. (2007). *Procedures for transportation workplace drug and alcohol testing programs.* Retrieved from http://www.dot.gov/ost/dapc/NEW_DOCS/part40.html?proc/

U. S. Department of Transportation (DOT), Office of Drug and Alcohol Policy and Compliance. (2011). *Best practices for DOT random drug and alcohol testing.* Retrieved from http://www.dot.gov/ost/dapc/testingpubs/final_random_brochure.pdf

RESOURCES
U.S. Department of Transportation
Drug and Alcohol Policy and Compliance Office.
Title 49: Transportation. Part 40—*Procedures for Transportation Workplace Drug and Alcohol Testing Programs*
Washington, DC 20590
http://www.dot.gov/odapc/NEW_DOCS/part40.html

WEB RESOURCES
Institute for s Drug Free Workplace
http://www.drugfreeworkplace.org
National Drug-Free Workplace Alliance
http://www.ndwa.org
National Institute on Drug Abuse
http://www.nida.nih.gov
Office of National Drug Control Policy
http://www.whitehousedrugpolicy.gov/prevent/workplace/index.html
Substance Abuse and Mental Health Services Administration
http://www.workplace.samhsa.gov

Workplace Injury Management

10

There is a significant inverse relationship between workers' compensation costs and business success. High injury rates and higher insurance costs can lead to lower profits. The occupational health nurse plays a key role in developing a strategic approach to managing workers' compensation costs, thus contributing to the profitability of the company.

(Guzik)

"I've fallen and I can't get up! Now what do I do?" This should never be a question in the minds of workers or their supervisors. A well-executed safety program should address the procedures and interventions related to work incidents and injuries. Through defined policies and procedures, coupled with education of management and workers, the employer can reduce risk and liability while maintaining a safe and productive workforce.

Workers' compensation laws were enacted in the early 1900s to cover the cost of medical care and benefits for workers who become injured or ill on the job. As a result, there are workers' compensation statutes, regulated by each state, providing rules and guidance for employers to provide certain benefits to workers when they are injured or become ill as a result of their jobs. These benefits cover the cost of medical expenses, death benefits, rehabilitation expenses, and time away from work related to the job injury. The workers' compensation statutes vary from state to state, and it is important for the employer and the occupational health nurse (OHN) to maintain keen knowledge of these regulations. Employers with workers in multiple states must abide by the regulations specific to each state in which workers are employed. These state regulations define specific criteria that constitute the workers' rights to the worker's compensation benefit and also define the parameters of payment through mandated fee schedules for healthcare providers who render services for the injured worker.

Failure to carry workers' compensation insurance or otherwise meet a state's regulatory requirements may expose the employer to not only paying for these

Essentials for Occupational Health Nursing, First Edition. Arlene Guzik.
© 2013 John Wiley & Sons, Inc. Published 2013 by John Wiley & Sons, Inc.

benefits out of pocket, but also to paying penalties levied by the state. Most state workers' compensation regulations require the employer to provide benefits as long as the incident arises out of the worker's employment and the injury occurs during the course and scope of performing job duties. Unlike other types of insurance coverage, such as health benefits or automobile coverage that have deductibles and dollar limits, workers' compensation insurance does not require the worker to share any cost and does not have a maximum dollar amount limit. Once a claim is filed, the employer is obligated to cover unlimited expenses as long as the costs fall under the purview of the state's requirement for covered benefits. Income replacement as payment for lost work time under workers' compensation is usually calculated as a percentage of the average weekly wage and is not subject to federal income tax for the employer or worker.

A fault of many employers is viewing this benefit as only a regulatory requirement or as a "necessary evil" and therefore leaving the management of the claims to those they pay to provide this service. On the other hand, the selection of partnerships with consultants, insurers' claims administrators, healthcare providers, and legal counsel is critical to a successfully executed program. Employers who take an interest in not only preventing injuries, but also in actively participating in the worker's recovery and return to work find, in most cases, a high degree of both worker and employer satisfaction. The strategy for success, however, starts way before the injury occurs. This chapter outlines the key components to managing workers' compensation benefits.

WORKERS' COMPENSATION INSURANCE
Most employers are required to provide workers' compensation benefit coverage for their workers. Employers exempt from this requirement include sole proprietors and partnerships (unless they have workers who are not owners) and employers whose workers are paid solely by commission. Some state laws also exempt certain categories of workers from coverage, such as domestic workers, agricultural workers, and manual laborers. The burden is on employers to know who is covered under the definition of "employee" in their specific state's workers' compensation regulations. And it is important to note that employers should be aware of how the state views coverage for independent contractors and leased workers. Employers must also maintain an awareness of coverage provided for workers when they establish business relationships with employee leasing agencies, contractors, and subcontractors. The terms of the agreement with these types of workers should define the obligations of coverage for workers' compensation benefits that is consistent with state regulations, and an astute employer will not only define the obligation in the contract, but will also require proof of up-to-date coverage by providing a copy of the coverage certificate that will be kept on file with the contract.

Types of Insurance Coverage

There are currently three systems in place for states to design their worker's compensations programs. Monopolistic states have special legislation that requires workers compensation coverage be provided exclusively through the state's workers compensation funded program. Insurance through private insurance companies is not permitted, and the workers' compensation system is administered by the state. This includes the processes of monitoring data and trends, setting insurance rates, and sometimes settling disputes. The second system is where states have their own independent bureau of workers' compensation rules and regulations that govern insurance classifications, premium computation, and experience ratings, thus allowing employers to choose between private insurance companies or a state-administered workers compensation fund.

Most states, however, manage their workers' compensation insurance programs based on data from the National Council on Compensation Insurance, Inc. (NCCI). NCCI is a national agency that manages the largest database of workers' compensation insurance information by analyzing industry trends. The agency also prepares workers compensation insurance rate recommendations, calculates proposed insurance rates, develops experience and retrospective ratings plans, analyzes the potential cost of changes in legislation, and provides a variety of services and tools to maintain an effective Workers Compensation system (NCCI, 2011).

Employers in non-monopolistic states have the choice of purchasing workers' compensation insurance in a variety of ways. The insurance may be purchased through commercial insurance carriers, through a state purchasing fund, or the employer may choose to set up a self-insured fund. There are certain benefits, risks, and considerations to each option.

Traditional Commercial Plan

Employers choosing to insure through a commercial insurance product have a variety of insurance carriers from which to choose. This sets the stage for a competitive market in that the insurance companies each vie for the opportunity to provide the employer coverage. In this case, the insurance product or coverage is consistent across insurers but is dependent on the type of policy selected. Under a fully insured commercial plan, the insurance company is responsible for the costs of all claims that arise under the employer's workers' compensation benefit in the states covered by the policy.

Guaranteed Plan

Under a guaranteed plan, the employer's premium rate remains consistent and predictable and is calculated based on the standard classification code (SIC) of the business, taking into consideration payroll data and an experience modification factor (mod factor). The employer has no control over the SIC classification

193

Table 10.1 Effect of workers' compensation costs on company profitability.

	COMPANY A	COMPANY B
Company's Annual Revenue		$10,000,000
Company's Expected Percent of Profit from Revenue (revenue minus expenses)		10% ($1,000,000)
Manual premium cost*	$200,000	$200,000
Multiplier: Mod Factor	× 0.5	× 1.5
Actual premium cost (% of annual revenue)	= $100,000 (1.0%)	= $300,000 (3.0%)
Variance	− $100,000 Savings for employer	+ $100,000 Additional cost to employer
	Adds $100,000 to bottom line	Loss of $100,000 from bottom line

*Considers the classification code for each type of business and an expected loss representing the cost of workers compensation insurance.

since the assignment is based on the nature and risk of the business operations. Payroll data is based on the average number of workers and the average wage of all workers covered under the plan. The mod factor is an equation based on actual claims versus expected claims for the employer's industry. The published NCCI data is typically used to establish the expected claims experience for the employer's particular industry. In calculating the mod factor, the expected claims experience (or average) is factored at 1.0. If the company has more claims than the expected industry standard, the calculated mod factor will be greater than 1.0, or greater than average. If the employer has incurred a lower number of claims than expected, the mod factor will be less than 1.0, or less than average. Therefore, an employer with less experience (i.e., fewer injuries or less severe injuries) will be rated at a lower premium cost. Conversely, an employer with high rates and/or high severity of injuries will be rated with a much higher premium cost.

Table 10.1 provides a comparison example of how workers' compensation costs can have a direct effect on profitability of the company, comparing two companies of similar service with very different insurance mod factors. As you can see, there is tremendous incentive to the employer to maintain a safe workplace in order to control workers' compensation benefit experience. Some insurance carriers also offer incentives designed to return a portion of the premium to employers that have controlled their losses during the policy period.

Under a guaranteed plan, the employer also has the right to choose a deductible. A small deductible plan includes the option to self-pay the first portion of cost (usually $100–$1,000) for each individual claim up to a predefined amount after which the additional claims costs are paid by the insurer. These deductibles, however, can cause a wide variation in the out-of-pocket expenses by the employer and are based on the number of claims incurred, thus are unpredictable. Employers may also choose to have a large deductible plan that requires the employer to pay out-of-pocket costs for the total aggregate of all claims up to a predefined amount. These amounts are usually upward of payment for the first $100,000 or more of all claims cost, after which the insurer assumes responsibility for the costs. Under this type of plan, the employer assumes responsibility for the initial payment of claims, as for a self-insured plan, yet gambles on the fact that the total claims cost will not exceed the deductible amount. The advantage to the employer is that out-of-pocket expenses are capped at the predefined amount, and the insurer assumes payment for costs thereafter. This is particularly effective in the event of a catastrophic claim or group of claims where costs may escalate beyond the employer's ability to assume payment out of the business' operating budget.

Retrospective Rating
Employers who focus on controlling claims costs may find retrospective rating to their advantage. This type of rating takes a look back, usually over a prior 3-year period, at the volume and cost of claims actually incurred and uses this value as a basis for establishing premium cost. Since the employer has some control over the mod factor, this plan provides the employer an opportunity to reduce its premium costs and reap reward by establishing and maintaining a safe workplace sustained over a longer period of time.

Assigned Risk Pool
An assigned risk pool is designed by each state for those employers who may find the purchase of an individual commercial product too expensive. Under this premium plan, the employer joins a pool of other businesses for the purposes of purchasing a more affordable plan. This approach is sometimes advantageous for small businesses, since the employer can often purchase the same policy at a more reasonable rate, just by nature of the fact that they have joined a group purchasing pool. Most times, employers in similar industries are assigned to the same purchasing pool since the premium is gauged on similar industry risk.

Self-Insurance
Employers can choose to be self-insured, rather than purchase insurance, which involves setting aside funds from their operating budget in anticipation of paying workers' compensation claims. Each state has regulations through its department of insurance with established standards for the employer to set aside financial bonds to assure financial security as a self-insured plan. Under this type of plan, instead of paying premiums to an insurance company, employers are able to use their own funds to directly pay claims costs. This strategy, when managed effectively, can reap a significant return on investment for the business.

Since funds to cover the costs incurred by claims directly impact the cash flow of the business, one must realize that a single catastrophic (high dollar) claim could result in unlimited expense for the employer. For this reason, most self-insureds choose to limit financial exposure by purchasing an "excess policy," which provides protection for the employer by shifting the costs for high dollar or catastrophic claims to an insured product. For example, the employer may choose an excess policy that covers costs for a single claim that exceeds $250,000 or more. Inherently, under a self-insured plan, employers have more choices and more control over how their money is spent.

Most times, the employer chooses to use the service of a third-party administrator (TPA) to adjudicate and manage claims, and less often, the employer handles the claims administration using employed staff through the company's internal risk management department. Under the self-insured plan, employers also may establish direct relationships with service providers in the workers' compensation industry to care for their injured workers. This type of coverage is sometimes seen as a cost-saving method for employers with a strong and effective safety philosophy and low claims experience.

The self-insured option is also available to small businesses in the form of a group purchasing pool, where like employers form groups to insure themselves. The disadvantage of this approach is that all employers share the risk of every other employer in their same group. Therefore, if one employer has increased claims experience, the effect is felt by all members of the group despite the fact that those employers may have less than average experience.

Other Factors to Consider

In deciding how a workers' compensation program is funded, the employer must realize that the insurance industry is a competitive market and should look for the most cost-effective option; however, quality cannot be overlooked.

The insurer/TPA should also offer services for the employer that are of additional value. These include safety inspections and hazard analysis, often conducted by safety specialists or engineers employed by the insurer. The insurer/TPA should also assign dedicated staff, adjusters, and case managers, who will consistently handle the employer's claims. It is of great value to have those individuals managing the claims also conduct a walk-through of the workplace in order to have a full understanding of the operations and associated jobs. The employer has the right to establish expectations for how communication flows to and from the claims administrators and to establish the frequency of meetings between the employer and representatives of the insurer/TPA. The employer must address expectations to engage with these services on a regular basis as terms of the insurance coverage.

The employer and assigned insurer/TPA representatives should also agree as to how injured workers access healthcare services to ensure quality. In some states, the employer has the right to direct the worker to a preferred healthcare provider, whereas in other states, the injured worker reserves this right and has free choice of his or her healthcare provider. It is important for the employer to understand how access to care is defined by specific state workers' compensation statutes. If the employer has the right to choose the healthcare provider, it is important that the employer and insurer/TPA agree to the preferred list of providers.

Insurers often offer discounts, rebates, and other options and the employer should explore all such options. Employers may be eligible for credits under the state's programs for such things as being a drug-free workplace. Merit ratings may also be available consisting of adjustments for good performance. Some options for discounts, however, may seem enticing to the employer, yet drive costs in an adverse fashion. For instance, the insurer/TPA may encourage the employer to use certain healthcare providers because of a "network affiliation." By using these network providers, the cost of healthcare services may be lower. The reason for this is that the insurer/TPA uses providers who agree to take a discount for the services provided. Discounts, however, do not ensure quality. Nor do they assure appropriate utilization. For example, an MRI performed by an in-network provider may cost less, but could also be of lesser quality. Healthcare providers in the network may agree to discounts for office visits; however, they will see the injured worker more often than necessary, thus increasing utilization. Insurer/TPAs often use managed care organizations (MCOs) as third parties to schedule and manage ancillary services in return for a percentage of "savings." Common services include diagnostics, rehabilitation and physical therapy services, transportation and translation services, etc. In this case, the MCO strikes an agreement with the service provider (e.g., medical clinic, diagnostic center, physical therapy provider) for a discounted rate. However, the rate billed to the claim is at a higher cost. As a result, the "middleman" (MCO) reaps the benefit of a percentage of the discount, typically between 15% and 22% (Pennachio, 2009). For example, if a provider normally charges $100 for a service, and the MCO negotiated the charge down to $60, it shows the employer a savings of $40. The MCO then takes a percentage of that $40 as its fee. The result is that the service provider is paid less. Yet, the employer does not pay the actual cost of the service, but pays a fee somewhere between the usual charge and the negotiated rate. An astute employer will scrutinize and question these practices in regard to the overall effect on the workers' compensation program.

The employer should also request a copy of any audits performed by the insurer/TPA to assure the ratings system used to determine the premium was appropriate. For example, errors in payroll computation or assignment of SIC codes may make a significant difference in premium cost. Additional strategies used by employer to assure a cost effective program include review of data through an analysis of claims conducted by the insurer/TPA. The employer should maintain astute awareness of the frequency, severity, and cost of claims, as well as legal and administrative costs associated with claims management. The engagement of employers in this regard is important in that the employer is ultimately held accountable for the information used to compute policy premiums. Issues of underreporting the number of workers covered in the plan or the number of claims can be viewed as insurance fraud.

In addition to selecting the appropriate insurance plan, several other strategies are required to ensure an effective workers' compensation program. These include the following:

- Focus on a safe workplace
- Education of workers and management on the proper procedures to use to report incidents and injuries and how to access healthcare
- Open communication with the assigned claims administrator on status of open claims, making sure the insurer/TPA maintains consistency by assigning the same adjuster to all the employer's claims
- Manage claims data, identify trends, and initiate the appropriate interventions to reduce frequency and severity of claims to assure the most appropriate outcomes

WORKPLACE INJURY AND ILLNESS CALCULATION

In order for an employer to determine how their workplace injury rate compares to average, they need to know some numbers. Knowing that workers' compensation insurance premium calculations also use these numbers, it is important to benchmark against industry standards. An annual report published by the U.S. Bureau of Labor Statistics (BLS) defines the number, types, and specifics of injuries that occurred the prior year for specific industries. This report provides a valuable benchmarking tool for employers to identify how their injury and illness rates compare to industry standards. The BLS report published for 2010 data reported that nearly 3.1 million nonfatal workplace injuries and illnesses were reported among private industry employers, resulting in an incidence rate of 3.5 cases per 100 equivalent full-time workers. This means that an employer with 100 workers can expect to have three to four workplace injuries in a given year. The BLS report also identifies that more than one-half of the 3.1 million private industry injury and illness cases reported nationally in 2010 were of a more serious nature that involved days away from work, job transfer, or restriction (commonly referred to as DART cases). These cases occurred at a rate of 1.8 cases per 100 full-time workers. Using this data, the employer can benchmark the number of cases that resulted in modified or lost work time in comparison to the industry average.

By calculating incidence rates, an employer can demonstrate the relative level of injuries and illnesses within its workplace. These rates assist in determining both problem areas and opportunities for preventing work-related injuries and illnesses. Incidence rates are meaningful for an employer when their specific injury and illness experience is compared with that of other employers doing similar work with workforces of similar size. In addition, workers' compensation premiums are calculated using similar information. The Bureau of Labor Statistics (2011) has developed the following instructions to provide a step-by-step approach for employers to evaluate their firm's injury and illness record. This calculator an also be found online at http://data.bls.gov/iirc/?data_tool=IIRC.

The incidence and injury rate (I&I rate) is computed using the following formula:

- Number of injuries and illnesses in 1 year multiplied by 200,000 (200,000 hours in the formula represents the equivalent of 100 employees working 40 hours per week, 50 weeks per year.)
- Divided by the actual number of employee hours worked that same year
- Equals the company's I&I rate for that specific year

BENEFITS FOR THE INJURED WORKER

The level and scope of benefits provided to injured workers under the workers' compensation system is guided by state regulations. Changes to these regulations require statutory reform by the state government, an, as a result, political forces and lobbying efforts of special interest groups may come into play (Balge & Krieger, 2000). The workers' compensation laws provide some protection for the employer by limiting liability regarding the employer's responsibility for benefit payment and compensation.

Although regulations are decided at the state level, most are very similar in defining parameters of coverage. Each state law provides definitions related to compensability and coverage. If the injury meets the definition of being work-related under the state regulation, medical benefits are covered in full for evaluation and treatment of the injured worker, without limits and without contribution from the injured worker in the way of copayments or deductibles. Few states allow the injured worker free choice of his or her medical provider, while most allow the employer to make the designation or require selection by the injured worker or employer from a network panel. Covered medical benefits include office visits, hospitalizations, surgical and interventional procedures, diagnostic procedures, rehabilitation services, pharmaceuticals, durable medical supplies, and other support services.

The injured worker is also entitled to wage-replacement benefits for lost work time, although some states require an eligibility waiting period before wage replacement goes into effect. The wage-replacement benefits are usually calculated as a percentage of the worker's wage; however, this income is not subject to state or federal taxation for either the worker or the employer. Depending on the worker's income level, the earnings under workers' compensation may be quite comparable to the worker's regular take-home pay after taxation.

Injured workers are also entitled to disability benefits based on the level of impairment as a result of the work injury. If the worker incurs a temporary

Table 10.2 Common workers' compensation disability classifications.

Disability Classification	Description	Example
Permanent total disability	The worker is totally incapacitated for an indefinite period of time, unable to do any work (including sedentary work) and is unlikely to return to gainful employment equal to the preinjury state	Injuries resulting in paralysis, severe brain trauma, permanent loss of sight, loss of limb with resultant loss of function.
Permanent partial disability	The worker has a permanent impairment or loss of function, is partially incapacitated, and impairment may affect future earning capacity. May be able to return to preinjury job, but if not, is able to obtain gainful employment with some physical limitations	Injuries resulting in herniated discs, partial hearing loss, fractures of bones, minor amputations, derangement of function, occupational asthma.
Temporary total disability	The worker is totally incapacitated for a temporary period of time, usually of short duration. Is unable to return to work even in a reduced labor capacity.	Recovery from injuries or illnesses during the acute phase, recovery post surgery, medical procedures, or infectious diseases.
Temporary partial disability	The worker has a temporary impairment or loss of function, is partially incapacitated, and can perform only certain aspects of his or her regular job. Is able to return to work in a limited capacity (modified duty), but is expected to return to full capacity.	Recovery from injuries or illnesses during acute and subacute phases, such as sprains and strains, and other common occupational injuries and illnesses.

permanent disability or impairment, he or she is entitled to financial compensation to replace lost income or to supplement a reduced earnings capacity. Table 10.2 lists common definitions of disability classifications. If the worker is unable to return to the same occupation after maximum recovery, he or she may also be eligible for vocational rehabilitation benefits for retraining and job placement assistance.

Since benefits under workers' compensation provide the worker with unlimited medical care and wage replacement (as long as medically necessary), the employer must be aware that it may be perceived as a better option for the worker who does not have healthcare insurance or for those who face copays and large deductibles under their group health plan. Therefore, incident investigations to assure the validity of the nature and extent of the injury are of prime importance. Chapter 7 outlines the principles of incident investigation. Once the incident that contributed to the worker's injury has been validated, a structured approach to claims management will assure the assignment of a fair and balanced benefit for all.

MANAGEMENT OF CLAIMS

The selection of key partnerships in the management of the workers' compensation program is critical to its success. As mentioned earlier, the selection of insurance consultants, brokers, and advisers sets a foundation for the program. Claims administrators, such as adjusters and case managers, are on the front lines dealing with injured workers and coordinating efforts with the healthcare provider managing the care. A synergy must exist among all individuals, considered stakeholders, who interact with the injured worker. The company's workers' compensation benefits administrator, along with the OHN, should set the tone for expectation with stakeholders. This includes department, safety, and human resources managers since interaction with the injured worker within the company can significantly influence the outcome of the claim. The employer's corporate and labor law attorneys must also share the same philosophy since often other employment-related issues may surface during the course of the claim. The employer must secure a solid legal workers' compensation defense attorney to represent the employer in adjudicating claims and defending the employer's stance regarding benefits eligibility and entitlement.

Stakeholders outside the company include any service provider who touches the injured worker during the course of the claim. These providers should share the philosophy of providing excellent service and quality care to the injured worker in a cost-efficient manner. Any opposing force in regard to this philosophy by any stakeholder can have an adverse effect on the attitude of the injured worker and on the outcome of the claim. For instance, if the healthcare provider has assigned medically appropriate restrictions and released the injured worker back to modified duty, the employer should support a return to work philosophy and provide accommodation for medically appropriate work restrictions related to the injury. This means they will keep the worker productive and on the job.

Case in Point

An injured worker is seen and treated by the company's workers' compensation healthcare provider, and the injured worker is returned to work with appropriate physical limitations (modified duty/work restrictions) related to the worker's job functions. The injured worker returns to work and provides his manager with the written work status form identifying the work restrictions. The manager proceeds to tell the worker that he would recover better if he took 2 weeks off work. The injured worker now becomes confused and loses confidence due to the conflict in expectations. In this case, the manager may be focused on the productivity of the department, considering the adverse effect of having a worker with limitations as being counterproductive to achieving production goals. Under a well-integrated workers' compensation program, managers and front-line supervisors understand the value of keeping the injured worker engaged and productive as part of the recovery process, realizing the ultimate positive effect on workers' compensation costs.

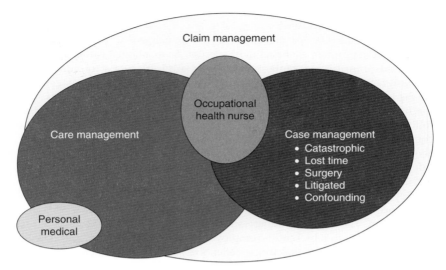

Figure 10.1 Dimensions of workers' compensation case management.

THE ROLE OF THE OHN

The OHN plays a key role in the success of the employer's workers' compensation program in a variety of capacities. Often, the clinical management of claims is a primary responsibility of the OHN. Once the insurance coverage in secured, the OHN should play a central role in identifying all stakeholders and defining roles and responsibilities. The OHN should assume responsibility for the development of company policies and procedures for incident reporting and access to healthcare for injured workers. Unlike other stakeholders in the company, the OHN holds content expertise and experience in identifying quality healthcare providers who will support the philosophy of the company's program. The OHN should also assume responsibility for monitoring the quality of care and its effect on the overall success of the program. The OHN plays a significant role in case management for the injured worker, communicating with adjusters and contracted case managers in coordinating care and bringing cases to closure.

Engagement of all stakeholders with a consistent philosophy is critical to success of the recovery of the injured workers and to the successful management of claims (Figure 10.1).

KEY PRINCIPLES IN MANAGING CLAIMS

After the injury occurs, the OHN should follow a consistent process in investigating the incident and providing the worker with appropriate healthcare intervention (as outlined in Chapter 7). Consistent management of each workers' compensation claim can be achieved by following a set of key principles.

Determining Mechanism of Injury

There must be a causal connection between injury/illness and employment in order for the medical findings to be considered work-related. The term *mechanism of injury* is used to describe the events or incident that led to the injury or illness. In other words: How did the injury or illness occur? Was there some risk incidental to or connected with employment? Did the injury/illness flow from employment as natural result? Did the injury occur within a period of time when the worker was where they were reasonably expected to be while performing essential duties related to their work? Was the worker doing what they were supposed to be doing at the time and place they were supposed to be doing it? These key questions must be considered in order to determine compensability of the claim under workers' compensation. A thorough investigation of the incident and point of contact with the workers involved in the incident will provide information regarding the mechanism of injury. Since a thorough interview and documentation of mechanism of injury can prove valuable in determining compensability of the claim, these key questions should be addressed during the interview and investigation process.

Defining the Diagnosis

It is the responsibility of the healthcare provider to interview and clearly define the subjective complaints of the worker and to conduct an objective evaluation of the clinical symptoms and complaints. A thorough, focused, and well-documented examination of the injured body parts will provide clinical information that supports medical decision making in regard to work-relatedness. The healthcare provider should obtain diagnostic tests that are appropriate to the injury or illness, that are widely accepted among practicing providers, and that are based on scientific criteria. The injured worker's subjective complaints should correlate with abnormal anatomical findings and diagnostic test results. Subjective complaints, in the absence of objective relevant medical findings, should not be considered the sole criteria for the diagnosis. The diagnosis and its relationship to the mechanism of injury set the foundation for determining compensability.

Rendering Opinion of Work-Relatedness

Some state workers' compensation statutes require the healthcare provider to render opinion in regard to major contributing cause and work-relatedness. Some states also require the healthcare provider to render opinion in regard to the influence of any preexisting, coexisting, and comorbid conditions and their relation to the findings. In other words, do the clinical findings relate to mechanism of injury and to what degree do other conditions influence the clinical findings? Determination of causation is usually straightforward; however, this requires careful analysis of mechanism of injury and clinical findings. The healthcare provider must weigh all causal or associated factors and use clearly defined terminology to describe findings as part of the medical record. The opinion of the healthcare provider is key to the determination of whether the workplace is the only cause, among other contributing causes, or one of several possible causes contributing to the injured worker's symptoms.

Healthcare professionals involved in the care of injured workers have an obligation to the worker, the employer, the workers' system, and to their professions to have an astute body of knowledge related to about state-specific rules on compensability (Foster, 2009). Questions to consider that support decisions in regard to work-relatedness include: Do the symptoms fit the injury? Do the physical findings correlate with the injury and symptoms? Are there preexisting, coexisting, or comorbid conditions that should be considered?

Providing Quality Care

Any medical service, prescription, or medical supply that is used to treat an illness or injury must be appropriate to the diagnosis. Ongoing treatment must be based on the status of recovery and must be supported by applicable practice guidelines. The healthcare provider must initiate only the medical and pharmaceutical interventions that are appropriate for the level of injury or illness. Treatment, using a sports medicine approach of high-intensity and short-duration, focusing on early recovery and restoration of function, is important. The treatment plan must be appropriate and must match the documented physiological and clinical problem.

Managing Work Status

Return to work is an integral part of the treatment plan. The assignment of work status should focus on the worker's capabilities. Work restrictions should be assigned that remove essential job functions or physical demands that are appropriate to the injury or illness and would have an adverse effect on recovery. The role of the healthcare provider is to determine restrictions that are appropriate to the level of injury. Advancing work status by removing restrictions and limitations as early as appropriate should be considered at each visit and should be a part of the treatment plan on a continuous basis. The assignment of restrictions and limitations should be reviewed with the injured worker at each visit and upon receipt of new information such as reports from physical therapy and specialty providers. The healthcare provider must communicate with the employer and insurance carrier any information regarding the treatment plan and the injured worker's work status for the timely and appropriate management of the workers' compensation claim. The OHN should assist with the assignment of modified duty and transition work assignments for the injured worker compatible with medically appropriate physical restrictions, assuring the restrictions are based upon the presence or absence of objective relevant medical findings. These processes are key to managing return to work and to facilitating maximum recovery.

STRATEGIES FOR SUCCESS

The engagement of all involved to employ *SMARTER** strategies help to create an effective workers' compensation program that meets the needs of injured workers while providing a high-quality, cost-effective benefit. By instituting these strategies, the employer is able to demonstrate value for both the injured workers and for the company.

Select Key Partnerships

It is common to use benefits consultants or insurance agents when securing coverage for workers' compensation benefits. The consultant or agent assists the employer in choosing the appropriate insurance coverage for workers' compensation. The consultant/agent should have the employer's best interests in mind and share the philosophy of recommending the most cost-effective option for the coverage, based on company size and history of experience.

The consultant/agent should hold comprehensive knowledge regarding other aspects of the employee benefits program, such as group health benefits and disability insurance since there is often significant interplay. Although the calculation of such benefits is dependent on the makeup of the workforce, work hazards, and wage levels, many other influences may come into play. Negotiated terms of labor unions may also influence worker entitlement and coverage under certain benefits. And, decisions to increase copays and deductibles under the group health benefits may influence workers to perceive workers' compensation benefits as a much more attractive benefit. The consultant/agent must take all influencers into consideration when providing guidance to the employer.

Performance expectations should be considered during the selection process for the insurer or TPA. The insurer/TPA must provide the employer with an efficient means for reporting claims and should also have an efficient internal process for administering claims. The adjusters assigned to the claims are on the front lines in regard to administrative management of the claims, with responsibility for claim investigation by obtaining information from the injured worker, witnesses, the employer, the workers' compensation medical providers, and they should obtain information related to the current and past health history of the injured worker. The claims adjuster also holds the power to authorize medical treatment and makes decisions related to assignment of benefits and claims settlements. Case managers may be assigned to certain claims to direct medical care by developing appropriate recovery plans for the injured worker. This is of particular value with complex and catastrophic claims or troublesome cases. Being the prime communicators with other stakeholders, adjusters, and case managers holds significant potential to influence the outcome of the claim by holding responsibility for managing claims without harassment, coercion, or intimidation toward the injured worker, the employer,

*Note that SMARTER is a proprietary brand owned by Dr. Arlene Guzik.

or the healthcare providers. Therefore, the selection of adjusters and case managers as key partners, with their agreement to subscribe to the company's philosophy related to claims and case management, is of vital importance.

The selection of key partners who will render care and services to injured workers has significant positive impact on the outcome of the claim. As long as statutory guidelines permit, the employer should engage in securing relationships with healthcare providers who render consistent, high-quality service in an efficient manner. These providers should be able to articulate a comprehensive knowledge of the state's workers' compensation system and execute their services accordingly. Healthcare providers should render care consistent with that authorized by the adjuster and within the parameters of care that are medically indicated for the level of the injury or illness, founded on scientific evidence-based guidelines. Appropriate and timely documentation of diagnostic results, medical findings, recommended treatment, and the injured worker's response to treatment assist the adjuster and case manager in handling the claim. Of utmost importance, these providers should demonstrate a willingness to openly communicate with the employer and other stakeholders involved in the claim, knowing there is always "another side to the story."

The employer's workers' compensation defense attorney plays a key role in providing advice related to the management and settlement of litigated claims. However, there is a role for the defense attorney to take a more proactive part as a key partner providing advice to the employer related to insurance coverage, hazard and risk reduction, and claims management based on analysis of potential exposure. The defense attorney should be involved up front in regard to development of the philosophical decisions related to policies and procedures for the overall workers' compensation benefit program to assure consistency with their approaches to claims defense. Of additional value is the integration of philosophical agreement between defense attorney and the company's labor law attorney since there is significant interplay between workers' compensation and employment labor laws.

Key partnerships must also be engaged within the company. The human resources and risk managers must work together to assure a firm, fair, and consistent approach to investigation of incidents and injury management. Management at all levels of the company should strive to consistently apply policies and procedures and maintain a safe work environment. Managers should be well versed in the steps to take when an incident or injury arises and provide appropriate guidance and intervention. And not of least importance are the workers. All workers must be made aware of the proper steps to take to report incidents and injuries that occur in the workplace. Appropriate notice should be posted to direct workers what to do should they be in need of medical intervention. Through the engagement of stakeholders at all levels within the company, acknowledging and understanding the importance of a safe and healthy workplace, the employer can reap the benefit of support at all levels.

Through the selection of key partnerships, the employer is able to engage a comprehensive philosophical approach to managing workers' compensation benefits shared by stakeholders from all perspectives. By taking charge early in the life of a claim and securing healthcare services focused on quality, injured workers will receive appropriate and timely benefits focused on positive outcomes and a swift recovery.

Managing Health and Safety

The employer's fitness for duty program provides the foundation for the workers' compensation program. Employers who conduct preplacement health evaluations gain benefit from documenting a baseline of the worker's health history at the time of placement, as well as assuring that the worker is the right fit for the job. The establishment of a drug-free workplace also serves to support a safe and healthful work environment. Health and wellness initiatives, through education, screening, and disease management assist workers in achieving high levels of safety and health, and as a result the employer benefits from reduced risks and a more productive workforce.

Philosophical support for developing and maintaining focus on health and safety must start at the top of the organization. A top-down expectation for reducing hazards and risks, for regulatory compliance, and for a safety-first management approach is vital. A focus on incident reporting, rather than just injury reporting, enables the employer to gain insight into near misses and trends that may prove a threat, thus creating an expectation for focus on intense investigation aimed at eliminating or minimizing injuries.

The selection of healthcare providers focused on quality that will provide care to workers under both group health and workers' compensation serves to support the workplace philosophy of good health. Although some employers focus on healthcare cost containment, an outcome-focused approach for quality care and efficient return to work will result in improved health and productivity of the workforce.

Assess Effectiveness

The assessment of organization effectiveness focuses on responsibility for health and safety at all levels. For all stakeholders there should be a keen awareness of the impact of incidents, injuries, and worker absences on company profitability. All workers should be knowledgeable about safety procedures, and management must maintain keen attention to incident and injury reporting, while staying engaged in all cost-containment efforts. Chargebacks to the department level for costs related to incidents and injuries serves to create awareness among managers of the cost implications and may provide additional motivation for department managers and supervisors to remain engaged in incident investigation procedures and the return-to-work process for injured workers.

Program effectiveness is assessed through consistent collection of data aimed at identifying the true cost drivers and should be coupled with the intent to

Table 10.3 Key Performance indicators.

- Number of incidents reported
- Number of injuries/illnesses reported
- Number/frequency of actual claims reported
- Total cost of claims
  - Costs per claim average
    - Medical costs
    - Indemnity costs
    - Legal costs
- Restricted/lost work days
  - Modified duty work days
  - Days away from work (lost time)

implement strategies for potential savings. This can be accomplished through benchmarking the company's performance with prior history of claims experience, comparison to industry standards, and identification of best practices that will lead to improved cost effectiveness. Establishment of key performance indicators at all stakeholder levels, such as business units, division, or locations, provides the employer with objective information on measuring performance and the effect on the workers' compensation program. See Table 10.3 for common key performance indicators.

Return to Work

Keeping workers healthy and on the job should be the focus of any employer wishing to maintain a productive workforce. Research and experience tell us that injured workers who remain off work recover less quickly and have poorer clinical outcomes as compared to those who maintain the social connection with the workplace and with coworkers (ACOEM, 2006).

The injured worker's ability to work should be assessed based on three factors (ACOEM, 2006):

- Functional capacity: What can the injured worker do today?
- Functional impairments or limitations: What can't the injured worker do now that he or she normally could do?
- Medically appropriate restrictions: What should the injured worker not do to avoid more harm?

The employer should strive to have a plan for return to work for all injured workers. A modified duty or transitional work assignment should be available that supports the worker's physical abilities while honoring the medically appropriate limitations or restrictions. This is accomplished by removing certain essential functions or by placing the worker in a different job where the limitations can be better accommodated. The assignment of modified or transitional duty should maintain respect for the worker's abilities while also maintaining compliance with regulatory standards and requirements, company policies, and respect for all safety concerns. Of utmost importance, in order to maintain a sense of self-fulfillment, the worker should be assigned to work that is meaningful and contributes to workplace productivity.

A strong return-to-work philosophy supports the employer's workers' compensation program by mitigating loss by keeping the worker gainfully employed and reducing indemnity benefits. While this is a very positive approach, one must be mindful of inherent risks as well, such as reinjury of the injured worker, aggravation of the condition, and varying attitudes of coworkers. Therefore, the employer must institute strategies for evaluating the effectiveness of the work assignments and should be aware of the need to garner support among all stakeholders for this strategy. This can be accomplished by staying in close communication with the injured worker (even when he or she is taken off work), the adjusters and case managers, and healthcare providers.

Training and Communication

Safety first. This should be communicated loudly and clearly to all levels of the organization. The employer must have written policies and procedures for safety and for incident and injury reporting. This is made clear by using a variety of communication vehicles, including wall posters, brochures, web messaging, e-mail messages, company newsletters, and wallet card reminders for those who may work in remote locations. Communication of expectations cannot be understated and cannot be overdone. One must only look at how workers' compensation plaintiff attorneys get their messages across through the use of billboards, television and radio ads, Web messaging, and the phone directory. If this is the first message workers remember at the time they are injured, surely they will be drawn to that resource for direction.

Training for workers must be at the reading level of the user and must be mindful of language preferences. Training material should also be attractive to the reader in order to stimulate interest. Efforts should clearly communicate expectations at all levels and should be reinforced through ongoing training for workers, supervisory staff, and managers at all levels.

Early Engagement

The RIMS Benchmark Survey (2010) established a direct correlation between early return to work and lower experience modification factors. Additionally, focus on prompt attention to the needs of the injured worker and access to appropriate services in the early part of the life span of the claim have proved successful. Early intervention at all stages of the claim proves effective: early incident investigation, early medical attention, early legal intervention.

Early engagement means the employer should make it easy for the worker to access the workers' compensation system when needed, for instance, report forms that are easy to find and easy to complete and communication regarding use of the worker's system that is easy to read and understand. Otherwise, the employer fails to obtain the information it needs regarding incident investigation, and the worker fails to get the appropriate message regarding his or her rights and responsibilities.

Early engagement also includes getting the injured worker quick and efficient access to the appropriate healthcare provider. Successful strategies used by employers include using the OHN as the first point of contact to provide immediate intervention and assess the need for further evaluation and treatment. Engagement with the OHN or other telephonic nurse case managers provides an efficient means of triage that gets the injured worker the care most appropriate for the level of injury. Most often, this serves to avert costly emergency room charges and avoids allowing the injured worker to navigate his or her own way through the system in search for medical care. Once the injured worker gets lost in the system, the claims most likely will have an untoward outcome. The engagement of select healthcare providers will lead to better outcomes. Providers should offer efficient appointments, establish appropriate diagnosis and treatment plans, and define appropriate apportionment of the injury when necessary. This leads to a faster recovery for the injured worker and efficient closure of the claim. With time as the enemy, early engagement by all stakeholders is good for all.

Responsibility and Reliability
All stakeholders hold certain responsibilities under the workers' compensation program, and in order to have positive outcomes, everyone must be held accountable for those responsibilities.

Worker Responsibilities
The worker holds the responsibility to report incidents and injuries in a timely manner, consistent with company policy. The worker then holds responsibility for following company policies and procedures, as well as guidelines established by the state's workers' compensation program, in accessing the system for benefit entitlement. Once the claim is filed, the claims administrator sends the injured workers information regarding their rights and responsibilities, and the workers hold the obligation to follow those guidelines.

The injured worker is responsible for open communication with other stakeholders, providing the claims administrator and medical providers with accurate information related to the incident. As well, the worker is responsible for accurately describing the resultant physical complaints or injuries, providing information related to past health history, and for accurately describing the effects of treatment modalities. The worker is also responsible for interaction with the employer, following the appropriate steps to communicate his or her assigned duty status and for returning to work as assigned. Once returned to work, the worker holds the responsibility for reliably showing up for work as scheduled and for working at his or her full potential, within the assigned medical limitations, thus remaining a productive contributor to the workplace.

Employer Responsibility

The employer holds responsibility for posting all notices related to the state's workers' compensation system and for communicating and reinforcing all aspects of company policies and procedures related to incident and injury reporting. The employer is responsible for ensuring workers know what to do when an injury occurs and must post the approved workers' compensation healthcare providers in those states in which the employer selects the medical provider or noting the workers' right to select their own provider if they choose to do so.

The employer is obligated to conduct a full investigation of all incidents, obtaining written statements from the injured worker, from all witnesses, and from the worker's supervisor. The employer is responsible for gathering reliable information that will assist in claims administration, including copies of any preplacement health history forms; identifying patterns of absences or patterns of other workers' compensation claims; and providing the appropriate payroll information.

It is the employer's responsibility to then file the claim with the insurer/TPA, and there is usually a state mandate regarding the time frame for reporting. This notice is the trigger to initiate the injured worker's access to benefits, knowing that failure to do so causes delays in authorizations for medical care and treatment.

The employer's responsibility for communication starts the day of the incident and continues throughout the life of the claim. The employer should stay in contact with the injured worker and with the claims administrator. Maintaining communications provides reliability that the worker is obtaining the appropriate benefits for recovery and may reduce the risk of the development of any adversarial relationship between stakeholders, thus reducing the chance the claim will become litigated.

The employer is also responsible for having an effective return-to-work program, providing modified duty assignments or transitional work plan. Training of supervisors provides assurance that the injured worker will be welcomed back into the workplace as a productive contributor, despite having been injured. The OHN is often responsible for establishing the return to work plan with supervisors and is responsible for evaluating the effectiveness of the plan. Having more than one option available for the modified or transitional duty provides reliability that the worker can return to work and remain productive.

Healthcare Provider Responsibility

Appropriate medical management is crucial to controlling claim costs and effecting claim outcomes. Appropriate medical management means that the healthcare provider is responsible for making the correct diagnosis, defining causal relationships, rendering appropriate treatment, and assigning the appropriate level of impairment or disability, if indicated. The medical provider is responsible for defining the diagnosis while addressing coexisting and preexisting conditions that may come into play. This diagnosis is based on relevant, objective evidence and should be consistent with the explained mechanism of injury. Treatment should be criteria-based and appropriate to the work-related injury. The medical provider should focus on returning the worker to duty on the first visit, unless medically contraindicated. According to ACOEM studies on preventing needless disability (2006), only a small fraction of medically excused days off work are medically necessary, and injured workers can generally work at something productive as soon as there is no specific medical condition to keep them from working.

The employer and claims adjuster need to know that they can rely on all healthcare providers to deliver services in an efficient, cost-effective, and consistent manner, providing injured workers exactly what they need – nothing less and nothing more than medically necessary. Decision making needs to be consistent and reliable across all claims to provide a reliable product for the employer that supports the company's philosophy. All healthcare providers, including medical, diagnostic, and rehabilitation, should support the injured worker's need for efficient access to services. All providers should also provide reliable, accurate documentation that will support decision making for the claim.

Claims Administrator Responsibilities

The claims administrator should be willing to meet face-to-face on a regular basis with the employer to evaluate the effectiveness of the program and to identify opportunities for improvement. Quarterly claims reviews with employer should include the workers' compensation medical provider and defense attorney in this meeting. This sets the tone for effective interaction and review of open claims while serving to reinforce stakeholder commitment to the company's philosophy for treating injured workers and managing claims.

In managing claims, the adjuster is responsible for initiating a three-point contact, usually within 24–48 hours from the time of claim notice. Contact is made with the three primary players that the adjuster will be in touch with during the course of the open claim: the injured worker, the employer, and the medical provider. Exchange of information takes place during this contact as the adjuster strives to investigate the claim in a timely and through manner. The use of consistent intake questionnaires to gather the same information on each claim provides the adjuster with reliable information that will assist in setting aside appropriate reserve funds anticipated for the claim. The adjuster is responsible for identifying workers with preexisting risk factors for prolonged disability and managing these cases more intensively from the onset (ACOEM, 2006).

Through the life of the claim, the claims administrator is responsible for maintaining open communication with stakeholders with the intention of providing the injured worker with a swift recovery and closing the claim. Reliability is achieved through consistent handling of every claim, adhering to the steps of the plan.

SUMMARY

Although employers must assume the costs of injuries, illnesses, and deaths that occur on the job, without regard to fault, several strategies can be employed to provide a quality, cost-effective benefit for injured workers. Stakeholder involvement and commitment at all levels is vital for success.

The employer should have policies and procedures to direct workers on what to do when an injury or illness occurs as a result of their work, and the procedures should provide clear direction on how to access healthcare services under the workers' compensation system. When a worker becomes injured or ill as a result of his or her work, the employer or insurer should provide authorization for an efficient referral to the most appropriate healthcare provider as defined in the state workers' compensation statute.

The employer should strive to align incentives for all stakeholders in the system, while holding them accountable for performance and adherence to expectations. Claims administrators should be held accountable for managing the finances of the claim in the best interest of the employer. All must understand that it is the employer's money that is being spent, and careless use of financial resources can have a lasting effect on the employer's experience modification factor and insurance rating. Additionally, bad decisions in regard to compensability for claims can have an effect on the company. If a claim is accepted for one employee for a health condition that is not supported by scientific evidence or state statute to be work-related, it may cause an epidemic in the workplace for other workers who perceive entitlement to the same benefit. It must be clearly acknowledged that workers' compensation claims can become a contagion in the workplace, so fair and balanced decision making is required at all levels.

Healthcare providers rendering services under the workers' compensation system must have an excellent understanding of the statutory regulations. Being familiar with the criteria of the workers' compensation statutes of the state in which the injury or illness occurs is of vital importance. Besides providing the healthcare services that are medically indicated, the healthcare provider is often required to render opinion on whether the injury or illness is related to work. Because healthcare provider decisions are critical to the quality and cost of workers' compensation claims, the healthcare provider must render care in a quality-oriented, cost-conscious manner using cognitive expertise related to the specialty of workers' compensation.

On-the-job recovery holds a valuable role by keeping the injured worker engaged and productive, yet requires a determined commitment by management at all levels of the company. Supervisors must be held accountable for supporting modified duty assignments with an attitude of caring for the injured worker. One of the strongest predictors of untoward outcomes from a workers' compensation claim is job dissatisfaction, or a lack of support from coworkers and supervisors. Home and family considerations are also factors that lead to concern from the injured worker since the injury may have a significant impact on their personal life, as well. By keeping the injured worker engaged, the employer is able to identify and investigate workplace and social issues that may have an impact on the claim and institute appropriate intervention and support (ACOEM, 2006).

Human reactions will revolve around all aspects of the claim, not just with the injured worker, but with all stakeholders. For example, if the injury was a result of a safety violation, supervisors, managers, and even the company can be held accountable. If company policies define such, workers who are injured as a result of failure to use proper safety devices can be faced with disciplinary action, up to and including termination of employment. Some state statutes also allow for a reduction in covered benefits for the worker under this circumstance. Workers who are found to be under the influence of drugs and alcohol may face denial of benefits and even termination of employment. These types of situations set an entirely different set of circumstances that have profound effects on the claim. The employer needs to address bad behavior at all levels with issues related to worker performance, attitudes of supervisors and managers, issues of professionalism and ethics in regard to claims administrators and healthcare providers, and even attempted interference from labor union representatives.

Criminal violations up to and including felony indictments can be imposed on stakeholders for violation of the workers' compensation statutes. A worker who files false claims, provides misleading information, or exaggerates injuries can be considered to have intent to defraud or deceive the employer or insurer and may be subject to punishment. Employers who knowingly fail to provide workers' compensation insurance coverage or who intentionally provide inaccurate information that misclassifies or fails to define accurate payroll or employee information are also subject to punishment. Healthcare providers who knowingly conspire with or assist individuals with the intent to commit fraud or those who submit fraudulent billing are subject to punishment and may lose rights to provide further services under the state's workers' compensation system.

Penalties can be assessed against the insurer for failure to report claims to the state's insurance division or to disallow or provide late payment of benefits or fees. Penalties can be assessed by the state's division of insurance for untimely reporting, inaccurate calculation of benefits and payment, or failing to meet audit standards.

Despite every effort by the employer to establish and maintain a quality-oriented health and safety program, workers will continue to get injured on the job. It is expected that future claims will be driven by three major factors: obesity, the aging workforce, and distracted driving. Statistics indicate that obese workers are twice as likely to file a workers' compensation claim. With individuals

214

working beyond the typical retirement age, this aging workforce will bring a host of challenges to the workers' compensation landscape. Preexisting and coexisting health conditions confound the claims and impact recovery, having an effect on lost time, claim age, and cost of claim. Highway accidents and incidents related to the use of mobile equipment continue to create challenges in regard to safety. Highway incidents are the leading cause of occupational deaths and also represent a significant risk to public safety (Fuge, 2009).

As the employer strives to establish an effective workers' compensation program, decision making should be focused on controlling costs, improving outcomes, and maintaining productivity. Despite the negative reputation and horror stories conveyed throughout the workers' compensation arena, the benefit it brings to the employer and to injured workers is exceptional. Aligned philosophies are important, and a philosophy of caring can make the difference.

REFERENCES

Adams, S. (2001). Risk management methods to reduce your workers' compensation rates. *Occupational Hazards, 63*(3), 1.

American College of Occupational and Environmental Medicine (ACOEM). (2006). *Preventing needless work disability by helping people stay employed.* Retrieved from http://www.acoem.org

American College of Occupational and Environmental Medicine (ACOEM), Improvement Committee. (2006). ACOEM Guideline: Preventing needless work disability by helping people stay employed. Stay-at-work and return-to-work process. *Journal of Occupational and Environmental Medicine, 48*(9), 9.

American College of Occupational and Environmental Medicine (ACOEM). (2007). Retrieved from http://www.acoem.org

American College of Occupational and Environmental Medicine (ACOEM). (2011). *Scope of occupational and environmental health programs and practice.* Retrieved from http://www.acoem.or

Balge, M. A. & Krieger, G. R. (2000). *Occupational health and safety* (3rd ed., pp. 409–430). Chicago: National Safety Council.

Brown, D. N. & Sliski, S. K. (2007). How can case managers develop positive and effective relationships with clients by phone? *AAOHN Journal, 55*(9), 349–350.

Bender, K. & Fritchen, B. (2008). *Government-sponsored health insurance purchasing arrangements: Do they reduce costs or expand coverage for individuals and small employers?* Retrieved from http://www.oliverwyman.com/ow/pdf_files/health_ins_purchasing_arrangements.pdf

Colledge, A. L. & Johnson, H. I. (2000). The S.P.I.C.E. model for return to work. *Occupational Health and Safety, 69*(2), 64–69.

Dasinger, L. K., Krause, N., Deegan, L. J., Brand, R. J., Rudolph, L. (2000). Physical workplace factors and return to work after compensated low back injury: A disability phase-specific analysis. *Journal of Occupational and Environmental Medicine, 42*(3), 323–333.

Dasinger, L. K., Krause, N., Thompson, P. J., Brand, R. J., Rudolph, L. (2001). Doctor proactive communication, return-to-work recommendation and duration of disability after a workers' compensation low back injury. *Journal of Occupational and Environmental Medicine, 43*(6), 515–525.

Delk, K. L. (2012). Occupational health nursing interventions to reduce third-party liability in workplace injuries. *Workplace Health & Safety, 60*(3), 107–109.

DiBenedetto, D. V. (2003). Informatics: Finding disability related information on the web. *AAOHN Journal,* (January), 10–12.

Foster, D. (2008). Occupational health nurse practitioners' roles in workers' compensation. *AAOHN Journal, 56*(5), 185–187.

Foster, D. (2009). When is an injury compensable? *AAOHN Journal, 57*(11), 443–444.

Fuge, C. (2009). *Workers' compensation issues and trends 2009—The NCCI perspective.* Retrieved from http://www.irmi.com/expert/articles/2009/fuge05-insurance-workers-compensation.aspx

Guidotti, T. L. & Rose, S. G. (2001). *Science on the witness stand.* Beverly Farms, MA: OEM Press.

Guzik, A. (2007). What you should know about work-comp claims. *Arthritis Practitioner, 3*(6), 26–30.

Guzik, A. (2008). Strategies for effective occupational health case management. *Professional Case Management, 13*(1), 48–52.

Haag, A. B., Kalina, C. M., & Brown, N. D. (2007). What role does the case manager play in a litigated case?, *AAOHN Journal, 55*(3), 93–96.

Kalina, C. M., Haag, A. B., & Brown, N. D. (2007). How can occupational health nurses get buy-in from management and unions for case management services? *AAOHN Journal, 55*(6), 221–224.

Matheson, L. N. (1988). How do you know he tried his best? *Journal of Industrial Rehabilitation Quarterly, 1,* 10–12.

National Council in Compensation Insurance. (2005). *Scopes manual.* Boca Raton: National Council of Compensation Insurance.

National Council on Compensation Insurance, Inc. (NCCI). (2011). *NCCI Holdings.* Retrieved from http://www.ncci.com

Pennachio, F. (2009). *Misaligned contracts drive comp costs. The self-insurer.* Retrieved from http://www.workcompadvisorygroup.com/Libraries/In_the_News_-_PDFs/Misaligned_Contracts_Drive_Comp_Costs.sflb.ashx

The Risk Management Society (RIMS). (2010) Rims *benchmark survey book.* http://cf.rims.org/Template.cfm?Section=RIMSPublications&Template=/Ecommerce/ProductDisplay.cfm&ProductID=1137

Rosenstock, L. & Cullen, M. (1994). Textbook of clinical occupational and environmental medicine. Philadelphia: W.B. Saunders.

Salazar, M. (2001). *Core curriculum for occupational & environmental health nursing.* (2nd ed.). Philadelphia: W.B. Saunders.

Shaw, W. S., Robertson, M. M., Pransky, G., & McLellan, R. K. (2006). Training to optimize the response of supervisors to work injuries—needs assessment, design, and evaluation. *AAOHN Journal, 54*(5), 226–235.

Servan-Schreiber, D., Kolb, N. R., & Tabas, G. (2011). Somatizing patients: Part I. Practical diagnosis. *American Family Physician*. Retrieved from http://www.aafp.org/afp/2000/0215/p1073.html

U.S. Department of Labor, Bureau of Labor Statistics (BLS). (2010). *Workplace injury, illness and fatality statistics*. Retrieved from http://www.osha.gov/oshstats/work.html

U.S. Department of Labor, Bureau of Labor Statistics (BLS). (2011). *Injuries, illnesses, and fatalities: Incidence rate calculator and comparison tool*. Retrieved from http://data.bls.gov/iirc/?data_tool=IIRC

U.S. Small Business Administration. Employment & Labor Law. Retrieved from www.sba.gov/content/workers-compensation

Walker, J. M. (2003). Disabler: A game occupational health nurses cannot afford to play. *AAOHN Journal, 51*(10), 421–424.

Zichello, C., & Sheridan, J. (2008). Occupational health nurses and workers' compensation insurance programs. *AAOHN Journal, 56*(11), 455–458.

WEB RESOURCES

American Association of Occupational Health Nurses
http//www.aaohn.org
American College of Occupational and Environmental Medicine
http//www.acoem.org
Occupational Health & Safety
http//www.ohsonline

Managing Health

11

> It is clear that health, as measured by health status, has an impact on worker prosperity and working skills that ultimately influence productivity.
>
> (Berger et al., 2001)

The principle of health and disability management proposes that health status is one of the important underlying factors in enhancing or maintaining productivity in the workplace. Personal health status, therefore, directly affects both the quantity (time worked) and quality (productivity) of workers, having an indirect effect on both human and financial capital (Berger et al., 2001). This chapter addresses the role of the occupational health nurse (OHN) in health and disability management, with a focus on the long-term benefits and rewards. These rewards, when managed appropriately, benefit the worker and the employer and lead to a healthier workplace.

WORKPLACE HEALTH AND PRODUCTIVITY

The term *"absenteeism"* has traditionally been used to account for the number of days or hours a worker has missed work. Although, when all factors are taken into consideration, absences from work can take on a variety of implications, some of which the worker can control, and others not. Table 11.1 lists the common factors associated with health-related workplace absences. Benefits associated with each of these factors can include workers' compensation, short-term disability, long-term disability, sick leave, Family Medical Leave Act (FMLA), paid time off (PTO), unpaid leave, and death. Add to this the costs associated with worker replacement, training, and compromised productivity, and we can then see that workers who are absent from work have a significant negative effect on the bottom line (Goetzel et al., 2001).

Direct costs associated with health-related absences include the medical, pharmaceutical, disability benefits, workers' compensation premiums, and other insurance benefits–related costs. And the indirect costs associated with

Essentials for Occupational Health Nursing, First Edition. Arlene Guzik.
© 2013 John Wiley & Sons, Inc. Published 2013 by John Wiley & Sons, Inc.

Table 11.1 Factors related to workplace absences.

- Workers' compensation
- Short-term disability
- Long-term disability
- Sick leave
- Family Medical Leave Act
- Paid time off
- Unpaid leave

Source: Table created from information found in:
Goetzel et al. (2001).

Table 11.2 Costs of employee benefits.

Traditional View: Costs of Employee Benefits
Group Health: 63%
Incidental absence: 16%
WC: 9%
STD: 8%
LTD: 4%

Comprehensive View: Total Costs of Employee Benefits
Lost productivity from absence: 71%
Employee WC and GH medical care: 19%
Wage replacement: 10%

Source: Table created from information found in Parry, T., Schweitzer, W., & Molmen, W. The Business Case for Managing Health and Productivity. Results from IBI's Full-Cost Benchmarking Program. Research by the Integrated Benefits Institute. June 2004. http://www.acoem.org/ uploadedFiles/Career_Development/Tools_for_Occ_Health_Professional/Health_and_ Productivity/IBIFull-CostResearch.pdf
WC, workers' compensation; STD, short-term disability; LTD, long-term disability, GH, group health

absences include the cost of replacement workers, overtime premiums, productivity losses related to unscheduled absences, and productivity losses of workers while on the job (Berger et al., 2001). Using a more comprehensive view, one can see that the influence of these factors has a significant economic impact on productivity in the workplace. See Table 11.2.

Even while working, the health status of the worker or a significant other can affect performance and productivity. The term *presenteeism* is used to describe situations in which the worker is physically present at work, but is limited in some aspect of job performance as a result of health-related problems (ACOEM, 2011). This may affect the quantity and quality of work and may also have an impact on others in the workforce. Workers with certain health conditions or those taking certain medications may be prone to the effects of presenteeism. Many health conditions are known to hamper one's ability to perform, thus

Table 11.3 Factors associated with presenteeism.

- Quality of Work
  - Incidence and severity of errors
  - Limited creativity
  - Impact on executive functions
- Quantity of Work
- Decreased amount of work output
  - Increased time on task
  - Diverted attention (in the workplace, but not working)
  - Reduced capacity for peak performance
- Interpersonal Factors
  - Social function (impact on morale)
  - Addictions (manipulative behaviors)
  - Personality disorders (interpersonal problems, criminal behaviors)
  - Mood disorders (irritable with co-workers and customers)

Source: Table created from information found in ACOEM (2011).

have an effect on fitness for duty. Medications that cause drowsiness or other side effects, both prescription and nonprescription, may have a deleterious effect on performance. Those workers with social or family concerns may have their attention diverted while thinking of their needs or issues outside the workplace. Something as elementary as a child's performance in school can divert a worker's attention when focused on a family issue. Table 11.3 outlines common factors associated with presenteeism.

There are various benefits programs and services that workers may access when sick, injured, or have family or social issues, including healthcare benefits, disability and workers' compensation benefits, employee assistance programs (EAPs), paid sick leave, and family medical leave. In addition to keeping workers healthy and on the job, the indirect benefits of managing health may result in enhanced morale and reduce turnover of the workforce (Schultz et al., 2002). Therefore, the OHN's involvement in planning and managing these programs can provide great value to the business.

There is increasing evidence that the work environment and the overall health, safety, and well-being of the workers are strongly connected (NIOSH, 2011), acknowledging that the overall effect of worker health not only impacts the individual, but may also have an effect on the work culture. Traditional safety programs have demonstrated effectiveness by addressing physical and organizational work environment concerns, leading to safer workplaces, reductions in hazards, and lowered injury rates. At the same time, workplaces can implement and develop programs in their organizations that integrate health and wellness activities that address the personal health-related decisions and behaviors of individual workers. This allows us to take the same concepts used in workplace safety management and apply them to the health of workers. The joint management of safety, health, and wellness benefits and programs is intended to create a work–life balance for the worker. There are four key goals in successful management of the health of workers: (1) identifying risk, (2) enhancing access to and the provision of quality healthcare, (3) maintaining productivity for the workplace by keeping the worker on the job, and (4) cost control.

WORKERS' COMPENSATION

Inappropriate management of worker's compensation claims can be one of the greatest cost drivers related to workplace disability. As covered in previous chapters, employers should have written policies and procedures concerning work-related injuries, medical care, lost time, and return to work. A proactive approach is to require "incident" reporting rather than "injury" reporting. By focusing on the incidents that lead to injuries or illnesses, an employer is able to track and trend incident reporting as a proactive measure. Along with written policies and procedures, postings in conspicuous places throughout the workplace defining the worker's rights and responsibilities under the state's specific workers' compensation laws are essential. Supervisor and worker training should be conducted to ensure everyone is informed on what action should be taken in the event of an incident or injury. Procedures for injury management should also be posted throughout the workplace giving workers and supervisors specific direction on managing worker incidents and injuries.

The company procedure should give clear direction regarding the worker's responsibility for notifying a designated company representative when an injury/illness occurs and for completing a written incident report. Additional procedures requiring a supervisor's written statement, witness's written statement, and prompt incident investigation and corrective action are essential. Table 11.4 outlines the key principles for successful management of a workers' compensation claim.

The OHN should objectively assist in the valuation of occupational causation of illness; provide content expertise regarding available medical resources, rehabilitation programs, and other healthcare facilities; and interact with healthcare providers and claims managers to facilitate return to work based on familiarity with the worksite and input from supervisory/management personnel (ACOEM, 2011). Responsibilities for the OHN include conducting the medical evaluation, authorizing and assuring quality medical care, and providing verbal and written procedural guidelines to the individual at the time of the injury. Remember the goals: a follow-up phone call, a walk to the workstation, a call or e-mail to the supervisor sends a goodwill message that will influence satisfaction.

The OHN should act as team leader by managing these cases until they reach maximum medical improvement (MMI). The OHN should also be a liaison with representatives of the insurer or third-party administrator (TPA). Often the adjuster for the insurer or TPA is several miles away. The OHN has the advantage of knowing local healthcare providers and developing good partnerships to assure quality medical care.

Table 11.4 Key principles in management of workers' compensation claim.

- Prompt action and appropriate medical care
- First aid/EMS response
- Authorization for treatment
- Appropriate documentation of the incident
- Written incident report by worker
- Supervisor's statement
- Witness's statements
- Prompt investigation and corrective action
- Safety investigation
  - Failure to follow safety procedures
  - Equipment malfunction
- Facilitation of modified duty assignment
- Avoid lost time
- Keep the injured worker productive and on the job
- Case management until maximum medical improvement (MMI) is achieved
- Assure worker attends all medical appointments
- Assure prompt and efficient claim closure

Healthcare providers under workers' compensation should not determine return to work. A company with good support for return to work will provide accommodations for all restricted duty, thus maintaining productivity of the injured worker. The healthcare provider should determine only medically appropriate work restrictions and limitations, allowing the OHN or other employer representatives to assign work within the scope of the restrictions. This is a key concept that influences reduction in lost work time and needless disability. Invite the healthcare provider for an orientation to the operations of the company. This will enable the healthcare provider to better understand the ability to accommodate certain work restrictions. This also provides the medical professional a perspective that assists in determining worker's compensation compensability issues in regard to the injury.

As an aspect of case management, the OHN must maintain communication with healthcare providers and know the status of the worker's treatment plan at all times, arranging for job modification and documenting all interventions. The role of the OHN is to also communicate with the supervisors and managers to advise them regarding the status of the injured worker. The OHN should assure that accommodations or work within the restrictions is being provided (Guzik, 1999).

The American College of Occupational and Environmental Medicine (ACOEM) has established an initiative that targets the prevention of needless disability. The initiative is based on the principle that "keeping people productively employed is good for them and for society" (ACOEM, 2006). There is great value in improving the access and utilization of services available to injured workers and in avoiding the overutilization of unnecessary resources and practices that result in losing personal and workplace productivity. The OHN plays a valuable role in this respect.

Role of the OHN in Case Management

Case management is a term used to describe an approach for managing complex medical care in a cost-effective manner (Ramos, 2006). According to Ramos, when administered through workplace case management programs, OHNs can manage the needs of workers with occupational and nonoccupational work injuries to accelerate recovery and minimize work days lost. The role of the OHN provides employers the ability to deal with the complexities of managed care and increasing pressure to manage healthcare costs, and as a result, can achieve average absence rates of 1.4% as compared to 5.3% for employers without a program. The American Association of Occupational Health Nurses describes case management as "a process of coordinating an individual client's total health care services to achieve optimal quality care delivered in a cost effective manner" (2003). The Case Management Society Association defines case management as a "collaborative process which assesses, plans, implements, coordinates, monitors, and evaluates the options and services to meet and individual's health needs through communication and available resources to promote quality cost effective outcomes" (1995). Figure 11.1 shows the overlay of stakeholders involved in managing the health of the worker. Together, they must strive to coordinate efforts based on a consistent philosophy of returning the worker to maximum productivity.

When is Case Management Necessary?

Case management is employed most often with workers' compensation cases, yet can also be employed to assist any worker in navigating the healthcare system, assuring appropriate care, and facilitating a return to work. The OHN, acting as case manager, should maintain an awareness of the status of all workers' compensation claims to assure the claim is brought to closure. Additionally, it is the responsibility of the case manager to assure quality, appropriate care for the worker. Case management is sometimes used in other disability cases, such as Family and Medical Leave Act (FMLA) or those workers out on short- or long-term disability. Since these situations employ company sponsored benefits, it is in the best interest of the company to assure that care is appropriate and work to facilitate a timely and effective return to work for the worker.

There are certain red flags that signal the need for case management. These include those workers who incur lost work days, those with concerning diagnoses, and those with potentially long recovery phases. Workers with certain social or language deficits can also benefit from the assistance of a case manager in order to successfully navigate the healthcare arena. In workers' compensation, those workers who display noncompliant behavior and those

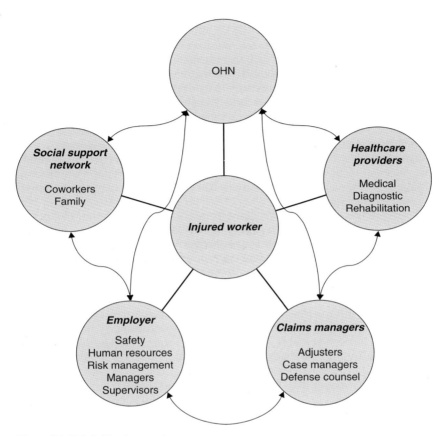

Figure 11.1 Stakeholders in managing care.

suspected of fraud should have an assigned case manager. Situations of distrust can also be overcome with appropriate intervention of a case manager. This distrust can arise between the injured worker and the employer, between the injured worker and the healthcare provider, or between the injured worker and the employer/guarantor.

The OHN can provide effective case management through a variety of ways. Fostering a supportive workplace climate and establishing disability policies provides the foundation. The OHN also acts as the content expert to establish the appropriate communication and cooperation among the workforce, the healthcare professional, union or worker representative, and the workplace. This can be accomplished through educational programs for management and supervisors and ongoing evaluation of the program.

WORKPLACE DISABILITY MANAGEMENT

Disability severity and duration have an effect on insurance ratings for the employer as well as on healthcare benefits costs for the employer and for the worker; thus, the financial effects of workplace disability are not impacted by the direct claim cost alone. There are several other influencers that drive the cost of disability. Additional effects include cost to the employer for replacement workers and the effect on productivity in the workplace. Workplace disability can also have in indirect effect on the morale of workers that may, in turn, affect customer service. So, as one can see, the effects of workplace disability are far-reaching.

The OHN has the opportunity to have a significant impact on disability management in the workplace. The first step is to understand the impact of disability on the workplace perspectives. The second step is to recognize opportunities for intervention.

There are three elements affecting a person's ability to recover: biologic or physical stimulus, psychological distress, and social stress. These three elements form a triad for intervention, thus supporting the biopsychosocial model. All aspects (physical, psychological, and social) of the workers must be taken into consideration when managing disability cases and maintaining productivity. Developing interventions that support all three aspects may have positive implications for recovery. For example, Greico et al. (2003) propose that, from a healthcare perspective, back pain is not a disease but rather a symptom. The authors go on to state that back pain resulting in disability is more likely dependent on psychosocial factors, such as other co-morbidities, psychological and stress-related symptoms, and work-related or other social problems, rather than physical pathology.

There are certain red flag warnings that demand the attention to managing certain cases (see Table 11.5), some of which are personal in nature and some of which are job related. Since the OHN serves as the healthcare expert in the company, certain cases deserve expert attention and intervention. Relationships can be established with human resources professionals or insurance adjusters to consult the OHN on cases that exhibit red flag warnings. As case manager, the OHN is often faced with individuals who are convinced that there is something seriously wrong with them despite normal exams and diagnostics.

Table 11.5 Summary of red flags for disability management.

- Inconsistency of medical findings
- Noncompliance
- Patient behavior that promotes disability
- Patient with needs
- Employment issues
- Rumors about case among other workers
- Attorney involvement

Table 11.6 Presenting features suggesting somatization.

- Multiple symptoms, often involving multiple body systems
- Symptoms that are vague or out of proportion with the objective findings
- Chronicity and delayed recovery
- Presence of a psychiatric disorder or symptoms
- Requests for or history of extensive diagnostic testing
- History of seeing multiple healthcare providers, or frequent requests to change providers or to see specialists

In some cases, the case manager and the treating providers often suspect a hidden agenda. Two disorders often come into play when managing difficult cases: somatization and symptom magnification. Both disorders present a somewhat self-destructive behavior in which the individual reports or displays certain symptoms that seem to consume the case, making it difficult to manage. It is important for the OHN to identify these cases, understand the concepts and dynamics of the disorders, and implement the appropriate strategies for managing these cases with attention to cost effectiveness.

Somatization occurs when the individual reports multiple medical problems, often involving more than one part of the body, but no physical cause can be found. Although the individual denies any psychological disorders, he or she has complex subconscious mechanisms driving behavior to seek continuing medical care. Somatization should be suspected when the case seems to have confounding issues and delayed recovery. See Table 11.6 for clinical presentations that may represent somatization. Somatization can present in two forms. In one case, there are no objective physical findings and the symptoms are primarily psychogenic or in the mind. In the other situation, there truly exists objective clinic findings; however, the individual's response related to the findings is inappropriate or exaggerated (Servan-Schreiber, Kolb, and Tabas, 2000a, b). In both situations, the individual's on-going complaints of pain and other symptoms display a tendency to malinger and may result in significant impairment in work and/or social functioning. Somatization may present as a result of an acute situational stressor or be related to either an acute or chronic psychiatric disorder. It is important for the OHN to differentiate the underlying precipitators influencing the individual's behavior. Behaviors displayed with a workers' compensation claim may be acute, whereas behaviors displayed with a short- or long-term disability case may be chronic in nature. Another important element in dealing with somatization behavior is to remember that there is a subconscious component that drives the individual's need to "prove" that he or she is seriously ill or injured. Once this is acknowledged, the OHN can strive to establish a more therapeutic relationship with focus on the psychological component.

Symptom magnification is an increased sensitivity and concern about physical symptoms as a means of justifying continued disability. In this case, the physical symptoms are real; however, the subjective complaints of the individual are reported out of proportion with the objective findings. In other words, there is a real health condition, but the individual's complaints are not consistent with exam or diagnostic findings. Matheson (1988) first defined symptom magnification as "a conscious or unconscious self-destructive socially reinforced behavioral response pattern consisting of reports or displays of symptoms which function to control the life circumstances of the sufferer."

Individuals may display signs of symptom magnification when they perceive the behavior will benefit the situation. This is often the case when dealing with benefit continuance or cases that will result in assignment of disability ratings. It is the individual's attempt to try to control the situation by exaggerating complaints and behaviors that may benefit the case. Unlike somatization, symptom magnification behavior may be conscious or unconscious (Colledge et. al., 2007).

As case manager, the OHN often holds the ability to influence the outcome of the case. When dealing with maladaptive behaviors, it is important to not allow these disorders to control the case. The goal with case management is to bring the case to closure or to stability. Often, the term *maximum medical improvement* (MMI) is used to define that state when the underlying condition causing the disability has plateaued. In this case, nothing further in the way of medical treatment can reasonably be anticipated to result in measurable change in the individual's comfort, function, or impairment.

PRINCIPLES OF DISABILITY MANAGEMENT

Review of national statistics (Fuge, 2009) and recent studies strongly suggests that current administrative and medical systems, when applied to managing workers' compensation claims and other disability-related benefit programs, are often ineffective and costly and can even promote disability. This suggests the greatest opportunity to influence recovery is early on in the case, thus the value of case management can apply to a broad number of cases. Colledge and Johnson (2000) describe certain principles that, when applied to the management of cases, result in positive outcomes. These principles are based on the military's "forward treatment" methodology and extensive experience in managing trauma. The model addresses both the biological and the psychosocial components of managing cases. The intent is to establish interventions aimed at reducing claims costs by dealing with them in an efficient, fair, and timely manner. Known as the SPICE model (Table 11.7), these principles can be applied to both workers' compensation cases, as well as short- and long-term disability cases. SPICE, is the acronym standing for its five concepts: Simplicity, proximity, immediacy, centrality, and expectancy (Colledge & Johnson, 2000).

Simplicity

Overemphasizing the potential seriousness of an individual's symptoms can lead to the individual's overreacting to discomfort and may have a negative effect on recovery. Sophisticated diagnoses and diagnostic tests that have

Table 11.7 SPICE model.

- Simplicity—When simple benign conditions are treated in a complicated fashion, they become complicated.
- Proximity—The need to keep the worker emotionally and geographically tied to the workforce
- Immediacy—The need to deal with illnesses and injuries in a timely manner to avoid establishing "disabled" behavior
- Centrality—Using the right provider at the right time in order to decrease the potential for iatrogenic complications
- Expectancy—The ill or injured worker often fulfills the clinical and labeling expectations placed upon them

little clinical relevance may serve only to lead the individual to suspect a serious health condition and adversely affect the subsequent clinical course. As a result, diagnostic tests should be reserved for use when only medically appropriate to confirm or refute a suspected diagnosis. Prescribed medications should be medically appropriate. Medication and splints, when not medically necessary, can also lead the individual to suspect a serious condition.

In keeping it simple, diagnostic tests, prescriptive medications or splints, and physical restrictions should be reserved for medically necessary purposes, and should not be implemented at the individual's request. Interventions prescribed at the request of the individual may result in adverse consequences of an overly concerned individual thinking his or her condition is more serious that it actually is.

Encouraging the individual to maintain an active life style is one of the simplest and safest recommendations. A focus on maintaining a regular work schedule with assignments within the assigned restrictions is therapeutic. Assigned work restrictions should be medically appropriate and commensurate with the degree of the injury or illness. Since exercise is one of the most therapeutic treatments, early return to occupational and nonoccupational activities should be encouraged.

Sophisticated testing procedures can have an adverse effect on the individual's illness behavior by reinforcing the severity of the "illness." Attention to a symptom amplifies it, whereas distractions diminish it (Colledge et al., 2007). Perhaps the most effective interventions that can be employed by the case manager is reassurance ... keeping it simple, realistic, and optimistic.

Proximity

This concept addresses the need to keep the injured worker emotionally and geographically tied to the workforce (Colledge & Johnson, 2000). Social support proves to be an important component in recovery. The support of family and social networks, as well as managers and co-workers, serves to reinforce the value of the worker to the workplace and provides psychological support. The goal of maintaining positive morale by keeping the worker engaged in a valuable role is both therapeutic and psychologically sound.

Studies have demonstrated that it is detrimental to keep the worker separated from the workplace, citing that cases where the worker who is no longer engaged in working usually result in more medical testing and treatment (ACOEM, 2009). The increased financial losses associated with lost work time may also encourage the worker to seek legal advice. Once there is attorney involvement, claims cost often skyrocket due to hopes for a more lucrative compensation (Colledge et al., 2009). Within weeks of attorney involvement, the individual sometimes begins to display negative psychosocial behaviors, along with increased physical complaints, that are now defining a more complex symptom overlay. There are associated undesirable psychosocial effects of lost work time that include increased psychological distress, depression, diminished income, and lack of socialization. In contrast, workers who return to work benefit from their ability to maintain their work status and gain improved conditioning These workers often display a more positive self-esteem and peer identity that may minimizes needless disability.

Immediacy

The concept of immediacy reflects the need to deal with illnesses and injuries in a timely manner to avoid establishing "disabled" behavior. Since delays in treatment significantly increase psychosocial issues, it also results in delayed recovery (Colledge & Johnson, 2000). The case manager should strive to meet the needs of the individual in an expedient manner, providing authorization for treatment and evaluation that is appropriate to the case. Focus should remain on increasing functioning to the maximal level, focusing on one's abilities rather than on disabilities. Should a disability exist, the case manager should work with the individual to adapt to his or her maximal potential and bring the case to closure.

The case manager should intervene during the acute phase of the injury or illness, offering reassurance about the nature of the condition and the plan of care. The earlier the intervention, the more successful the outcome. Individuals should be followed closely to ensure symptoms are properly interpreted, questions and concerns are addressed expeditiously, and fears and anxieties appeased (Colledge et al., 2007).

Centrality

Centrality focuses on using the right provider at the right time in order to decrease the potential for iatrogenic complications (Colledge et al., 2007). All providers involved with the injured worker must share a common vision and common goals for successful return to work and closure of the claim. In today's healthcare environment, it is not unusual for the individual to be treated by multiple specialists, with no one holding ultimate responsibility for directing care in a holistic manner. Medical services for ill and injured workers are sometimes fragmented and organized around various medical specialties.

The concept of centrality places value on the primary treating provider who provides the link into or establishes a network of providers willing to use established protocols, provide immediate communication, and establish uniform expectations in approaching the full spectrum of the injured worker's needs. Centralized medical management prevents exposure to confusing and threatening diagnostic tests, terminology, and treatments. Instead, the individual tends to get the correct treatment at the appropriate time (Colledge et al., 2007). The case manager is the facilitator of care and should make the assignment of the primary treating provider, maintain communication among all treating providers, and assist in the establishment of a coordinated plan of care.

Expectancy
This concept reflects the idea that the ill or injured worker often fulfills the clinical and labeling expectations placed upon him or her. Often, the case manager, and even the healthcare provider, may take on the character displayed by the individual, buying into his or her distress and negative outlook. Compassion and empathy overshadow objectivity. It is important, instead, that the healthcare provider and case manager maintain objective views of the case with a vision of case closure, moving toward MMI with each encounter.

Expectations for treatment and recovery should be clearly outlined, including treatment goals and expected timelines, and shared by all involved in the case, including the injured worker. The employer and the individual must develop a plan to facilitate compliance with the treatment plan that supports recovery. It is important that all involved subscribe to this same plan; otherwise, if only one person involved in the case verbalizes a different expectation, the result is confusion and mistrust on the part of the individual. In order to achieve optimum outcomes, it is important to minimize the chance of developing anger, suspicion, and distrust. Instead, encourage self-responsibility and motivation on the part of the individual by stating clear expectations at the start of and often throughout the course of treatment. The individual is responsible for complying with the treatment plan and must be held accountable for compliance with the prescribed care. Part of setting the expectation is to make sure the individual is aware that failure to comply with treatment may serve as evidence that he or she is not serious about getting better and thus have a negative impact on the claim. Under some state statutes, failure to comply with the treatment plan is considered noncompliance and could lead to termination of benefits.

BRINGING THE CASE TO CLOSURE
When a temporarily disabled worker recovers sufficiently to return to work, a fitness-for-duty (FFD) evaluation may be indicated. Such evaluations are important in the assessment of function and to determine an appropriate fit between the worker's capabilities and the essential functions of the job. The

FFD evaluation establishes objective evidence of what functions the worker is capable of performing, despite any residual disability or impairment.

Depending on the statutory entitlement under which the individual is being evaluated (such as workers' compensation, Social Security, military, etc.), there are varying definitions of impairment and disability. The most commonly used guide is published by the American Medical Association (AMA, 2008), although for workers' compensation, some states publish state-specific impairment rating guidelines. According to AMA, impairment is defined as "an alteration of an individual's health status; a deviation from normal in a body part or organ system and its functioning," whereas, disability is defined as "an alteration of an individual's capacity to meet personal, social, or occupational demands because of an impairment." In a broad sense, impairment takes into consideration the level of impact the condition has on the performance of certain bodily functions, and disability, therefore, is focused on the ability to engage in certain activities, one of which is the ability to work.

The ultimate goal of managing cases is to have the individual achieve MMI. MMI exists when the underlying condition causing the disability has become stable and has plateaued. It does not necessarily mean that the health condition was resolved or eliminated. It simply means that there is nothing further in the way of medical treatment that can reasonably be anticipated to result in measurable change in the condition, including comfort, function, or impairment.

In establishing MMI, measures of disability ratings are focused on objective findings, including physical impairments and limitations to function, resulting in the assignment of a disability rating. This takes into consideration any preexisting or coexisting conditions that may also interfere with full recovery. It is important that these objective findings equate with the individual's subjective complaints. Any discordance in subjective complaints that are not supported by objective findings must be measured and validated as part of the impairment evaluation. Usually one physician is responsible for determining MMI and associated impairment ratings. This is done through a thorough review of all medical records and medical examination, and it sometimes includes an aspect of functional testing to determine what the individual is physically capable of doing. The impairment evaluation addresses causality of the resulting health conditions and assigns apportionment for preexisting or coexisting condition.

The result is a disability rating. Since assignment of these ratings will have a significant impact on the individuals' future and ability to work, they must be performed in a prudent fashion. In some cases, these ratings are permanent in nature and have life-long implications for the individual's future earning capacity. The *AMA Guides to the Evaluation of Permanent Impairment* (2008) is the most widely used basis for determining impairment and may be used in federal systems, automobile casualty, and personal injury. Some state workers' compensation systems use this guide, while others may have state-specific guides specifically published for this purpose.

SUMMARY

According to data published by the World Health Organization (WHO, 2001), chronic health conditions are on the rise across all age groups in the United States, and it is expected that "conditions such as diabetes, heart disease, and cancer will add an enormous burden to already high costs of healthcare," WHO predicts that employers will be particularly challenged to provide medical benefits for workers in a cost-efficient manner while absorbing the costs of absenteeism and of long- and short-term disability claims.

The *Morbidity and Mortality Report* published by the Centers for Disease Control and Prevention (CDC, 2005) indicate the 21.8% prevalence of disability in 2005 remained unchanged from 1999. It is expected that this percentage will significantly increase due to the aging population. The three most common causes of disability continued to be degenerative diseases, spinal problems, and cardiovascular conditions, with women experiencing a higher prevalence of disability compared with men at all ages. The CDC estimates that 7 of the 10 leading causes of death in the United States are chronic diseases, and, nearly 50% of Americans live with at least one chronic illness. It is estimated that 80% of healthcare spending is expended on care for chronic conditions. (CDC, 2011). We can then expect that since health risks leading to chronic conditions are on the rise, employers will be faced with increasing issues related to disabilities and workplace productivity.

Colledge and Johnson (2000) propose that 85% of costs are usually incurred by 10% of cases and that delayed recovery points to ineffective management of cases, thus promoting disability.

A major emphasis for the future of healthcare is promoting health and wellness, with recovery as a key concept. Use of the biopsychosocial holistic approach may improve overall health, delay onset and limit the severity of chronic diseases, and promote "personal success in family, community, and work" (Manderscheid et al., 2010).

The CDC (2011) estimates that as the number of adults reporting a disability increases, there will be an increasing demand for available health services. Three aspects of the system that will affect the ability to promote health and reduce disability include: management of the *claim*, management of the *care*, and management of the *case*. Management of the claims is focused on primarily administrative issues, such as authorization for and payment of benefits. Care management aims to guide the utilization of healthcare resources in order to provide the appropriate provider at the right time during the course of the claim to assure quality outcomes. Management of the case takes these other two aspects into consideration, striving for a more holistic approach. The OHN as case manager has the potential to influence decisions related to both administration of the claim and appropriate utilization of healthcare resources. These interventions may positively impact the satisfaction of both the worker and the employer. OHNs are in a position of being able to facilitate an expanding reach within the workplace by establishing effective strategies and interventions aimed at promoting health and preventing disability.

REFERENCES

Adams, S. (2001). Risk management methods to reduce your workers' compensation rates. *Occupational Hazards*. (March).

American Association of Occupational Health Nurses (AAOHN). (2003). Position Statement. *The licensed practical nurse (LPN) in occupational health.* Retrieved from http://www.aaohn.org

American College of Occupational and Environmental Medicine (ACOEM). (2006). *Preventing needless work disability by helping people stay employed.* Retrieved from http://www.acoem.org

American College of Occupational and Environmental Medicine (ACOEM), Special Committee on Health, Productivity, and Disability Management. (2009). Healthy workforce/healthy economy: The role of health, productivity, and disability management in addressing the nation's health care crisis: Why an emphasis on the health of the workforce is vital to the health of the economy. *Journal of Occupational and Environmental Medicine, 51*(1), 117.

American College of Occupational and Environmental Medicine (ACOEM). (2010). *A guide to high value physician services in workers' compensation.* How to find the best available care for your injured workers. Retrieved from http://www.acoem.org

American College of Occupational and Environmental Medicine (ACOEM), Health and Productivity Management Center. (2011). *Elements of health-related productivity measurements.* Retrieved from http://www.acoem.org/Health ProductivityMeasurements.aspx

American Medical Association. (2008). *Guides to the evaluation of permanent impairment* (6th ed.), Chicago, IL, AMA Press.

Baicker, K., Cutler, D., & Song, Z. (2010). Workplace wellness programs can generate savings. *Health Affairs, 29*, 1–8.

Berger, M. L., Murray, J. F., Xu, J., & Pauly, M. (2001). Alternative valuations of work loss and productivity. *Journal of Occupational and Environmental Medicine, 43*, 18–24.

Burton, W., & Conti, D. (1999). The real measure of productivity. *Business & Health, 17*(11), 34–36.

Case Management Society of America. (1995). *Standards of practice for case management.* Little Rock, AK: Case Management Society of America.

Centers for Disease Control and Prevention (CDC). (2005). Prevalence and most common causes of disability among adults: United States. *Morbidity and Mortality Weekly Report, 58*(16), 421–426.

Centers for Disease Control and Prevention (CDC). (2011). *Healthy communities. Preventing chronic disease by activating grassroots change at a glance.* Retrieved from http://www.cdc.gov/chronicdisease/resources/publications/aag/pdf/2011/Healthy_Communities_AAG_Web.pdf

Colledge, A. L., et al. (2007). Cervical whiplash: Assessment, treatment, and impairment rating. *AMA: The Guides Newsletter*, pp. 1–3, 8–15.

Colledge, A. L., Hunter, B., Bunkell, L. D., & Holmes, E. B. (2009). Impairment rating ambiguity in the United States: The Utah Impairment Guides for Calculating Workers' Compensation Impairments. *J Korean Med Sci*, 24 (Suppl 2), S232–S241.

Colledge, A. L. & Johnson, H. I. (2000). The S.P.I.C.E. model for return to work. *Occupational Health and Safety*, 69(2), 64–69.

Dasinger, L. K., Krause, N., Deegan, L. J., Brand, R. J., & Rudolph, L. (2000). Physical workplace factors and return to work after compensated low back injury: A disability phase-specific analysis. *Journal of Occupational and Environmental Medicine* 42(3), 323–333.

Dasinger, L. K., Krause, N., Thompson, P. J., Brand, R. J., & Rudolph, L. (2001). Doctor proactive communication, return-to-work recommendation and duration of disability after a workers' compensation low back injury. *Journal of Occupational and Environmental Medicine*, 43(6), 515–525.

DiBenedetto, D. V. (2003). Informatics: Finding disability related information on the Web. *AAOHN Journal*, (January), 10–12.

Emmons, K., Linnan, L., Shadel, W., Marcus, B., & Abrams, D. (1999). The working healthy project: A worksite health-promotion trial targeting physical activity, diet, and smoking. *Journal of Occupational and Environmental Medicine* 417, 545–555.

Ensalada, L. H. & Brighan, C. R. (2000). Somatization. *AMA: The Guides Newsletter.* Retrieved from https://catalog.ama-assn.org/MEDIA/ProductCatalog/m1830650/2000.4.JulAug.pdf

Foster, D. (2009a). When is an injury compensable? *AAOHN Journal*, 57(11), 443–445.

Fuge, C. (2009). *Workers' compensation issues and trends 2009—The NCCI perspective.* Retrieved from http://www.irmi.com/expert/articles/2009/fuge05-insurance-workers-compensation.aspx

Goetzel, R. Z. (2005). Policy and Practice Working Group: Examining the value of integrating occupational health and safety and health promotion programs in the workplace. Retrieved from http://www.saif.com/_files/CompNews/CNexamining.pdf

Goetzel, R. Z., Guindon, A. M., Turshen, I. J., & Ozminkowskiet, R. J. (2001). Health and productivity management: Establishing key performance measures, benchmarks, and best practices. *Journal of Occupational and Environmental Medicine*, 43, 10–17.

Goetzel, R. Z., Shechter, D., Ozminkowski, R. J., Marmet, P. F., Tabrizi M. J., & Roemer, E. C. (2007). Promising practices in employer health and productivity management efforts: Findings from a benchmarking study. *Journal of Occupational and Environmental Medicine*, 49, 111–130.

Gregg, M. S., Muchmore, L. & Gardner, H. (2003). Quantifiable impact of the contract for health and wellness: Health behaviors, health care costs, disability, and workers' compensation. *Journal of Occupational and Environmental Medicine*, 45(2), 109–117.

Grieco, A., Fano, D., Carter, T. & Iavicoli, S. (Eds). (2003). *Origins of occupational health associations in the world*. Amsterdam: Elsevier Science.

Guidotti, T. L. & Rose, S. G. (2001). *Science on the witness stand*. Beverly Farms, MA: OEM Press.

Guzik, A., (1999). Workers' compensation, FMLA, and ADA: Managing the Maze. *AAOHN Journal*, 47(6), 261–274.

Guzik, A., (2007). What you should know about work-comp claims. *Arthritis Practitioner*, 3(6), 26–30.

Guzik, A., (2008). Strategies for effective occupational health case management. *Professional Case Management*, 13(1), 48–52.

Hymel, P. A. (2011). ACOEM guidance statement: Workplace health protection and promotion. A new pathway for a healthier and safer workforce. *Journal of Occupational and Environmental Medicine*, 53(6), 695–702.

Integrated Benefits Institute (IBI). (2001). *Linking medical care to productivity: Considering a new employer healthcare strategy*. Retrieved from http://www.ibi-web.org/do/PublicAccess?documentId=494

Manderscheid, R. W., Ryff C. D., Freeman E. J., McKnight-Eily L. R., Dhingra, S., Strine, T. W. (2010). Evolving definitions of mental illness and wellness. *Prevention of Chronic Disease*, 7(1), A19. Retrieved from http://www.cdc.gov/pcd/issues/2010/jan/09_0124.htm

Matheson, L. N. (1988). How do you know he tried his best? *Journal of Industrial Rehabilitation Quarterly*, 1, 10–12.

Musich, S., Napier, D., Edington, D. (2001). The association of health risks with workers' compensation costs. *Journal of Occupational and Environmental Medicine*, 436, 534–541.

National Council in Compensation Insurance (NIOSH). (2005). *Scopes manual*. Boca Raton, FL: National Council of Compensation Insurance.

National Council in Compensation Insurance (NIOSH), Commission on Health and Safety and Workers' Compensation. (2010). *The whole worker: Guidelines for integrating occupational health and safety with workplace wellness programs*. Retrieved from http://www.dir.ca.gov/chswc/WOSHTEP/Publications/WOSHTEP_TheWholeWorker.pdf

National Council in Compensation Insurance (NIOSH). (2011a). *Total worker health. Employer and employee resources*. Retrieved from http://www.cdc.gov/niosh/twh/essentials.html

National Council in Compensation Insurance (NIOSH). (2011b). *Total worker health: Integrating health protection and health promotion*. Retrieved from http://www.cdc.gov/niosh/TWH/

National Institute for Occupational Safety and Health (NIOSH). (2005). Workplace. Final Report. Retrieved from http://www.cdc.gov/niosh/TWH/history.html

Parry, T., Schweitzer, W., & Molmen, W. (2004). *The business case for managing health and productivity. Results from IBI's full-cost benchmarking program. Research by the Integrated Benefits Institute.* Retrieved from http://www.acoem.org/uploadedFiles/Career_Development/Tools_for_Occ_Health_Professional/Health_and_Productivity/IBIFull-CostResearch.pdf

Pennachio, F. (2009). Misaligned contracts drive comp costs. *The Self-Insurer.* Retrieved from http://www.workcompadvisorygroup.com/Libraries/In_the_News_-_PDFs/Misaligned_Contracts_Drive_Comp_Costs.sflb.ashx

Ramos, E. I. (2006). Occupational health nurses and case management. *Nursing Economics, 24*(1), 30–40, 3.

Randolph, S. A. *Occupational and environmental health nursing.* (2004). Retrieved from www.nsna.org/Portals/0/Skins/NSNA/pdf/Career_Randolf2.pdf

Rosenstock, L. & Cullen, M. (1994). *Textbook of clinical occupational and environmental medicine.* Philadelphia: W.B. Saunders.

Salazar, M. (2004). *Core curriculum for occupational & environmental health nursing* (3rd ed.). Philadelphia: W.B. Saunders.

Schulte, P. A. (2007). Work, obesity, and occupational safety and health. *American Journal of Public Health, 97*(3), 428–436.

Schultz, A., Lu, C., Barnett, T. E., Yen, L. T., McDonald, T., Hirschland, D., Edington, D. W. (2002). Influence of participation in a worksite health-promotion program on disability days. *Journal of Occupational and Environmental Medicine, 448*: 776–780.

Servan-Schreiber, D., Kolb, N. R., & Tabas, G. (2000a). Somatizing patients: Part I. Practical diagnosis. *American Family Physician, 61*(4), 1073–1078.

Servan-Schreiber, D., Kolb, N. R., & Tabas, G. (2000b). Somatizing patients: Part II. Practical diagnosis. *American Family Physician, 61*(5), 1423–1428.

Serxner, S., Gold, D., Anderson, D., Williams, D. (2001). The impact of a worksite health promotion program on short-term disability usage. *Journal of Occupational and Environmental Medicine, 431*, 25–29.

Serxner, S., Gold, D., Bultman, K. (2001). The impact of behavioral health risks on worker absenteeism. *Journal of Occupational and Environmental Medicine, 434*, 347–354.

U. S. Department of Labor, Bureau of Labor Statistics. (2010). *American time use survey.* Retrieved from http://www.bls.gov/news.release/atus.nr0.htm

Walker, J. M. (2003). Disabler: A game occupational health nurses cannot afford to play. *AAOHN Journal,* pp. 421–424.

World Health Organization (WHO). (2001). International classification of impairments, disabilities, and handicaps. Geneva, Switzerland: World Health Organization. Retrieved from http://www.who.int/classifications/icf/en/

WEB RESOURCES

American Association of Occupational Health Nurses, Inc. www.aaohn.org

American College of Occupational and Environmental Medicine www.acoem.org

Integrated Benefits Institute www.ibiweb.org/publications/research/15/>

Occupational Health & Safety www.ohsonline

U.S. Small Business Administration www.sba.gov/content/workers-compensation

WorkersCompensation.com www.workerscompensation.com

Managing Productivity

12

Occupational health nursing ... serving two masters ... the worker and the employer.

And the greatest impact of an occupational health nurse's role is to keep workers healthy, productive, and on the job. A significant principle in managing productivity is the focus on one's ability, rather than focusing on their disability.

The Occupational Health and Safety aspects of the U.S. *Healthy People 2010* are intended to promote the health and safety of people at work. There is an acknowledgment, however, that those workplace settings "vary widely in size, sector, design, location, work processes, workplace culture, and resources" (U.S. Department of Health and Human Services, 2010). In addition, the landscape of today's workforce varies greatly in terms of age, gender, training, education, cultural background, and health practices. In addition, access to and utilization of preventive healthcare services can vary widely among worker populations. Occupational health nurses (OHNs) have the opportunity to provide a partnership with benefits managers in order to tailor health benefits programs and services to specifically meet the needs of the population. In addition, the OHN serves as a content expert to assure regulatory compliance with a variety of regulations intended to protect and support the health of the workforce.

An integrated approach to health management focuses on reducing lost work time and maintains productivity of the workforce. Companies promoting health and wellness strive to develop strong relationships with their workers by acknowledging that they are the company's single most important investment. From prevention (wellness) to absence management, the OHN has the opportunity to establish a role that contributes greatly to the productivity and profitability of the workplace.

Workers often become engaged with one or more of the existing disability benefit systems and laws, for example, sick leave, workers' compensation,

Essentials for Occupational Health Nursing, First Edition. Arlene Guzik.
© 2013 John Wiley & Sons, Inc. Published 2013 by John Wiley & Sons, Inc.

short-term disability (STD), long-term disability (LTD), Social Security Disability Insurance (SSDI), the Family Medical Leave Act (FMLA), and the American's with Disabilities Act (ADA). As a result, the estimated total annual cost of disability benefits paid under all these systems exceeds $100 billion (ACOEM, 2010). A report on the Survey on Health, Productivity, and Absence Management Programs (Mercer, 2008) reported that 6.0% of the employer's direct business costs were related to sick, disability, and workers' compensation benefits. Yet when calculating both direct and indirect costs, the Mercer report calculated the costs at an average of 36% of the employer's payroll (25% for exempt workers, 36% for nonexempt salaried, 39% for nonunion hourly, and 49% for union hourly), including 9.2% for unplanned incidental and extended absences. The Mercer report notes that incidental unplanned absences result in the highest net loss of productivity for employers per day (Mercer, 2008).

Absences of workers have a significant impact on the profitability of the company, resulting in lost work time, reduced productivity, increased benefits costs, and decreased morale. Wages paid to absent workers, replacement costs of the worker, and the administrative responsibility to manage these benefits all contribute to the costs.

This chapter addresses the major components of productivity management within the realm of the OHN.

The profession of occupational health nursing is facing the need for rapid redevelopment as a result of demands and expectations from employers and workers with the advent of changes in the economic situation, social and health resources, and ever-changing health benefits offered in the workplace. As a result, it is important for the OHN to address the healthcare needs of worker populations in the context of the public health strategies, national health reform, and healthcare benefits laws and regulations.

According to Davis (2005), there are three general purposes that characterize disability management programs: Prevention of accidents or disabilities, initiation of coordinated strategies for return to work, and early intervention activities to decrease the effect of disability or illness risks in the workplace. In order to accomplish these purposes, the occupational health nurse needs to be confident and competent in responding to a wide variety of health-related issues in the workplace, providing the appropriate advice to both workers and their employer (Walker, 2003). The goal is to assist workers to maintain good health, maintain productivity, and to return to work with normal functioning after periods of disability.

The World Health Organization (WHO, 2001) defines the role of the OHN in workplace health management, stating that it is "important to note that the focus of the occupational health nurse's case managing is not restricted to workers' compensation injuries," since increasing numbers of employers are depending on the OHN to also manage non-work-related illnesses and absences. This approach is also intended to mitigate litigation surrounding statutory benefits, such as the FMLA and the ADA (Walker, 2003).

INTEGRATED ABSENCE MANAGEMENT

Integrated absence management aims to provide accountability for worker attendance by determining causation of the absence as being health related versus non-health related. The employer can then initiate the appropriate actions, recognizing that when workers are not at work, productivity is affected.

If the absence is identified as being related to a personal or family health situation, the OHN should become involved. Since confidentiality of health information in the workplace is a sensitive issue, the occupational health professional is best prepared to intervene. Retrieval of medical notes, medical records, and communication with healthcare professionals all fall within the realm of responsibility for the OHN. The employer should have specific written policies and procedures related to attendance and guidelines for workers on how to proceed if an absence is health related. The OHN can intervene in a number of ways to assure the worker receives the appropriate care to recover and return to work. This can be done simply by providing guidance and advice on intervention, including use of over-the-counter remedies and appropriate access to the healthcare system.

Benefit entitlement can also be addressed. The worker may be eligible for benefits under FMLA for either personal or family medical situations. It's important to expand the concept of wellness to include the total worker and not just the worker's health. Financial worries and job stress are two examples of non-health-related issues that can impact a worker's health and attendance. (Neftzger & Wallace, 2009).Other benefits may include access to an Employee Assistance Program or another community health service when appropriate. The OHN can also determine if the worker's issues are work related, and initiate the appropriate mechanisms for care under the workers' compensation system. Workers may also have health issues that can be alleviated with ergonomic interventions that will be conducive to recovery. And if the worker is expected to incur an extended period of absence, the OHN can assist in determining eligibility for short- or long-term disability benefits, and initiate the appropriate case management strategies to follow the case and establish a plan for return to work.

The impact of absenteeism in the workplace cannot be understated. Beyond the absence of the worker, the business is faced with reduced productivity, replacement workers (perhaps requiring addition training), and lowered morale, all of which can lead to decreased profitability. According to Commerce Clearing House Inc., a company that provides employment law information for human resources professionals, the 2007 survey on absenteeism in the workplace found that personal illness accounts for only 34% of unscheduled absences, while 66% of absences are due to other reasons, including family issues, personal needs, entitlement mentality, and stress (Bonacum & Allen, 2007). It has been reported that unscheduled worker absenteeism costs more than $700 per worker per year (Bonacum & Allen, 2005). According to a Mercer survey (2008), total direct and indirect costs of all major absence categories

Table 12.1 Key elements for managing absences.

- Gather the medical facts by reviewing the completed Certificate of Healthcare Provider form.
- Evaluate if the facts meet the FMLA criteria
  - Validate that the worker's condition meets the defined criteria as a serious health condition
  - Validate the need for the worker to provide assistance for basic needs or safety, for transportation, or to provide psychological comfort for a family member's serious health condition
- Establish the approximate commencement and probable duration of the serious health condition, including the probable duration of the present incapacity
- Consult with the worker to determine if an intermittent or reduced work schedule leave will be necessary
  - For intermittent leaves, determine the expected duration and anticipated frequency of periods of incapacity
- Obtain a general description of any continuing treatment regimen, including the probable number of treatments, the interval between treatments, or actual dates of treatment when known, and any period of recovery required following treatment
- Identify when the worker is able to perform work of any kind and/or when the worker is able to perform all essential functions of his or her position

average 35% of base payroll, and incidental unplanned absences have the greatest impact on productivity.

Greenhaus, Collins, & Shaw (2003) define work–family balance as the "extent to which an individual is equally engaged in and equally satisfied with their work role and family role." The National Institute for Occupational Safety and Health (NIOSH, 2009) reports that workers who work full time on evening shift, night shift, rotating shifts, work irregular schedules, or long work hours have been associated with health and safety risks. WorkLife, a program developed by the NIOSH, offers employers and workers information to promote the kinds of work environments and programs aimed at supporting a healthier and more productive workforce. NIOSH also offers suggested policies intended to result in reduced disease and injury and lower healthcare costs.

The OHN can assist human resource professionals in managing absences and productivity in the workplace. Table 12.1 offers key elements for managing absences. The OHN can provide a valued role by implementing programs and policies to both prevent and minimize the risk of health-related absences that will lead to a healthier and more productive workforce. NIOSH (2011) proposes that a most effective strategy to improve work–life balance for workers is by evaluating not only the physical and organizational work environment, but also addressing the personal health-related needs and decisions of workers and their families.

AMERICANS WITH DISABILITIES ACT (ADA)

The ADA was enacted in 1990 and was later amended with changes made by the ADA Amendments Acts of 2008 and 2010. The ADA states that employers are required to provide reasonable accommodations for workers with disabilities in order to assist the worker in performing the essential functions of the job. Employers with 15 or more workers, defined as covered entities, are required to abide by ADA law. Covered workers under the ADA include qualified individuals with disabilities and workers participating in any substance abuse rehabilitation program.

A statement from the ADA, Title 1, states " No covered entity shall discriminate against a qualified individual on the basis of disability in regard to job application procedures, the hiring, advancement, or discharge of workers, worker compensation, job training, and other terms, conditions, and privileges of employment" (USDOJ, 2005). The intent is to provide those with a disability fair and equal treatment as any other person without a disability. The Act prohibits discrimination in recruitment; restricts questions that can be asked about an applicant's disability before a job offer is made; prohibits discrimination in hiring, promotions, training, and pay; and prohibits discrimination in social activities along with other privileges of employment. (USDOJ, 2009).

It is essential for the OHN to understand the core components of the Act as a content expert to provide guidance and decisions related to situations requiring evaluation in respect to the need for accommodation. Frequent updates and interpretations of the Act occur, and the OHN holds the obligation to maintain current knowledge in this regard. Decisions related to reasonable accommodation must be sound due to the potential impact on the worker's ability to work along with the impact related to the employer's legal obligations and potential liability. Several definitions are provided in the Act that define core aspects of the law, as we discuss next.

Disability is defined as a physical or mental impairment that substantially limits one or more life activities (USDOJ, 2009). The worker must either have that disability, have a record of having a disability, or be regarded as having such impairment. An individual is regarded as having such an impairment if the individual "establishes that he or she has been subjected to an action prohibited under this chapter because of an actual or perceived physical or mental impairment whether or not the impairment limits or is perceived to limit a major life activity" (USDOJ, 2005). This last point is very significant and has potentially serious implications for the company. This point is more fully covered later in the chapter. The Act does not require employers to accommodate temporary or transitory impairments. The impairment is considered transitory if the impairment has an actual or expected duration of 6 months or less. On the other hand, if the impairment is episodic or in remission, it is a disability if it would otherwise substantially limit a major life activity when not in remission.

A *physical or mental impairment* is defined as a "physiological disorder, a condition, a disfigurement, an anatomical loss affecting one or more of the following body systems: neurological, special senses, muscular/skeletal, skin, endocrine, hepatic, genitalia, digestive, reproductive, cardiovascular, and respiratory systems." It also covers a mental or psychological disorder such as mental retardation, organic brain syndrome, emotional illnesses, mental illnesses, and learning disabilities (USDOJ, 2009). Since the inception of the Act, case law has ruled on several specific health conditions in regard to this definition, such as vision and obesity.

Major life activities include, but are not limited to, caring for oneself, performing manual tasks, seeing, hearing, eating, sleeping, walking, standing, lifting, bending, speaking, breathing, learning, reading, concentrating, thinking, communicating, and working. A major life activity also includes, but is not limited to, functions of the immune system, normal cell growth, digestive, bowel, bladder, neurological, brain, and respiratory systems. A disability does not include the following: environmental or cultural disadvantages, pregnancy, or personality traits that are not a result of a psychological disorder. Bad workplace behavior does not qualify under ADA (Anaclerio, 2005).

The term *substantially limits* means that the worker is unable to perform or has significant restrictions related to one or more life activity. These life activities include caring for oneself, walking, seeing, hearing, performing manual tasks, concentrating, breathing, learning, working, speaking, thinking, and interacting. The determination of whether an impairment substantially limits a major life activity must be made without regard to the "ameliorative effects of mitigating measures" (USDOJ, 2009), such as medication, medical supplies, equipment, or appliances, low-vision devices (which do not include ordinary eyeglasses or contact lenses), prosthetics including limbs and devices, hearing aids and cochlear implants or other implantable hearing devices, mobility devices, or oxygen therapy equipment and supplies. Decisions must also be made without regard to the use of assistive technology, auxiliary aids or services, learned behavioral or adaptive neurological modifications (USDOJ, 2009).

Case in Point

If an individual comes into human resources and has a hearing disability, yet wants to apply for a position as a telephone sales representative, the individual cannot be denied employment based on such disability. The employer is required to evaluate the ability to provide reasonable accommodations to enable the individual to perform the essential functions of the job. If a worker is required to take telephone orders, one envisions that the individual must be able to see, hear, talk, and type. That, however, is not the essential function of the job. The essential function of the job is "to take an order." It does not imply that the individual must be able to see, hear, talk, and type. If a person has a hearing disability, a TDD (telecommunications device for the deaf) system may be provided that enables the phone calls to come across the computer screen so they may be seen visually instead if heard. This may be considered a reasonable accommodation under ADA.

Essential job functions include those that are absolutely required to perform the job. The judgment of what qualifies as an essential function is basically defined by the employer and written in the job description. In order to evaluate the need for an accommodation, one must look at the amount of time spent on the function, the terms of the collective bargaining agreement, and past or current work experiences.

The duty to provide *reasonable accommodation* is an elemental statutory requirement of the ADA law that is intended to remove workplace barriers and resultant discrimination for individuals with disabilities. These barriers may be physical obstacles (such as obstacles related to facilities or equipment), or they may be procedures or policies. Reasonable accommodation includes modifications to how an individual applies for a job, modifications or adjustments to the work environment, or modifications or adjustments that enable a covered individual with a disability to enjoy equal benefits and privileges of employment" (EEOC, 2002). To provide reasonable accommodation, an employer would consider a change or adjustment to how a job is performed, such as modifying equipment, restructuring the job, adjusting work schedules, modifying training materials or processes, or making the workplace more accessible. Learning disabilities may qualify under ADA, and the provision of readers or interpreters would then qualify as a reasonable accommodation. The employer, however, is not obligated to remove essential functions or to compromise production standards in order to provide an accommodation under ADA.

Although the ADA places certain obligations on the employer to provide reasonable accommodations, the law is specific in its intent to define that the worker bears the responsibility of notifying the employer of the need for an accommodation as a result of a disability. Therefore, it is beneficial for the employer to have in place written policies and procedures for such requests, requiring that the worker's request be in writing. There are two common situations where this is beneficial. First, in order to fully determine fitness for duty, each new job candidate should be required to fill out a health history form that includes two questions: (1) Do you have a disability? and (2) Do you require an accommodation or any job modifications as a result of the disability? This form should be submitted directly to the OHN for review and intervention.

The second situation occurs when the worker, as a result of a covered condition, incurs difficulty performing the essential functions of the job and its requirements. The employer's policy and procedure should define a clear process for workers to create an awareness of the need for accommodation. The worker again should be required to submit a written request for accommodation along with supporting documentation from his or her healthcare provider. Appendix 21 provides a sample form that can be used for this purpose, Request for Workplace Accommodation.

Although the OHN should hold expert knowledge in the provisions of ADA, it is often necessary to obtain an additional opinion from another expert source, such as the company medical director or other physician with expert knowledge regarding ADA. A consultation with an occupational therapist or rehabilitation professional can provide the OHN with invaluable support in regard to the provision of medical accommodations in the workplace. The occupational therapist can offer recommendations for the use of assistive devices and physical plant improvements that will provide reasonable accommodations for the disabled worker. And although opinions may be rendered by healthcare professionals, the employer always holds the obligation to assure these recommendations are in accordance with ADA law. Therefore, consultation with a labor law attorney is often helpful. When there is a question regarding the validity of any request for accommodation, the employer has the right to a second medical opinion or review of the medical records. In order to obtain additional information or to hold a conversation with the worker's healthcare professional, a written release from the worker to obtain such information is required under the Privacy Act. This release may be obtained using the Request for Workplace Accommodation form in Appendix 21. When in doubt of the validity of any information, the employer may also request a second medical opinion at the employer's expense.

Once the request for reasonable accommodation is evaluated and all options are exhausted, there may be situations in which the employer is not able to provide the accommodation. At this point, the worker should be offered a vacant, budgeted position for which they are qualified and able perform the essential functions of the job. The worker must to be able to perform the essential functions of that job and have all of the qualifications that any other person would have in order to do that job. The employer is not obligated to create a position for a person with a disability.

There are a few situations when an employer could defend the denial to provide a reasonable accommodation. One reason is when the need for special accommodation was not known the employer. The worker may allege the employer was aware of the need and refused to accommodate, yet the employer was unaware. This is one rationale for requiring a written policy and procedure that requires the worker to submit requests for accommodation in writing. Another reason is based on business necessity, when the required job performance could not be accomplished by an accommodation. Additionally, when an accommodation would be a direct threat to the health or safety of other workers, the employer is not required to accommodate. These reasons may be defined as undue hardship, meaning that providing an accommodation would either be too expensive, too extensive, too disruptive, or actually alter the nature of the operations.

Table 12.2 defines the steps to determining the need for reasonable accommodation. The employer must take caution to follow these steps to maintain a formal process for accommodation. Workers and supervisors must know the proper procedures to the process. Otherwise, if a supervisor provides an accommodation for a worker, modifies the job, or takes away essential functions of a job as a result of a physical or mental condition, this action then justifies as

Table 12.2 Steps to determining need for reasonable accommodation.

1. Require a written request for accommodation from the worker
2. Evaluate the worker's job description and the essential functions of the job, including workplace demands, both mental and physical
3. Consult with the worker to identify the barriers to performing the job
4. Validate the presence or absence of a permanent impairment by requiring written documentation from the worker's healthcare provider defining the medical necessity of the requested accommodation
5. Evaluate the worker's capacity, both mental and physical, to perform the job functions and delineate workplace restrictions. A fitness for duty evaluation may be conducted, if necessary.
6. Ascertain the worker's ability to perform the essential functions of the job with, or without, accommodations.
7. Identify all possible reasonable accommodations.
8. Consider the accommodation of preference of the worker.
9. Document all interventions in the worker's human resources medical file.
10. Evaluate the effectiveness of the interventions after implementation.
11. Make appropriate adjustments as necessary.

a medical accommodation under ADA. This action qualifies the disability, whether or not the person has an ADA-protected disability. This, in effect, creates a "perceived disability" situation. In this case, the employer perceives the worker as having a disability and the accommodation is made despite the lack of supporting medical documentation. This may set the stage for potential liability for the company if the case comes into question in regard to the validity of the disability or need for the accommodation.

ADA protects workers while they are working. The employer is not required to provide transportation for a disabled worker. The employer is not expected to disregard attendance requirements for a worker with a disability. The employer is not obligated to assign another worker or supervisory staff to assist a disabled person with hygiene or personal matters, such as bathroom privileges or nutrition functions. The employer must assure that appropriate physical facilities are available for the disabled worker and, if further assistance is needed, allow provisions for assistance from a family member or a personal aid. Several states have specific legislation regarding substance abuse that the OHN must research. In general, a current user of illegal substances is not a protected disability. However, if that worker has entered or has completed a rehabilitation program, it is considered a covered disability. If the worker is required to be drug tested and tests positive, ADA protection ceases. Alcoholism, on the other hand, is a covered disability whether or not the worker is in a rehabilitation program.

ADA and Confidentiality
ADA law requires that medical information be filed separately from the personnel file. The law was enacted, in part, because workers were being discriminated against in regard to transfers or promotions. Before this time,

access to the personnel file also allowed access to medical information that may have influenced the hiring, transfer, promotion, or disciplinary decisions. Employers should also have a standard prohibiting discussion of medical situations in the workplace.

Annual training session provided by the OHN for managers and supervisors should cover confidentiality of protected health information. This assures appropriate triage of medical concerns to the OHN. If a worker attempts to disclose personal health information to the supervisor, the supervisor should refer the worker to the OHN. The nurse will then disclose, to the supervisor or appropriate entity, any business need regarding a medical accommodation.

Supervisors and managers are to be told about necessary restrictions and necessary accommodations, not about the specific health conditions. First aid and safety personnel may be told about a health condition if a worker might require emergency treatment, and government officials have the right to this information upon request. Otherwise, the OHN must assume the role of medical confidant and advisor.

Requests for reasonable accommodation must be addressed on a case-by-case basis. One worker may have a medical condition that interferes with one (or more) life activity that may be a qualifying condition under ADA. Another worker may have the same qualifying condition, but the condition may not interfere with any life activity. This being the case, it would not qualify for protection under ADA.

Table 12.3 outlines the OHN's role in determining reasonable accommodation. The OHN should develop partnerships with both internal and external resources in order to provide reasonable accommodations. Internal resources may include supervisors and managers, safety specialists, physical plant engineers, training and development specialists, information system specialists, and human resource managers. External resources include other occupational health professionals, vocational rehabilitation professionals, physical rehabilitation specialists, disability offices, and occupational therapists. Through a proactive approach, the OHN can assure regulatory compliance and assist with the evaluation and accommodation of workers with disabilities.

Table 12.3 OHN's role in determining reasonable accommodation.

- Assist with the establishment of policies and procedures for compliance with ADA
- Review all requests for accommodations
- Serve as the company liaison for communicating with the healthcare providers
- Approve or deny requests for medical accommodation
- Facilitate the provision of reasonable accommodations
- Evaluate the effectiveness of interventions

FAMILY AND MEDICAL LEAVE ACT (FMLA)

The FMLA, administered by the wage and hour division, requires employers of 50 or more workers to provide up to 12 weeks of unpaid, job-protected leave to eligible workers for the birth or adoption of a child or for the serious illness of the worker, their spouse, child, or parent. The FMLA law created many challenges for employers when the law came into effect, and we have now seen case law that provides a more clear definition for employers.

FMLA law was enacted in 1993 and is mandated at both federal and state levels. It is a federal law; however, some states have enacted state laws that interface with and sometimes supersede the federal law. For purposes of this chapter, the interpretation of FMLA law will be explained based on federal statute. The OHN must refer to the individual state laws for state specific regulations.

The FMLA law states that, if a worker has been employed with a company for at least 1 year, and has worked a minimum of 1,250 hours within the past 12 months, the worker is eligible for up to 12 weeks of unpaid leave time for personal or family medical leave, guaranteeing the worker same-job protection. At the end of the FMLA period, the worker must be reinstated to the same position, or an equivalent position with equal rights and benefits, working conditions, perquisites, and status (U.S. Department of Labor, 2008). Employers required to comply with the FMLA law include all public agencies, private schools, and public schools regardless of the number of workers. The law applies to private employers with at least 50 workers in one location or in various locations within a 75-mile radius (U.S. Department of Labor, 1993). If the company has satellite locations or subsidiary locations, this has a significant impact on the FMLA policies and procedures.

Because the law essentially provides every qualified worker up to 25% of their work time as FMLA leave, the company should have a solid attendance policy in place to capture absences that fall under FMLA. The company's attendance policy should interface with FMLA management and reinforce the importance of consistent medical management within the organization to assure validation of the medical necessity of FMLA leaves and appropriate application of the law.

General notice regarding FMLA benefits must be provided to workers. An FMLA poster must be in a conspicuous place. A summary of FMLA benefits must be provided in a worker handbook, or if the company does not have a handbook, a written summary must be provided to each worker. When a worker incurs 3 or more days of absence due to a health condition, the employer must notify the worker of eligibility for coverage under FMLA "as soon as practicable" (U.S. Department of Labor, 2008), usually within 2 business days of the request. The worker must be provided with oral and/or written notice of eligibility and FMLA qualification. If given orally, a written notice must follow by the next payday, unless the payday is within 1 week.

FMLA law requires the company to provide unpaid leave; however, based on company policy, workers may choose to take paid time in lieu of the unpaid time. This includes sick days, vacation days, short-term disability, or any other paid time-off benefit. FMLA should interface with any short-term disability benefit in providing wage replacement for time off, and FMLA should be integrated with vacation and short-term disability policies on how the leave will be managed and how the worker will be compensated.

The federal law states that the worker is obligated to notify the employer 30 days in advance of the leave or whenever practicable, specifically within 1 or 2 days of the worker learning of the need to take leave. The worker only has to request leave once, and it can be in the form of a verbal or written notice. For this reason, annual FMLA training for managers and supervisors is a must. The law does not state that the worker must notify human resources, the medical office, or the OHN. It states one must notify "the company," and if verbal notice is given to someone in a supervisory position, that verbal notice may be sufficient. The worker also does not have to mention or ask for FMLA protection. The worker is expected, however, to follow the established company policies and procedures for medical leave.

The employer may not require the worker to adhere to any stricter requirement for leave notice if state law or bargaining agreement allows for less advance notice. This would apply particularly if the company has a policy or a state law that states workers do not have to give 30 days advance notice. If the company has a statement in the policy book indicating that vacations can be requested 1 week in advance, the FMLA policy must be consistent with that statement. It is important that the company vacation policy mirror FMLA, thus assuring consistency. If not, and the worker chooses to take paid leave, the case must be managed under the policies and procedures for vacation or sick time.

For unforeseeable leaves, the law states that the worker must notify the employer as soon as practicable, which is defined as within 1–2 business days of learning of the need for leave (U.S. Department of Labor, 2008). It does not specifically state that the worker must be the one to make this call. The worker may notify by fax, phone, through a family member or significant other. Once notified, it is important to address the fact that the situation may qualify under FMLA, and FMLA procedures should start immediately.

The employer has the right to apply FMLA to all eligible workers' medical absences. Since the worker does not have to request FMLA, it is important to establish a system to verify reasons why workers call off work. If one knows that the absences are due to a medical situation, FMLA entitlement should be considered. A caution is that this must be applied fairly and consistently with every single worker within the organization in all company locations. Centralization of the management of FMLA in the human resources department or OHN's office assures the FMLA determination and application of the law consistently to every situation.

FMLA must be applied at the time the worker requests the medical leave. The employer does not have the right to retrospectively apply FMLA to any situation, except in the case when the company had not been advised that there was a serious health condition that interfered with the worker's ability to work. The company may retroactively apply FMLA as far back as 30 days. This again reinforces that the employer can designate FMLA after it ends only if the company did not know the reason for the leave at the time of the leave or because of a delay in obtaining medical certification. When a worker is off work, the federal law states that the company should be notified within 2 business days that the leave was because of a medical condition. The worker should give notice of the reason for the leave within 2 business days of returning to work.

Healthcare Provider
Medical certification is required for all FMLA leaves. Federal law states that when a worker misses work because of a serious health condition, a healthcare provider must certify the medical necessity of the leave. Healthcare providers can be licensed doctors, osteopaths, dentists, podiatrists, clinical psychologists, social workers, optometrists, nurse practitioners, midwifes, chiropractors and some Christian Science practitioners (U.S. Department of Labor, 2008).

Certificate of Healthcare Provider Form
The Certificate of Healthcare Provider form was devised by the U.S. Department of Labor and should serve as verification of the medical necessity of the leave. Once that form is completed, federal law prohibits the employer from asking for any additional information. The information required from the healthcare provider should relate only to the worker's reason for taking medical leave. The healthcare provider is not obligated or required to put any additional information on the form. The medical certification should indicate the worker's inability to perform any one or all of the job functions requiring the worker to be off work. If the leave is for a family medical situation, the healthcare provider must indicate the worker's need to care for the family member.

The employer's request for medical certification should be given to the worker within 1 or 2 business days of the worker giving notice of the need to be on leave. The worker is obligated to return the requested information within 15 business days in order to certify that the absence is related to a serious health condition.

Serious Health Condition
The burden is on the worker to notify the employer of a serious health condition that interferes with his or her ability to work. A serious health condition is defined as an illness or injury or an impairment of a physical or mental condition that involves hospitalization, hospice care, residential medical care or subsequent care in continuing treatment by a healthcare provider. It involves a period of incapacity for more than 3 consecutive days, two or more treatments by a healthcare provider, or one treatment by a healthcare provider with a continuing regimen or supervision. This includes one visit to the healthcare provider with prescription

medication. Sometimes it would also include treatment with over-the-counter medication, if it involves two visits to the healthcare provider. This is outlined on the third page of the U.S. Department of Labor form.

There are very specific definitions of how the healthcare provider is to complete the form. The healthcare provider must categorize the illness. If the illness does not fall into any of the stated categories, the healthcare provider marks "None of the Above," meaning it does not qualify under FMLA. If the form is not completed in entirety or if the healthcare provider does not check one of the qualifying categories, the form is not acceptable and the leave may be denied (U.S. Department of Labor, 2008).

There are some exclusions to a serious health condition, those being routine physical exams, eye exams, and dental exams. Along with those, about eight other conditions are excluded: the common cold, flu, earaches, upset stomachs, ulcers, and headaches (other than migraine headaches), routine dental ortho-dontia, and periodontal disease (U.S. Department of Labor, 2008). An exception would be the case in which these conditions are treated with prescription med-ications or involve more than one office visit, when they would be considered a serious health condition.

The healthcare provider is only obligated to give information related to the specific medical situation requiring medical leave. The company is not permitted to ask any additional information. The healthcare provider may be contacted only to clarify or authenticate aspects of the certification. As a rule of thumb, it is suggested the company accept only original copies of the Department of Labor form or fax copies directly from the healthcare provider's office. This reduces the potential for the form to be altered in any way.

If there is doubt of the authenticity of the medical certification, the employer has the right to challenge. That challenge must be at the employer's expense by covering the cost of the exam and reasonable transportation costs for a second medical opinion. That second opinion can be by a provider selected by the employer; however, it cannot be a medical officer that is regularly contracted or employed by the company.

If the second opinion differs from the first opinion, the FMLA decision may be made based on that second opinion. If the worker challenges the second opinion, the company may choose to have a third medical opinion. With a third medical opinion, it must be a healthcare provider that is jointly selected by the company and the worker. In this situation, a medical officer that is contracted or employed by the company may be selected because it is a joint agreement between the company and the worker.

The worker is entitled to provisional benefits under FMLA while the deter-mination is being made, which means that the worker can use the benefits to be off work. When the determination is made determining whether it is an FMLA qualifying event, the case must be managed appropriately. If it is not an FMLA qualifying event, FMLA hours cannot be applied to the period when the person has been off work and the worker cannot be penalized for this period.

There are only a few situations in which the employer may make a request for recertification of medical necessity. The first is at the end of that leave period when the worker asks for an extension of the leave or fails to return to work. The second situation is for a leave that is longer than 30 days. This would apply particularly to an intermittent medical leave. Another situation is when a certification is received that indicates that the worker needs to be off work for a defined period of time, but the medical situation changes, which may enable the worker to return to work with or without medical accommodations.

Denied Requests

FMLA requests may be denied, first of all, if the worker is not eligible—having not worked 1 year or 1,250 hours. The worker also does not qualify if the 12 weeks of FMLA leave has been exhausted. The leave may be denied also if the worker fails to provide adequate medical certification.

Once the worker gives notice that they do not plan to return to work because of the medical situation, FMLA benefits may be terminated. It is recommended that the employer require the worker's resignation in writing. This provides justification to the file of why FMLA benefits were terminated.

At this time, the company may choose to remove the worker from the rolls as an active worker; however, there are some situations in which an interface with the company's disability policy is appropriate. An integrated approach should be taken that supports the worker's benefits under FMLA, while adhering to company guidelines for STD and LTD benefits.

Reduced Hours or Intermittent Medical Leaves

The federal law states that a worker may also take FMLA leave on a reduced work hour basis or on an intermittent basis. A worker returning from medical leave may need reduced hours or an intermittent medical leave.

If the worker has to reduce the number of worked hours for a medical reason, it may apply to FMLA. It is important that the information system used to calculate FMLA time is based on hourly increments rather than daily increments because of intermittent medical leave. If the worker's work hours are reduced for a temporary period of time, the missed time is applied to FMLA. If the reduced hours leave is on a permanent basis, this should be considered a permanent medical accommodation evaluated under ADA. At this point, the worker may be offered a vacant, budgeted position within the company that meets the scheduling restrictions.

The intermittent medical leave means that the worker has occasional absences that interfere with the ability to work; missing an entire day, arriving to work late, or leaving work early because of the medical situation. This can be due to the worker's own personal medical condition or that of a family member who qualifies under FMLA for medical appointments, therapy, or periods of incapacity. It covers conditions such as heart disease, asthma, backaches, migraine headaches, physical therapy appointments, chemotherapy appointments, etc. It may also be used for prenatal visits for pregnancy, ill parents, or children who have medical conditions.

The intermittent medical leave becomes significant when a worker has attendance problems and is being counseled for the absences. If the worker attributes the absences to a medical situation, FMLA eligibility must be evaluated. Any medical condition that interferes with the worker's ability to work must be evaluated in relation to FMLA and ADA.

With intermittent medical leave, the absences can be foreseen or unforeseen. If the worker is aware of medical appointments in advance, the schedule may be changed to accommodate this need per standard company guidelines. If the absence is unforeseen, the intermittent absence may be covered under FMLA, as well. This has implications for workers whose medical symptoms interfere with the ability to work. It is important that these situations be managed appropriately to assure the medical necessity of the absence.

The company should not just assume that every absence the worker has is related to the serious health condition with FMLA protection. The worker is required to go through the process of applying for FMLA, establishing eligibility, and obtaining the medical certification. The worker is also obligated to notify the company within 2 business days of the absence that the absence is related to the serious health condition qualifying for FMLA. Each company should develop a form to be used as the worker's notice to the employer of intermittent absence. An example is provided in Appendix 22. This verifies that the intermittent absence is related to the serious health condition and has protection under FMLA. If the worker fails to submit the form within 2 business days, FMLA protection for the absence may be denied.

If a worker asks for an intermittent medical leave or reduced hours, the employer has the right to determine if the work schedule can be adjusted to allow the worker time from work before applying FMLA benefits. An example would be when the worker has physical therapy three times a week at 4:00 pm, but is scheduled to work from 8:00 am to 4:30 pm. The employer has the right to adjust the worked hours to accommodate this need, perhaps by having the worker work 7:00 am to 3:30 pm. This decision is based on business need in cooperation with management and human resources.

Although FMLA leave applies equally to exempt and nonexempt workers, caution should be exercised in regard to intermittent absences for an exempt worker. If the worker's position allows for flexibility of the work hours and the missed time may be offset by working additional hours, FMLA hours may be waived. If the exempt worker is able to work from home in order to make up the missed hours, this also must be taken into consideration in regard to company policy.

Pregnancy, Births, Adoption, and Foster Care

FMLA covers pregnancy and the prenatal condition, such as morning sickness and medical appointments, during the pregnancy. A significant point is that under normal conditions, pregnancy is not considered a serious health condition.

Pregnancy is not a disability, unless there is a medical complication. The Pregnancy Discrimination Act must also be taken into consideration. This means that pregnancy must be treated the same as any other medical condition qualifying for a disability. Care must be taken to apply all of these laws fairly and consistently to the pregnant person as you would with anyone else with another serious health condition. Although a normal pregnancy is not a disability and is not a serious health condition, one must consider the aspects of these laws when making decisions (Breckenridge, 1996).

The birth period or any period prior to birth when a physician certifies that the woman cannot work because of a disability qualifies for FMLA. Any qualifying time under FMLA that is used prior to birth counts toward the 12-week benefit and subtracts from any time available for use after the delivery. This should be made clear to the worker who applies for intermittent medical leave prior to the delivery date.

The prenatal period is covered under FMLA. If a pregnant worker has interference with the ability to come to work or has to leave work because of a prenatal visit, or morning sickness, or other medically appropriate situation, FMLA must be considered. The worker can be on an FMLA intermittent medical leave during the term of the pregnancy, and when the baby is born, the disability period starts, thus qualifying the worker for FMLA and/or short-term disability. With the pregnancy there is a period of physical disability when the new mother is not able to work due to childbirth. This is considered a disability and a serious health condition under FMLA. It requires a "fitness for duty" note before resuming work. However, the woman can choose to continue the leave to exhaust a total of 12 weeks to take care of the newborn child.

FMLA also covers absences from work for adoption and foster care. During the preplacement stage of the adoption or foster care, FMLA covers absences from work to attend any meetings or appointments to arrange the placement. FMLA time may also be used after placement in order to care for the child.

Both the father and the mother are eligible for up to 12 weeks of unpaid time under FMLA to care for the newly born, newly adopted, or newly placed child in the home. Importantly, if the same company employs both mother and father, they must share the 12 weeks for child care. For postbirth or postplacement care, the time may be taken either consecutively or in intermittent increments within the first 12 months of the birth or placement of the child.

Worker's Serious Health Condition

The FMLA policy should not conflict with any other company medical leave policy. These policies should interface with one another. A serious health condition means that the worker is unable to perform the functions of the job, and there is an associated period of disability. Because it is a period of disability for the worker, it is essential to require the worker to submit a "fitness for duty" release upon return to work. This is done for two reasons: (1) it verifies that the person is medically qualified to do the job, thus protecting the worker, and (2) it protects company from liability.

Any physical limitation or restriction must be evaluated under ADA. This may be done using the form in Appendix 23 as the "fitness for duty" form. The healthcare provider must indicate if the restrictions are temporary or permanent. If the restrictions are temporary, the employer is under no obligation to provide accommodations and is not required to grant return to work unless the worker is able to perform the essential functions of the job without accommodations. If the OHN is able to arrange a reasonable accommodation in order to facilitate return to work, this may benefit the company by reducing disability costs and increasing productivity, thus supporting the company mission.

If the restrictions are indicated as permanent, protection under ADA must be evaluated. A statement by the healthcare provider that the worker has a disability as defined by ADA obligates the employer to provide reasonable accommodations in order to assist the worker in performing the essential functions of the job in a safe and effective manner.

Parent, Child, or Spouse

Under the family situation, FMLA covers medical absences related to serious health conditions of the parent, child, or spouse. Leave to care for a domestic partner is not covered, unless covered by state law. Under the FMLA, the family medical situation is absence of an worker to provide physical or psychological support, including medical care, hygiene, nutritional support, transportation, psychological comfort, reassurance, or filling in for another caregiver (U.S. Department of Labor, 2008).

Documentation of a family relationship may be verified through four criteria:

1. The physician or the healthcare provider writes it on the medical certification.
2. A birth certificate to assure that they are under the age of 18.
3. A court document or a written statement from the worker as good faith.
4. Assumption that the worker is being honest unless reason to believe otherwise.

Parents are defined as biological parents. *In loco parentis* means that they acted as a parent to the worker as a child. It does not include in-laws except in three states: New Jersey, Connecticut, and District of Columbia. A child has to be under the age of 18, be a biological, adopted, or a foster child, stepchild, or a legal ward. In this case, in loco parentis means that the worker raised that child. It also covers a child over the age of 18 incapable to caring for himself or herself. A spouse is a husband or wife as defined by state law. Unmarried, domestic partners are not covered under the federal law, but they may be covered under state law (U.S. Department of Labor, 2008).

The family leave situation must be supported by medical certification. Because this leave does not involve a physical disability on the part of the worker, a fitness for duty note is not required.

Military Family Leave Entitlements
Eligible workers with a spouse, son, daughter, or parent on active duty or call to active duty status may use their 12-week leave entitlement to address certain qualifying requirements (such as attending certain military events, arranging for alternative childcare, addressing certain financial and legal arrangements, attending certain counseling sessions, and attending postdeployment reintegration briefings). FMLA also includes a special leave entitlement to care for a covered service member who has a serious injury or illness incurred in the line of duty while undergoing medical treatment, recuperation, or therapy, is in outpatient status, or is on the temporary disability retired list.

SUMMARY
To assure appropriate analysis of issues related to health conditions of workers, the OHN plays a valuable role as healthcare expert. While most benefits administrators still tend to view costs in their programs in regard to the direct costs per full-time worker, there are many other indirect benefits that can be derived from appropriate management of absences and ability to work. The lost productivity from absences and poor performance resulting from health conditions account for 71% of lost productivity, while 23% of lost productivity is attributed to actual absences from work (Stewart et al., 2003).
The OHN can demonstrate value by doing the following:

- Assisting with the establishment of written policies and procedures for health-related benefits and programs
- Reviewing all requests for medical leave
- Communicating with the healthcare providers
- Acting as the healthcare expert to make recommendations to human resources professionals on approving/denying medical leave requests
- Case managing and communicating with the worker while out on leave
- Coordinating efforts with short-term disability carrier, as applicable
- Facilitating return to work
- Addressing the need for work accommodations related to health conditions

Facilitating return to work is a key responsibility. When a worker is off work because of a personal medical disability, ADA considerations must be evaluated upon return to work. Respect the confidentiality of medical information and develop a standard practice requiring that all FMLA forms are handed directly to the nurse or directly to the medical office. In large facilities, install locked medical drop boxes in the central locations throughout the company for convenience. Supervisors and management staff must be educated regarding the confidentiality of medical information. This should be reinforced on an annual basis.
Key factors in the success of managing integrated absence and disability programs include centralized reporting of all absences and integration of all

available employee benefits. For this reason, the OHN has the opportunity to advise employers about regulatory compliance and strategies that will lead to decreased absences and disability. Remember that there are never two sides to a story, there are always multiple sides to a story. This includes the worker, the employer, coworkers, the treating healthcare providers, and rehabilitation specialists. It is important to consider input from as many sides as possible before rendering a final opinion or taking final action. The more information gained from the involved parties, the more effective the outcome.

According to Morris (2008), objective measures of the costs and outcomes of OHN strategies and interventions are critical and should be used to demonstrate the value of the role of the OHN. To address the issue of spiraling healthcare costs, initiatives that positively affect the costs of illness, lost work days, lost productivity, and disability claims can have a positive effect on the bottom line. The OHN has the opportunity to blend knowledge of occupational health with their nursing expertise to promote a safe, healthy, and productive work environment. OHNs possess a unique understanding of health and governmental regulations and compliance issues, which has quickly proven the OHN's value to the company.

REFERENCES

Agency for Healthcare Research and Quality (AHRQ). National Guideline Clearinghouse. Work Loss Data Institute. Official Disability Guidelines. (2005). *Fitness for duty.* Corpus Christi, TX: Work Loss Data Institute.

American Association of Occupational Health Nurses, Inc. (AAOHN).(2002). An in-depth look at FMLA: What is the OHN's role? AAOHN News, 22(7), 1.

American College of Occupational and Environmental Medicine (ACOEN). (2006). "Preventing needless work disability by helping people stay employed." *The Journal of Occupational and Environmental Medicine, 48*(9), 972–987.

Americans with Disabilities Act. Title 42–The Public Health and Welfare. Chapter 126–Equal Opportunity for Individuals with Disabilities. ADA Amendments Act of 2008 (P.L. 110-325), Americans with Disabilities Act of 1990, 42 U.S.C.S. § 12101 et seq. Retrieved from http://www.ada.gov/pubs/adastatute08.htm#12102

Anaclerio, N. (2005). *ADA no shelter for bad workplace behavior. Labor & employment update.* Retrieved from http://www.uhlaw.com/ada_no_shelter_bad_workplace_behavior/

Bonacum, L., & Allen, N. (2005). *CCH unscheduled absence survey: Costly problem of unscheduled absenteeism continues to perplex employers.* Retrieved from http://www.cch.com/press/news/2005/200510121h.asp

Bonacum, L., & Allen, N. (2007). *CCH 2007 unscheduled absence survey: CCH survey finds most employees call in "sick" for reasons other than illness.* Retrieved from http://www.cch.com/press/news/2007/20071010h.asp

Breckenridge, J. (1996). *Developments under the FMLA and How to Avoid the Pitfalls Which Trap the Unwary*. Tampa, Florida.

Centers for Disease Control and Prevention. (2011). Healthy Communities. *Preventing chronic disease by activating grassroots change. At a glance, 2011.* Retrieved from http://www.cdc.gov/chronicdisease/resources/publications/aag/pdf/2011/Healthy_Communities_AAG_Web.pdf

Davis, L. (2005). Disabilities in the workplace: recruitment, accommodation, and retention. *AAOHN Journal, 53*(7), 306–312.

D'Arruda, K. A. Supreme Court Update—*Toyota Motor Manufacturing v. Williams. AAOHN Journal, 50*(5), 210–212.

Denniston, P. L., & Whelan, P. (2005). Benchmarking medical absence: Measuring the impact of occupational health nursing. *AAOHN Journal, 53*(2), 84–93.

Goetzel, R. Z., (2001). Health and productivity management: Establishing key performance measures, benchmarks, and best practices. *Journal of Occupational and Environmental Medicine.* Retrieved from http://www.acoem.org/Page3Column.aspx?PageID=7351&id=1330

Goetzel, R. Z. (2005). Policy and Practice Working Group Examining the Value of Integrating Occupational Health and Safety and Health Promotion Programs in the Workplace: Final Report January 2005. National Institute of Occupational Safety and Health (NIOSH) #211-2004-M-09393.

Greenhaus, J. H., Collins, K. M., & Shaw, J. D. (2003). The relation between work–family balance and quality of life. *Journal of Vocational Behavior, 64*(3), 510–531.

Guzik, A. (2008). Strategies for effective occupational health case management. *Professional Case Management*, January/February, 48–52.

Guzik, A. (1999). Workers' compensation, FMLA, and ADA: Managing the maze. *AAOHN Journal, 47*(6), 261–274.

Guzik, A. (2008). Strategies for effective occupational health case management. *Professional Case Management*, January/February, 48–52.

Kravetz, S., Dellario, D., Granger, B., & Salzer, M. (2003). A two-faceted work participation approach to employment and career development as applied to persons with a psychiatric disability. *Psychiatric Rehabilitation Journal, 26*, 278–289.

Krieger, N. (2010). Workers are people too: Societal aspects of occupational health disparities—An ecosocial perspective. *American Journal of Industrial Medicine, 53*, 104–115.

Integrated Benefits Institute. (2004). *The business case for managing health and productivity. Results from IBI's full-cost benchmarking program.* Retrieved from http://acoem.org/uploadedFiles/Career_Development/Tools_for_Occ_Health_Professional/Health_and_Productivity/IBIFull-Cost Research.pdf

Matt, S. & Butterfield, P. (2006). Changing the disability climate: Promoting tolerance in the workplace. *AAOHN Journal, 54*(3), 129–133.

McCunney, R. J. (2001). Health and P\productivity: A role for occupational health professionals. *Journal of Occupational and Environmental Medicine.* Retrieved from http://www.acoem.org/Page3Column.aspx?PageID=7351&id=1366

Mercer. (2008). *The total financial impact of employee absences: Survey highlights.* Retrieved from http://www.kronos.com/AbsenceAnonymous/media/Mercer-Survey-Highlights.pdf

Miller, C. (2011). An integrated approach to worker self-management and health outcomes: Chronic conditions, evidence-based practice, and health coaching. *AAOHN Journal, 59*(11), 491–501.

MorningStar Health, Inc. (2008). FMLA absenteeism and costs. Unpublished raw data.

Morris, J. A. (2008). Integrated absence management and the Family and Medical Leave Act. *AAOHN Journal, 56*(5), 207–214.

National Institute for Occupational Safety and Health (NIOSH). (2009). Centers for Disease Control and Prevention. Work Schedules: Shift Work and Long Work Hours. Retrieved from http://www.cdc.gov/niosh/topics/workschedules/

National Institute for Occupational Safety and Health (NIOSH). (2010). Centers for Disease Control and Prevention. Stress . . . At Work. Retrieved from http://www.cdc.gov/niosh/docs/99-101/

National Institute for Occupational Safety and Health (NIOSH). (2011). Total Worker Health: Essential Elements of Effective Workplace Programs. Retrieved from http://www.cdc.gov/niosh/twh/essentials.html

Neftzger, A., & Wallace, S. (2009). Society for Human Resource Management. Why Employee Well-Being Matters to Your Bottom Line. Retrieved from http://www.shrm.org/hrdisciplines/benefits/Articles/Pages/EmployeeWellBeing.aspx

Rector, B. (2006). *Selected recent FMLA developments.* Paper presented at the Grand Rapids Bar Association Labor & Employment Law Section, Grand Rapids, MI.

Salazar, M. (2004). *Core curriculum for occupational & environmental health nursing* (2nd ed.). Philadelphia: W.B. Saunders.

Stave, G. M., Muchmore, L., & Gardner, H. (2003). Quantifiable impact of the contract for health and wellness: Health behaviors, health care costs, disability, and workers' compensation. *Journal of Occupational and Environmental Medicine, 45*(2), 109–117.

Stewart, W. F., Ricci, J. A., Chee, E., Morganstein, D., Lipton, R. (2003). Lost Productive Time and Cost Due to Common Pain Conditions in the US Workforce *Journal of the American Medical Association, 290*(18), 2443–2454.

U.S. Department of Health and Human Services. (2010). *Healthy people 2010.* Retrieved from http://healthypeople.gov/2020/topicsobjectives2020/overview.aspx?topicid=30

U.S. Department of Justice. Civil Rights Division. (2005). *A guide to disability rights laws.* Retrieved from http://www.ada.gov/cguide.pdf

U.S. Department of Justice (USDOJ). (2009). Americans with Disabilities Act of 1990, as amended. Current text of the Americans with Disabilities Act of 1990 incorporating the changes made by the ADA Amendments Act of 2008. Retrieved from http://www.ada.gov/pubs/adastatute08.htm#12112a

U.S. Department of Labor. (1993). *The Family and Medical Leave Act*. Retrieved from http://www.dol.gov/whd/regs/statutes/fmla.htm

U.S. Department of Labor (2008). Wage and Hour Division. The Family and Medical Leave Act of 1993, as amended. Retrieved from http://ecfr.gpoaccess. gov/cgi/t/text/text-idx?c=ecfr&sid=48d6ee3b99d3b3a97b1bf189e1757786& rgn=div5&view=text&node=29:3.1.1.3.53&idno=29

U.S. Department of Labor. (2009). *The Family and Medical Leave Act of 1993*. USDOL Publication, Federal Regulations Part 825. Washington, DC: US Government Printing Office.

U.S. Department of Labor. (2011). Employee Benefits Security Administration. Consumer Information on Healthplans. Retrieved from http://www.dol. gov/ebsa/consumer_info_health.html

U.S. Department of Labor. *Title 29 Part 1630—Regulations to implement the equal employment provisions of the Americans with Disabilities Act*. Retrieved from http://www.ecfr.gpoaccess.gov/

U.S. Equal Employment Opportunity Commission (EEOC). (2000). *Enforcement guidance: Disability-related inquiries and medical examinations of employees under the Americans with Disabilities Act*. Retrieved from http://www.eeoc.gov/ policy/docs/guidance-inquiries.html

U.S. Equal Employment Opportunity Commission (EEOC). (2002). *Enforcement guidance: Reasonable accommodation and undue hardship under the Americans with Disabilities Act*. Retrieved from http://www.EEOC.gov

Walker, J. M. (2003). Disabler: A game occupational health nurses cannot afford to play. *AAOHN Journal*, pp. 421–424.

Wallace, M. A. (2009). Occupational health nurses—The solution to absence management? *AAOHN Journal*, 57(3), 122–127.

Weiss, M. D. (2011). Creating Health connections for vulnerable working populations: Goodwill North Central Wisconsin's Circles of Good Care Model. *AAOHN Journal*, 59(12), 519–524.

World Health Organization (WHO). (2001). *The role of the occupational health nurse in workplace health management*. Copenhagen: WHO Regional Office for Europe. Retrieved from http://www.who.int/occupational_health/regions/ en/oeheurnursing.pdf

RESOURCES

Publications and information on EEOC-enforced laws may be obtained by calling the Job Accommodation Network:

(800) 669-3362 (voice)

(800) 800-3302 (TTY)

For information on how to accommodate a specific individual with a disability, contact the Job Accommodation Network at:

West Virginia University
PO Box 6080
Morgantown, WV 26506-6080
(800) 526-7234 (voice/TTY)

http://www.jan.wvu.edu

Promoting Health and Well-Being

13

"Hire them well, teach them well, and keep them well".

(Guzik, 2012)

Each year in the United States, chronic disease such as heart disease, stroke, cancer, and diabetes affects nearly 50% of the population and causes 7 in 10 deaths, accounting for about 75% of the $2 trillion spent on medical care (CDC, 2011c). The U.S. Bureau of Labor Statistics estimates that workers spend an average of 8.6 hours, nearly 50% of their waking time, at work (see Figure 13.1), and states that private health insurance obtained through the workplace continues to be the major source of insurance, covering 157.9 million people or 61.6% of the population. Together, chronic illnesses (e.g., cancer, obesity, depression) cause Americans to miss 2.5 billion days of work each year, resulting in lost productivity totaling more than $1 trillion (Kessler et al., 2001). By focusing on the prevention and control of chronic diseases, workplaces can support the National Prevention Strategy: America's Plan for Better Health and Wellness, established by the Centers for Disease Control and Prevention (CDC). One strategic direction of the National Prevention Strategy is that of building healthy and safe community environments (CDC, 2011a): One community environment can be the workplace.

The wellness movement started back in the 1970s and has continued to evolve through the years to better address the needs of workers in a variety of ways. Although there are many definitions of wellness, a few fundamental definitions are addressed here. Dr. Bill Hettler, cofounder of the National Wellness Institute (NWI) and early pioneer in wellness, defined an interdependent model consisting of six dimensions of wellness: physical, emotional, spiritual, intellectual, social, and occupational. The model created a foundation for wellness strategies that was holistic in nature. The NWI defines wellness as "an active process through which people become aware of, and make choices toward, a more successful existence" (Hettler, 1976). Even in those early years,

Essentials for Occupational Health Nursing, First Edition. Arlene Guzik.
© 2013 John Wiley & Sons, Inc. Published 2013 by John Wiley & Sons, Inc.

	Hours
Working and work-related activities	8.8
Sleeping	7.6
Leisure and sports	2.5
Other	1.7
Caring for others	1.2
Eating and drinking	1.1
Household activities	1.1
Total	24.0

Figure 13.1 Time use on an average work day for employed persons age 25–54 with children. *Note*: Data include employed persons on days they worked, ages 25–54, who lived in households with children under 19. Data include nonholiday weekdays and are annual average for 2010. *Source*: Bureau of Labor Statistics, American Time Use Survey. http://www.bls.gov/tus/charts

the occupational dimension was a significant factor, recognizing that a healthy workplace contributes to one's wellness. The concept of wellness has more recently been defined by the National Wellness Association as "an active process of becoming aware of and making choices toward a more successful existence."

More recent definitions continue to focus on a holistic model, encompassing the individual, the workplace, and the community as significant factors. Berry et al. (2010) define workplace wellness as "an organized, employer-sponsored program that is designed to support employees (and, sometimes, their families) as they adopt and sustain behaviors that reduce health risks, improve quality of life, enhance personal effectiveness, and benefit the organization's bottom line." Hymel et al. (2011) define workplace health protection and promotion as the "strategic and systematic integration of distinct environmental, health, and safety policies and programs into a continuum of activities that enhances the overall health and well-being of the workforce and prevents work-related injuries and illnesses."

Through the past several years, despite the evolving definitions of health and wellness and despite multiple wellness strategies, we still struggle with having a consistent, measurable product with which to enhance the health of the workforce that leads to minimizing disability and promoting productivity. Many methods have been implemented in various work settings that aim to positively impact the health and wellness of workers and their families. Access, utilization, and cost of care continue to be a challenge. However, there is no one-size-fits-all model that can be implemented across workplaces that demonstrates consistent results.

Access to Care

The workplace continues to be the primary source of health insurance accessing the health system through an employer-funded or employer-sponsored product (Main, 2008). But because of variations in eligibility requirements and variations in health plans offered by employers, we are faced with a lack of consistency in what workers and their families can expect as a valued benefit. In most workplaces, workers must work a minimum number of hours to be eligible for participation in the group health benefits program. Often, part-time or temporary workers are not eligible for participation. Workers are also frequently required to complete a waiting period before they can enroll in the employer's health benefit program, usually between 30 and 90 days. During this period, many go without health insurance coverage. Once eligibility requirements are met, the worker is then faced with making choices regarding the type of benefit program that will best meet his or her healthcare needs; however, it is often difficult for the worker to understand the various options presented. The options usually have variances related to the co-premium cost (how much the employer contributes versus how much the worker contributes toward the cost of the premium) and variances in copays associated with the use of healthcare services. These options are often confusing to the worker and hold great meaning for those who have existing health conditions requiring healthcare visits or the use of pharmaceuticals on a regular basis. The worker often wonders: Should I choose the plan where I pay more in monthly premiums and less in copays, or should I choose the plan where I pay less in premiums and more for copays and deductibles? Variances in deductibles are often confusing. Certain covered services related to preventive healthcare may not involve a monetary deductible, but services required for illness-related services often require the worker to pay the first contributing dollars to reach the threshold of the deductible before the plan begins to cover the services. The worker then gambles on decision making based on current healthcare needs, running the risk that it will continue to provide a valued benefit should their healthcare needs change. The option to carry supplemental insurance is often offered to workers as well. This includes insurance that supplements the coverage paid by the primary plan for certain health conditions, such as cancer, or offers additional options for coverage for dental and vision plans. Some options provide additional financial support by helping to pay for services the standard insurance doesn't cover. Pharmacy plans may also differ under the available options, limiting pharmacy choices and limiting coverage for certain pharmaceuticals. Copays may vary for generic versus brand-name pharmaceuticals or for the use of community pharmacies versus mail-order pharmacies. All of these choices affect the pocketbook of plan holder: the worker. Once the worker

265

becomes familiar with the plan, and may be established with a primary care provider, specialist(s), and pharmacy vendor, it is not uncommon for the employer to change the plan at the end of the benefit year. This usually occurs because the employer is faced with increases in cost of premiums. As a result, the employer jockeys to evaluate other plan options that pose a most affordable choice for both the employer and the worker in order to mitigate rising costs. The end decision may require workers to change healthcare providers or service vendors because they are not participants in the new plan. Disruption of continuity of care and established relationships occurs for workers and their covered family members.

Utilization of Care
Although the worker may be covered under the health insurance benefit, many fail to use the healthcare system in a proactive manner. Many fail to have established primary care providers and fail to participate in annual preventive checkups. The insurer fails to require primary care evaluations as incentive to promote health and well-being as an eligibility requirement. As a result, care becomes episodic in nature—illness-related rather than wellness-related. Some primary care providers will not provide care to the ill person unless the person is an "established" patient. Now required copays and deductibles become a disincentive to use the benefit, until the covered individual is acutely ill. Entry into the healthcare system then becomes catastrophic, and the common entry is through use of the most expensive option: the emergency department. This often is one of the primary drivers of increasing cost under the insurance plan.

The healthcare system is attempting to mitigate this situation with the proliferation of urgent care centers that are an intermediary option between primary care and the emergency department. The urgent care center will accept unscheduled, walk-in appointments and take care of those conditions that do not require true emergency intervention. Conditions commonly encountered in the urgent care environment are self-limiting conditions that are not of a chronic nature.

Cost of Care
Employers, faced with rising health insurance premiums year after year, are strategizing on ways to mitigate this erosion to profits, as well. According to Mercer (2011b), healthcare benefits costs are expected to increase by 5.4% in 2012, well over the general rate of inflation of 3.9%. As a result, employers again may be strategizing on ways to shift the burden of this cost increase to workers. Over the years, we have seen the evolution of health benefits plans to include multiple options, such as health maintenance organization (HMO) plans or preferred provider organization (PPO) plans. New on the forefront of benefits plans that strive to shift cost and drive healthy behaviors are consumer-directed health plans (CDHPs), involving high deductibles and a health savings account. The health-savings account (HSA) is a tax-deferred account that permits a

set-aside fund that can be used for qualified medical expenses that are not covered as a as results of a deductible, copay, or other noncovered expenses. The contributions to the fund may be made by either the employer or the worker. It continues to grow year after year as a tax-deferred fund, and it is portable. The intent is to encourage the covered individuals to become a savvier healthcare consumer, considering they are now spending money out of their own savings account. (HSA Resource Center, 2003).

The Mercer survey 2011b) also found that healthcare use seems to be slowing. Several reasons for this were proposed, such as the hard economic times and the increased use of workers covered under HSAs, which may have an influence since they are spending their own money. Or, another thought is that workplace health and wellness promotion strategies may be more effective. However, there is no objective data available that can prove the reason for this trend.

WELLNESS IN THE WORKPLACE

Access to wellness programs through group health benefits has typically ranged from 23% to 31% (USDOL, 2010a), with worksites with more than 100 workers being three times more likely to offer wellness programs to their workers. Access to health and wellness programs vary significantly based on worksite size (see Figure 13.2). Those who work for state and local government and those worksites with the presence of collective bargaining agreements are

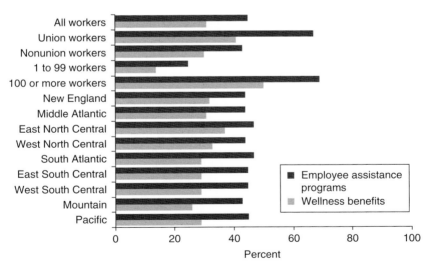

Figure 13.2 Percentage of workers with access to employee assistance and wellness programs, by census division, size of establishment, and union status, private industry, National Compensation Survey, 2012.
Source: U.S. Bureau of Labor Statistics. http://www.bls.gov/opub/cwc/cm20110519ar01p1.htm

more likely to offer health and wellness programs; however, there is not much variation based on geographic location of the worksite across the United States (Mayfield, 2011). The number of individuals with chronic diseases is increasing, yet health systems continue to be specialty focused on acute health problems leading to fragmented care (Marcy, 2010). The individual ends up being treated by multiple specialists, without the value of having a single healthcare provider managing his or her care. Diseases thus are also often unmanaged.

The use of incentive programs to encourage worker participation in health and wellness programs is rising (Mercer, 2011b). In years past, it was common for employers to offer small financial perks (such as gift cards) or small gifts and tokens. Employers have recently shifted those incentives to impact the amount of premium contribution to the health benefit made by the employer. For example, in order to participate in a health benefits plan with a lower deductible, the covered individual may be required to participate in certain health promotion activities. These may include biometric screenings, annual physical exams, preventive health screenings, etc. The use of health risk assessments (HRAs), as a requirement for participation, has also become popular. The HRA aims to identify modifiable lifestyle behaviors that may lead to health risks. This information is then used to provide the covered individual with information that would lead to a healthier lifestyle by modifying behavior to eliminate or reduce risk of disease or accident. Examples include smoking cessation, use of seatbelts, increased exercise, etc. The HRA can be completed annually and provides a measure of health improvement and risk reduction as a result of this health promotion strategy. The information gleaned from the HRA also provides the insurer or employer with aggregate data from the covered population that can also serve to predict risk and measure the impact on health and wellness strategies over time. By using this aggregate data, the employer/insurer can initiate specific programs that would have the greatest interest and benefit to the covered population.

Another strategy by employers to attempt to control healthcare costs is the development of employer-sponsored on-site health clinics (Mercer, 2011c). Traditionally, company based on-site clinics have been staffed by occupational health nurses (OHNs) with a focus on delivering occupational health services, such as regulatory exams, medical surveillance, and injury management. An evolution to expand those services to include urgent care, primary care, and even specialty and ancillary services is becoming popular, mostly with large employers. The rationale is to provide convenient, efficient access to a cost-effective means of healthcare delivery that focuses on appropriate use of the healthcare system. In other words, the employer is now in control of the delivery of healthcare for their population.

Some employers choose to establish these on-site clinics as part of the business strategies by expanding existing occupational health clinics. Most are large employers whose program is under the supervision of a corporate medical director, and the expansion of services is simply an extension of the existing structure of healthcare services offered to workers. Other employers choose to contract with third-party vendors to establish and/or staff the on-site clinic. The decision to establish an on-site clinic relies on the structure of the employer's health benefits program, requiring a self-funded program rather than one that is fully insured under an insurance carrier. Obviously, a large, nondispersed workforce is also a key aspect since the on-site clinic is tailored to support population-based healthcare. This same approach works for smaller employers as well. Strategies to solicit the resources of a community health system to provide on-site services can produce the same effect. In some cases, coalitions of small or mid-size employers have developed employer-sponsored clinics through a cost-sharing approach.

The clinic may provide urgent care, primary care, and/or specialty medical care. Pharmacy, physical therapy, and laboratory services are usually amenities that can provide an early and measurable means of cost containment since it eliminates choice of service vendor by the covered member. A comprehensive program will include occupational health services, urgent and primary care services, on-site pharmacy and laboratory, physical therapy and fitness center, employee assistance services, case management, and health education and coaching. Directed access to within a limited network of medical specialists, diagnostics services, and out-patient and in-patient services provides a further extension of a comprehensive program. Cost and quality are then able to be controlled in a very broad fashion by "hiring them well, teaching them well, and keeping them well."

Certain risks are inherent in establishing an employer-sponsored clinic. Along with management support, support from the workers is vital to assure participation in the benefit design using the employer-sponsored clinic. When the doors open, you want workers and their covered dependents to benefit from a welcoming, professional environment that is nonthreatening. The most common concern of workers is that the employer will have access to their health information. The assurances of privacy along with the development of a trusting environment are key underpinnings for success. The long-term success of the program depends on the worker making the choice to participate in the benefit plan that includes use of the employer-sponsored clinic and the willingness to participate in the health and wellness strategies that are required components of the program. Because the employer is investing financial and human capital in the program, a long-term strategy for measureable success is most important. Therefore, careful planning and the inclusion of workers in the conceptual phase of the program development are important. The value to the employer is not the only deciding factor to be considered. The perceived value to the workers and their covered dependents is sometimes most important.

WELLNESS—HOW DOES IT REALLY WORK?
Guiding Principles
The foundation of a successful occupational health and safety program is built on the principles of public health, with the underpinning foundation being senior management support and expectation for a safe workplace and protection of workers. Working with a fixed population of workers, the program is then built around applied science principles of the specialties of safety, industrial hygiene, toxicology, and epidemiology to identify risks and determine prevention strategies. Through our experience with safety initiatives, we have found that management support is demonstrated through financial support and allocation of resources needed for a successful program. The guiding principles are supported by senior management, and an environmental health and safety manager is held accountable for the establishment and outcomes of the program. Strategies are then implemented that are intended to reduce risk and increase safety, leading to a reduction in accidents, injuries, and illnesses as a result of an unsafe workplace. Metrics are measured to demonstrate success of the program, specifically to validate the financial return on investment, thus assuring accountability. Over the years, we have seen clear evidence that an emphasis on workplace safety makes a difference.

Truly integrated programs that comprehensively address both health promotion and health protection in a systematic fashion are most effective. These programs blend the "wellness community" and the "safety community" with the same focus on safety and health awareness that companies adopted over the last 40 years in response to workplace illness and injuries. Employers of any size can engage a strategy that systematically integrates their health promotion and safety programs, policies, and processes (Hymel et. al., 2011).

The same principles used to reduce workplace illness and injury, when applied to the establishment of a health and wellness promotion program, should also make a difference (Tables 13.1 and 13.2).

Support from leadership that includes a strong philosophy of supporting the health of the population serves as a foundation of the program. By working with a defined group of workers and health benefits program dependents, a fixed population exists. Guiding principles are supported by senior management and a worksite health and wellness manager is held accountable for the establishment and outcomes of the program. The applied science of preventive health, using guiding principles grounded in evidence-based interventions, becomes the focus. Strategies for risk identification and stratification are implemented, with focus on identifying and preventing the leading cost drivers, the causes of disability and their underlying factors. Programs can then be established, aimed at identifying those at risk. Interventions are prioritized with emphasize on those that prove effective, have an impact, and that are sustainable. Lastly, accountability is ensured by specifying goals, defining metrics,

Table 13.1 Comparative principles of safety and wellness programs.

Environmental Health and Safety Principles	Health and Wellness Promotion Principles
Know Your Workforce	Know Your Population
• Age	• Age
• Gender	• Gender
• Culture	• Culture
• Health & Safety Issues	• Health & Safety Issues
Know Your Workplace	Know Your Community
• Hazards	• Hazards
• Risks	• Risks

Table 13.2 Comparative structure of safety and wellness programs.

Safety	Wellness
• Leadership—Principles are supported by senior management, and an environmental health and safety manager is held accountable for the establishment and outcomes of the program	• Leadership—Principles are supported by senior management, and a worksite health and wellness manager is held accountable for the establishment and outcomes of the program
• Fixed Population—Workers	• Fixed Population—Workers and health plan dependents
• Apply Best Science—Environmental health and safety, industrial hygiene, toxicology, epidemiology	• Apply Best Science—Preventive health and disease management
• Financing—Operative expenses are supported and are a part of the annual fiscal budget	• Financing—Operative expenses are supported and are a part of the annual fiscal budget
• Strategies—Based on prevention; to include administrative, engineering, and work practice controls, along with personal protection that proves effective	• Strategies—Based on prevention and early intervention; to include planning, assessing, implementing and evaluating program effectiveness

and establishing methods to evaluate the effectiveness of the program (NPHPPHC, 2011). Figure 13.3 provides a figurative overlay of the financial impact of the safety and health continuum.

Leadership and a Culture of Support

Leadership support is vital for the success for any health and wellness program. According to Mercer (2011c), workplaces that have strong supportive culture established by senior leadership tend to have higher participation by workers in health and wellness activities. Although discussed later in this chapter, the need for leadership support must come first. Many attempts are often made to establish health and wellness programs without gaining leadership support, only to find that despite interest by the workers, the funding of the program was not supported by top management. So it must start at the top in order to have the greatest effect.

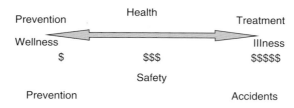

Figure 13.3 Safety and health cost continuum.
Source: Guzik, A. (2003). Maximizing the Value of Your Occupational Health Program. PowerPoint presentation in New York, NY.

Table 13.3 Role of health and wellness committee.

- Evaluate current programs, services, and policies that are available at the workplace.
- Develop a health promotion operating plan, including a vision statement, goals, and objectives.
- Develop strategies for assessing worker needs and preferences.
- Assist in implementing, monitoring, and evaluating health and wellness promotion activities.

Source: Centers for Disease Control. *Healthier Worksite Initiative*. (2010). http://www.cdc.gov/nccdphp/dnpao/hwi/programdesign/wellness_committees.htm

    The culture must exist and be supported at the highest level of the organization. This support not only provides the financial funding for the health initiatives, but incorporates the expectation of health promotion as a core requirement in business objectives. The attitude of health and wellness must exude throughout the organization and trickle down from management and their support of health and productivity. A common philosophy that health supports productivity must be a core theme of the business. Members of the leadership team should be visible supporters and participants in health and wellness strategies.

    The strategies for health and wellness promotion should be governed by a core group of workers as part of the health and wellness committee, otherwise known as ambassadors of health and wellness. As part of the Healthier Worksite Initiative, the CDC (2010a) proposes certain roles of a health and wellness committee (Table 13.3). Cost calculators are also available through the CDC website to help estimate the costs of lifestyle factors and preventable diseases. This type of information can be quite useful in establishing baseline information and for planning intervention strategies.

    The establishment of a health and wellness committee mimics the same strategy and approaches used in promoting safety. For years, we have used safety teams or committees, comprised of grass-roots members representing all aspects of the workplace, to establish and promote a culture of safety in the workplace. And it has proven quite beneficial in changing attitudes and driving safe practices through the workplace. The same can happen with health and wellness promotion.

Framework

The National Institute for Occupational Safety and Health (NIOSH) believes that the engagement of management in the well-being of its workforce will lead to having the safest and healthiest workers in an environment that is free of hazards, an environment in which workplace policies and interventions encourage healthy choices. In other words, the workplace is focused on the total health of both the workplace and the workers.

The National Prevention Strategy recognizes that the achievement of optimal health comes not just from receiving quality healthcare, but also from "clean air and water, safe outdoor spaces for physical activity, safe worksites, healthy foods, violence-free environments and healthy homes" (NPHPPHC, 2011). It cites the workplace as having a role in creating a healthier nation. With better health, individuals are more productive at work and miss work less often. The U.S. Department of Health and Human Services estimates that asthma, high blood pressure, smoking, and obesity each reduce annual productivity by between $200 and $440 per person (USDHHS, 2011c). So by knowing that the prevention and control of disease can increase productivity, targeted interventions that focus on risk reduction and health maintenance become vital to the work population.

Preventable health risks such as tobacco and excessive alcohol use, insufficient physical activity, and poor nutrition contribute to the development and severity of many chronic diseases. For example, tobacco use is known to be the single most avoidable cause of disease and disability. By effectively addressing chronic disease through health and wellness promotion efforts, the program provides parallel support for improving the health of our nation (CDC, 2011a).

Several templates and models for health and wellness promotion exist and have been an established priority for policy makers and for public and private health insurance plans. The Agency for Healthcare Research & Quality's (AHRQ) Prevention and Chronic Care Program (2012) provides a list of prevention and chronic care resources available for health care professionals, researchers, consumers/patients, and communications professionals, intended to improve primary care practice and assist with evidence-based decision making. The Prevention and Chronic Care Program focuses on the establishment of clinical–community linkages to better coordinate healthcare delivery in the context of public health in order to promote healthy behavior. The workplace can form partnerships and relationships among clinical, community, and public health organizations to serve as strategic partners in health and wellness efforts. By using community services, families can also be included in health and wellness promotion activities.

The Prevention and Chronic Care Program guidelines focus on individuals being active healthcare consumers and participants in managing their health. Initiatives include (1) exercise and fitness; (2) healthy eating and nutrition; (3) healthy lifestyle focused on weight loss, tobacco cessation, and accident prevention; (4) age-appropriate vaccinations and health screenings through primary care initiatives; and (5) healthy environments, including the workplace.

These same initiatives can serve as the structure for workplace health and wellness programs (AHRQ, 2010).

The Healthy People Initiative (USDHHS, 2012a) provides a 10-year initiative for improving the health of the nation. The Healthy People 2020 leading health indicators (LHIs) place emphasis on specific strategies that will be monitored over the course of the decade in support of improving the health of the nation. These LHIs can be also used as the foundation of a worksite health and wellness program that focuses on indicators specific to the workplace population, consistent with Health People 2020 mission and goals (Table 13.4). Examples of such initiatives include access to health services; focus on preventive service;

Table 13.4 Healthy People 2020.

Healthy People 2020 strives to:

Mission
- Identify nationwide health improvement priorities.
- Increase public awareness and understanding of the determinants of health, disease, and disability and the opportunities for progress.
- Provide measurable objectives and goals that are applicable at the national, state, and local levels.
- Engage multiple sectors to take actions to strengthen policies and improve practices that are driven by the best available evidence and knowledge.
- Identify critical research, evaluation, and data collection needs.

Overarching Goals
- Attain high-quality, longer lives free of preventable disease, disability, injury, and premature death.
- Achieve health equity, eliminate disparities, and improve the health of all groups.
- Create social and physical environments that promote good health for all.
- Promote quality of life, healthy development, and healthy behaviors across all life stages.

Leading Health Indicators
- Physical activity
- Overweight and obesity
- Tobacco use
- Substance abuse
- Responsible sexual behavior
- Mental health
- Injury and violence
- Environmental quality
- Immunization
- Access to health care

Source: U.S. Department of Health and Human Services, http://www.healthypeople.gov/2020/about/default.aspx

improving environmental health and safety; improving nutrition, activity, and preventing obesity; tobacco cessation and substance abuse. These LHIs can prove beneficial as the basis for worksite health and wellness promotion programs. For example, the CDC has established a public health campaign to improve cardiovascular health that helps communities, worksites, and individuals engage in strategies to reduce the prevalence of heart disease and stroke. Worksite health and wellness programs can be tailored through educational and awareness campaigns based on these strategies. (See Sample Wellness Program, Appendix 24.)

Population Focused Initiatives

So many worksite wellness efforts focus on strategies aimed at individuals, offering isolated health education or screening activities. Little value is reaped from a single event. The only value served is to perhaps increase the awareness of the individual regarding an associated health risk (such as blood pressure screening, cholesterol screening). In order to achieve the far-reaching goal of having a healthy workforce and improving productivity, the program must encompass a consistent and sustainable process based on education, screening, and prevention and based on a comprehensive effort that promotes preventive health as the foundation of the health benefits program. A worksite health and wellness program should strive to create a culture of health of all individuals, despite their participation in the company-sponsored benefits program, and health of the environment in the workplace as well as in the community.

The CDC's (2011d) Worksite Health Promotion platform defines four elements necessary for a comprehensive health and wellness program:

1. Individual—focused on lifestyle and health behavior changes that impact health risk and health status
2. Interpersonal—focused on social networking within the workplace, within the family, and within the community that provides an atmosphere of social support
3. Organizational—focused on providing the structure and support for workplace safety and health programs that strive to support healthy individuals and a healthy work environment
4. Environmental—focused on providing the facilities and resources for workers to access quality healthcare programs and health promotion activities

The CDC (2011d) also defines elements of a comprehensive health and wellness promotion program, included in the Health People 2020 framework.

1. Health education that enhances awareness and is focused on lifestyle behavior change
2. Social and environmental support that encourages and expects health behaviors

Table 13.5 Essential elements of effective workplace programs.

Guiding Principles
- Develop a "human-centered culture" built on trust, not fear.
- Demonstrate leadership built on a commitment to worker health and safety, reflected in words and actions.
- Engage mid-level management as a link to integrating the culture though motivating and communicating with workers

Framework
- Establish clear principles focused on prevention of disease and injury that supports worker health and well-being.
- Integrate a program design that is consistent with all programs and policies relevant to safety, health, and well-being within an overall health and safety management system.
- Eliminate recognized occupational safety and health hazards.
- Be consistent in your expectations for workers to engage in worksite safety and health-directed programs
- Promote participation by encouraging workers to be actively engaged, to identify relevant health and safety issues, and to contribute to program design and implementation.
- Tailor programs to the *specific* workplace and the diverse needs of workers, recognizing that one size does *not* fit all—flexibility is necessary.
- Consider individual incentives and rewards aligned with accomplishment of program objectives.
- Find and use the right tools to measure success. Optimal assessment of a program's effectiveness is achieved through the use of relevant, validated measurement instruments.
- Adjust the program as needed based on the results of the program evaluation results.
- Make sure the program is sustainable, with a long-term outlook to assure responsiveness to changing workforce and market conditions.
- Ensure confidentiality, and make sure that the communication to employees is clear on this issue.

Program Implementation and Resources
- Be willing to start small and scale up. Be willing to abandon pilot projects that fail.
- Provide adequate resources. Take advantage of credible local community and national resources. Allocate sufficient resources, including staff, space, and time, to achieve the results you seek.
- Effective communication is essential for success. Communicate strategically to assure that those with a stake in the safety and health promotion program know the intent and rationale for the program. Maintain program visibility at the highest level of the organization.
- Build accountability into program implementation reflective of leadership at the highest levels. Reward success.

Program Evaluation
- Measure and analyze. Develop objectives and a selective menu of *relevant* measurements, and integrate data systems across programs and among vendors.
- Learn from experience. Adjust or modify programs based on established milestones and on results you have measured and analyzed.

Source: The National Institute for Occupational Safety and Health (NIOSH). (2012.) Total worker health: Essential Elements of effective workplace programs. http://www.cdc.gov/niosh/TWH/essentials.html

3. Integration of the health and wellness program into the vision and mission of the organization
4. Integrating holistic programs that include physical, mental, and behavioral health to promote healthy work and family balance
5. The development of screening programs linked with appropriate healthcare referrals for follow-up and intervention
6. A sustainable screening program that supports individual behavior change and follow-up
7. A structured process for program evaluation and improvement focused on effectiveness and efficiency

The framework and initiatives can be established based on these or other elements that have proven to provide a solid structure for the health and safety programs. By establishing a framework based on national or community strategies, the initiatives are then not only targeted at establishing a healthy and safe workforce, but also become a part of a larger initiative that supports a broader scope. The program takes on a community population focus.

Planning

The hallmark of every successful safety and health program is top management's active and aggressive commitment. However, once the commitment is made, support for the commitment must be demonstrated through words, actions, and examples. The establishment of a written policy statement endorsing the commitment to safety and health of the workforce is the first step, and this must be communicated to every worker. The expectation for management support must be stressed as a top priority. The policy statement must be endorsed in the employee handbook and be included as a part of orientation for all workers. Additionally, communication, both verbal and written, is sustained that provides a continuous message regarding the priority for health and well-being. The actions and examples of leadership support are also necessary in order for workers to see that company leaders not only establish the policy, but also set the example by actively participating in health and wellness events. The willingness to put health and well-being as a priority professes the commitment; however, actions and example forcefully and clearly proclaim the policy. The NIOSH (2008) Worklife Health and Wellness Initiative has published the Essential Elements of Effective Workplace Programs (Table 13.5) and provides the following example as a policy statement: *The protection, preservation, and improvement of the health and well-being of people who work are goals shared by workers, their families, and their employers.*

Goals and objectives must then be established that are intended to lead to the desired result of creating a sustained culture of health and wellness. The goal statement establishes a vision of what you wish to achieve. The goal statement should be established by the health and wellness committee and endorsed by leadership. See Table 13.6 for a sample goal statement. Once the goal statement

Table 13.6 Sample goal statement.

To assist individuals to achieve their full potential at work and in the community by:
- Providing resources that will assist workers and their families in making informed healthcare decisions
- Providing education and resources that will guide access and utilization of quality and appropriate healthcare services

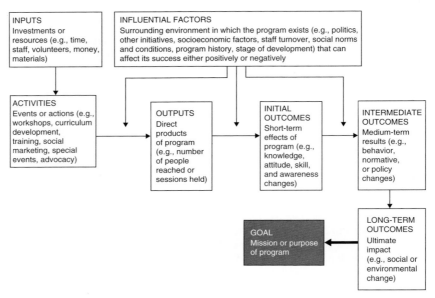

Figure 13.4 Components of a basic logic model.
Source: Centers for Disease Control and Prevention. http://www.cdc.gov/nccdphp/dnpao/hwi/programdesign/logic_model.htm

is established, identifying what you wish to achieve (point B), it is important to assess where you are now (point A). These two points establish the map that will provide the direction of getting from point A to point B. As we know, there are several ways to get from one point to another, and this is where a specific plan with clear objectives and initiatives is necessary. Just as you would map directions to get from New York to California, with milestones to achieve along the way, things to do, and alternative routes, your health and wellness initiatives must have this same, clear direction. Where are we now? Where do we wish to be? What are the obstacles? The use of a specified logic model (see Figure 13.4 and Table 13.7) helps to create structure in three dimensions of the program (CDC, 2002). It is first used to describe the core components of the program,

Table 13.7 Use of a program logic model.

- Clarifies program strategy.
- Justifies why the program will work.
- Assesses the potential effectiveness of an approach.
- Identifies appropriate outcome targets (and avoids overpromising).
- Sets priorities for allocating resources.
- Incorporates findings from research and demonstration projects.
- Makes midcourse adjustments and improvements in your program.
- Identifies differences between the ideal program and its real operation.
- Specifies the nature of questions being asked in the evaluation.
- Organizes evidence about the program.
- Makes stakeholders accountable for program processes and outcomes.
- Builds a better program.

Source: http://www.cdc.gov/nccdphp/dnpa/physical/handbook/pdf/handbook.pdf

illustrating the connection between program components, strategies, and expected outcomes. The logic model also includes pertinent information regarding program framework.

During the process of establishing goals and objectives, it is important to now determine how you will measure the effectiveness of the program and the achievement of the desired outcomes. Several markers of success can be established by measuring participation rates, worker satisfaction, reduced healthcare costs, reduced individual risk factors, enhanced morale, reduced absenteeism, and perceived individual health. Be definitive in setting the criteria that will be measured, at what points the measures will be made, and what is expected to be achieved. The evaluation design must define the methods and tools that will be used, along with the data that will be gathered. Examples would include written surveys (handout, telephone, fax, mail, e-mail, or Internet); personal interviews (e.g., individual or focus groups, structured or simply conversational); observation; and data measurements. The sources for evaluation must provide credible evidence using specific indicators, both qualitative and quantitative, to describe and measure program effects. Remember, you cannot manage what you don't measure. Therefore, it is important that measures be established that will evaluate the effectiveness of the program for individuals, the workplace, and the population.

Implementation

A clearly defined process is necessary for implementation. Consider using the same process that is used within the business for other new ventures or program initiatives. A business-case proposal must be developed and presented to management. As the leader, the OHN must strive to meet two specific objectives related to the health and wellness initiatives: (1) to set a path, goal, or vision for the program for management and (2) to motivate the worker population to pursue and eventually achieve the goal. How the program is communicated can make all the difference.

The first step is to conduct a business cost analysis in order to sell the program scope, involving those persons responsible for the decision making and/or those who will be affected by the program. Foster input and participation from a variety of sources in conducting the analysis. Data gathering is required to define a cost-benefit analysis for the proposal and to measure results. The data should include a combination of both quantitative and qualitative information. Quantitative data includes that which can be objectively measured in a numerical fashion or on a scale. Qualitative data, such as interviews and observations, describe meaning and is often used when describing attitudes or behaviors. In other words, quantitative data defines whereas qualitative data describes. Also, quantitative is numerical (measures) and qualitative is narrative (tells a story).

For each program activity, identify what outputs or targets you aim to achieve. Identify the short-term and long-term outcomes you expect for each activity. For example, a wellness screening event might aim to have 30% participation from the workforce. Describe the impact you anticipate with each activity, such as increasing awareness, identifying risk, or diagnosing health concerns. Describe each of the activities you plan to conduct in the program, along with the internal and external resources available to support the program activities.

Market, market, and market some more. Participation is enhanced by getting the word out. Establish a plan that includes all members of the health and wellness committee and other key workers. Publish information in the workplace newsletter and intranet, and use e-mail blasts. Establish an expectation that health and wellness activities become an agenda item on every department's meeting agenda. Assign individuals from each work area as champions of the cause, responsible for garnering interest and participation from coworkers. Incentivize participation and create team challenges. Reward participation and risk reduction. Encourage participation in walk-a-thons and community events that will provide exercise and social opportunities that will promote healthy community relationships. Host workshops and invite speakers to present educational or informative topics. Develop support groups and support memberships to local health clubs. Think broadly in terms of wellness, not only physical and mental health, but also social, financial, and spiritual health. The health promotion activities that you plan should be tied to your data (surveys, risk reports, claims) and to goals and objectives. They should address existing risk factors in the population and be in line with what both management and workers desire as an intended result of the programs and initiatives. Success varies. While some businesses have implemented very comprehensive health promotion programs, others have achieved goals, reaped savings, or increased productivity with just a few activities.

Table 13.8 Four general purposes of program evaluation.

- To gain insight and provide useful information
- To change practice that leads to refining the program in order to improve quality and effectiveness
- To assess the effects of the program and establish accountability
- To provide feedback to management and participants related to the program impact

Source: CDC, 1999.

Evaluation

Evaluation will include measuring how well the initiatives are working and if the program is achieving the expected results. Program evaluation should always engage a variety of stakeholders, including participants, management, and even nonparticipants, those involved in program development and implementation, and those served or affected by the program. Evaluation should aim to gather credible evidence that will validate conclusions and lead to quality improvement (CDC, 1999) (see Table 13.8). As mentioned earlier, the evaluation criteria should be decided when establishing the goals and objectives of the program. The health and wellness committee members should be involved in establishing the evaluation criteria by addressing the following:

- What do we wish to learn from the evaluation?
- What is the best way to evaluate? What information will be gathered and how?
- How will the information be used?
- How will the information be communicated?

There are always lessons learned when a program is evaluated in a comprehensive manner. According to the Kellogg Foundation (2004), information gathered during program evaluation should lead to the following:

- Improving the effectiveness of current activities by helping initiate or modify program activities
- Providing support for maintaining the program over the long term
- Providing insight into why certain goals are or are not being accomplished
- Helping program leaders make decisions

There are several aspects to address when evaluating programs. One aspect focuses on the individual. Participant-focused evaluations address how individual lives will improve as a result of the program. The types of outcomes that are expected to be achieved at the individual level might include changes in circumstances, status, quality of life, or functioning. Change is expected to occur based on the content area of the program and can occur in four general areas: knowledge, attitude, skills, and behavior. Program evaluations should address these four areas. Was new knowledge gained? Was there a change in attitude as a result of participation? Was a new skill learned? Did participation affect behavior? Participation rates, participant evaluations, and surveys are the most effective evaluation tools and are easy to define. Success is not just about participation. The goal is to discover how workers felt about the program: if they attended, why they attended, and if they did not attend, why? A worker may choose to attend an event, yet not find benefit.

Evaluation criteria should also address a broader perspective related to system-specific goals. These criteria should focus on the outcomes you are trying to achieve for the program and for the company or population (e.g., decreased absenteeism, increased productivity, lower healthcare costs). Also measure results by reviewing each program goal and determining if it has been achieved. Outcomes should be measured from the focus of the intended results: financial, health, morale, productivity. It is important to acknowledge that intended outcomes may not be achieved for many years, especially when focused on changing attitudes, changing behaviors, and impacting cost. Therefore, it is important to establish early on the timelines associated with the intended goals and objectives. Many of the desired outcomes may also be difficult to measure, such as improved morale, yet sometimes these initiatives hold the greatest promise and return on investment, making a significant difference in the workplace environment and population.

A program evaluation should strive to provide information from a variety of perspectives that will communicate information about the program. The information must be perceived as balanced, unbiased, and credible by all stakeholders. Credible evidence strengthens the judgments and recommendations for continuing, expanding, redesigning, or eliminating the program (CDC, 1999).

A calculated and deliberate effort must be undertaken to communicate findings, and the information must be communicated appropriately. Communicate results, not only to management, but also to the workers. It is important for workers to understand the intended goals and outcomes. Celebrate successes while sharing the results. This requires measuring and evaluating whether the interventions worked and determining why they worked or failed. This may lead to further fine-tuning of the program to attain continuous improvement and outcome achievement.

WORK—A PLACE TO CALL HOME

"Home is not where you live, but where they understand you" Christian Morganstern.

A new conceptual model for health and wellness has recently been proposed—the patient-centered medical home (PCMH), with an emphasis on improving the health of individuals and populations. The model encourages healthcare providers to coordinate health and wellness initiatives through integrated goals, both individual and population-based goals, emphasizing the central role of a primary care provider. The model also proposes the facilitation of partnerships among the patient, family, and healthcare providers and integrates care along a spectrum of wellness to illness. The model is intended to establish a process whereby the individual plays a greater role in healthcare decision making and aims to achieve better health outcomes at lower cost.

Occupational health professionals can play a valued role by adopting these precepts and integrating the PCMH concept as a part of the occupational and environmental health program (McClellan et al., 2012).

The workplace provides the perfect atmosphere for the coordination and comprehensiveness of care, with the ability to manage individuals with multiple health care needs. And the OHN is the perfect healthcare professional to understand the individuals and their specific health needs as well as that of the population and their associated health risks. This approach mirrors the efforts proven successful in identifying and reducing workplace safety and health risks, and a well-established infrastructure of paralleled strategies can be initiated to affect the health (not just the safety) of the individual worker and the population workforce. McClellan et al. (2012) propose the use of "key quality improvement practices, including health information technology, to overcome geographic, cultural, language, and other barriers through a team-based approach to care that starts in the workplace … a place where millions of Americans spend the major portion of their daily lives." The extension of a well-organized occupational health program can now embrace the delivery of primary and preventive care and disability management for the nonoccupational components of the health and benefits program.

The same steps used in managing the traditional occupational health program can be initiated through the OHN's involvement, as the healthcare expert, in the decisions related to the design of the health benefits program. By understanding the population, the OHN's expert knowledge is key in identifying health needs of the population and coordinating care. This can be achieved by implementing the appropriate screening and preventive services and directing the use of the appropriate healthcare provider at the most appropriate time. The health and wellness program will serve as a motivation for change, promoting health and positive outcomes. Health and wellness awareness becomes a part of the work philosophy with targeted health initiatives. Risks are identified through health risk assessments of the worker population, and targeted initiatives are implemented specific to the identified health risks. These initiatives become a part of health benefits reform, wellness initiatives, and disease-focused management strategies. And, as workplaces develop and implement health and wellness strategies, the advice of legal counsel should be sought to assure compliance with all applicable workplace and disability regulations (Brigham, 2010).

The medical home concept, when applied in the occupational setting, should parallel the NIOSH WorkLife Initiative. This initiative is intended to "identify and support comprehensive approaches to reduce workplace hazards and promote worker health and well-being" (NIOSH, 2008). The initiative applies comprehensive practices and policies that take into account the work environment—both physical and organizational—as well as the personal health risks of individuals; the combination of which is "more effective in preventing disease and promoting health and safety than each approach taken separately" (NIOSH, 2008). Health is the central concept and is applied in a holistic manner: addressing the quality of health and safety at home, at work, and in one's life (see Figure 13.5).

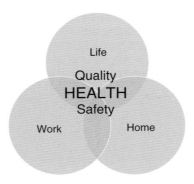

Figure 13.5 Hallmarks of the medical home.

The medical home concept, when applied to the occupational setting, must take on a variety of structures in order to meet the needs of various sizes of workplaces (see Figure 13.6 and Figure 13.7). Typically, mid- and large-size businesses are able to support an on-site occupational health clinic. When incorporating the medical home concept, these clinics expand their scope to include the provision of nonoccupational health services, such as urgent care or primary care. Smaller workplaces can adopt a variety of models that achieve the medical home concept by coordinating efforts with community resources to achieve the intended outcomes of providing a comprehensive health and wellness model that achieves the balance of health at home, at work, and in life.

The principles discussed in this chapter require significant change—both organizational and individual change. This change must encompass changing philosophies, changing attitudes, and changing behaviors. All this, along with a change in the structure of health benefits program, will lead to changes in health—at home, at work, and in life.

SUMMARY

Employers can gain efficiencies and achieve greater impact by integrating their health, safety, and worker productivity management programs (Goetzel, 2005a), and several program elements have proven effective. Yet, there is no magic bullet, no magic wand, no miraculous approach to establishing and maintaining a worksite health and wellness program. The program must be uniquely tailored to meet the needs of the population base of workers and dependents. To be effective, it must be established based on population-specific strategies, similar to the principles and underpinnings of the public health model, and it must be sustained. It is only then that workplace health programs can lead to change at both the individual and the organizational levels (CDC, 2011d).

For individuals, workplace health and wellness programs have the potential to impact the health of the worker by influencing health behaviors that reduce

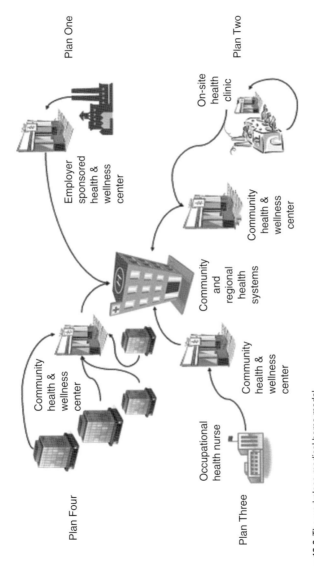

Figure 13.6 The workplace medical home model.
Source: Guzik, A. (2011). The Concept of Medical Home. Where Will You Call Home? PowerPoint presentation in Tampa, FL.

Plan One

- Large business (1,000 + employees)
  - ☐ On-site employer-sponsored health and wellness center (health clinic)
    - Formalized occupational health and safety program
      - ☐ Comprehensive occupational health services
      - ☐ On-site comprehensive primary care (employees and dependents)
      - ☐ On-site health and wellness initiatives
    - Corporate medical director
      - ☐ Physicians
      - ☐ Health nurse(s) and/or nurse practitioner(s)
      - ☐ Safety/IH team
    - Health benefits program
      - ☐ Includes services at employer-sponsored health and wellness center
      - ☐ Formalized network of specialists and support services
      - ☐ Contractual arrangement with community health system

Plan Two

- Medium-size business (500–1,000 employees)
  - ☐ On-site employer-sponsored health and wellness center (health clinic)
    - Formalized occupational health and safety program
      - ☐ Comprehensive occupational health services
      - ☐ Limited on-site primary care/urgent care
      - ☐ On-site health and wellness initiatives
    - Consultant medical director
      - ☐ Health nurse(s) and/or nurse practitioner(s)
      - ☐ Safety/IH team
  - ☐ Health benefits program
    - Includes services at employer-sponsored health and wellness center
    - Includes services at community health clinic
      - ☐ Primary and urgent care
      - ☐ Formalized network of specialists and support services
    - Services within community health system

Plan Three

- Mid-size business (250–500 employees)
  - ☐ On-site employer-sponsored health and wellness center (health clinic)
    - Formalized occupational health and safety program
      - ☐ Occupational health services
      - ☐ Limited on-site health care by the health nurse
      - ☐ On-site health and wellness initiatives

Figure 13.7 The workplace medical home model.
Source: Guzik, 2011.

- Consultant medical director
  - ☐ Health nurse(s) and/or nurse practitioner(s)
  - ☐ Safety/IH consultant
- Health benefits program
  - ☐ Includes services at employer-sponsored health and wellness center
  - ☐ Includes services at community health clinic
    - Limited primary and urgent care
    - Formalized network of specialists and support services
  - ☐ Services within community health system

Plan Four

- Small business (<250 employees)
  - ☐ Use of the community health center
    - Basic occupational health and safety program
      - ☐ Occupational health services
      - ☐ On-site health and wellness initiatives
    - Consultant
      - ☐ Health nurse(s)
      - ☐ Safety/IH
    - Health benefits program
      - ☐ Includes services within the community health system
      - ☐ Includes
        - Occupational health services
        - Primary and urgent care
        - Formalized network of specialists and support services
        - Services within community health system

Figure 13.7 *(Continued)*

health risks for disease and have a positive effect on the health and productivity of the worker. For organizations, workplace health and wellness programs hold the potential to reduce healthcare costs, lower absenteeism, and increase productivity. Many health and wellness programs aid in recruitment and retention of workers by creating a desirable work culture and enhanced morale within the workplace. The community then benefits by having healthy individuals and families that influence the prevention of disease and injury and achieve a higher level of sustained health (CDC, 2011a).

The American health system has been a system focused on providing care, caring for one individual at a time. As we move to reform the health of our populations, the workplace becomes the perfect catalyst for change. By adopting a public health approach, the workplace can become a system of caring for populations, hundreds or thousands at a time. A population-based approach, with accountable financing and analysis built on best evidence and best practice, can and will transform health.

REFERENCES

Agency for Healthcare Research and Quality (AHRQ). (2010*). Guide to clinical preventive services, 2010–2011.* (Publication No. 10-05145). Retrieved from http://www.ahrq.gov/clinic/pocketgd.htm

Agency for Healthcare Research and Quality (AHRQ). (2012). *Prevention and chronic care program.* Retrieved from http://www.ahrq.gov/clinic/ppipix.htm

American Cancer Society (ACS). (2010). *Partnerships for a healthy workforce 2010: An essential health promotion sourcebook for employers, large and small.* Retrieved from http://www. acsworkplacesolutions.com/documents/ Healthy_Workforce_2010.pdf

Berry, L. L., Mirabito, A. M., & Baun, W. B. (2010). What's the hard return on employee wellness programs? *Harvard Business Review, 88*(2),104–112.

Brigham, C. L., Association of Corporate Counsel. (2010). *Wellness programs: A quick overview.* Retrieved from http://www.acc.com/legalresources/quick-counsel/wpaqr.cfm

California Commission on Health and Safety and Workers' Compensation. (2008). *Summary of July 16, 2008. Workplace Wellness Roundtable.* Retrieved from http://www.dir.ca.gov/chswc/Reports/CHSWC_SummaryWorkplace WellnessRoundtable.pdf

Centers for Disease Control and Prevention (CDC). (1999). Framework for program evaluation in public health. *Morbidity and Mortality Weekly Report, 48*(RR11), 1–40. Retrieved from http://www.cdc.gov/mmwr/preview/ mmwrhtml/rr4811a1.htm

Centers for Disease Control and Prevention (CDC). (2002). *Physical activity evaluation handbook.* Retrieved from http://www.cdc.gov/nccdphp/dnpa/ physical/handbook/pdf/handbook.pdf

Centers for Disease Control and Prevention (CDC). (2005). *CDC evaluation working group: Resources online.* Retrieved from http://www.cdc.gov/eval/ resources.htm#logic%20model

Centers for Disease Control and Prevention (CDC). (2010a). *Healthier worksite initiative.* Retrieved from http://www.cdc.gov/nccdphp/dnpao/hwi/ index.htm

Centers for Disease Control and Prevention (CDC). (2010b). *The guide to community preventive services glossary.* Retrieved from http://www.the-communityguide.org/about/glossary.html

Centers for Disease Control and Prevention (CDC). (2011a). *National prevention strategy: America's plan for better health and wellness.* Retrieved from http:// www.cdc.gov/Features/PreventionStrategy/

Centers for Disease Control and Prevention (CDC). (2011b). *New million hearts tools announced by partners.* Press release. November 3, 2011. Retrieved from http://www.cdc.gov/media/releases/2011/p1103_Million_Hearts.html

Centers for Disease Control and Prevention (CDC). (2011c). *Rising health care costs are unsustainable.* Retrieved from http://www.cdc.gov/workplace-healthpromotion/businesscase/reasons/rising.html

Centers for Disease Control and Prevention (CDC). (2011d). *Workplace health promotion: Making a business case.* Retrieved from http://www.cdc.gov/workplacehealthpromotion/businesscase/index.html

Chapman, L. S. (2005). Presenteeism and its role in worksite health promotion. *American Journal of Health Promotion, 19*(4), Suppl 1–8.

Chenowith, D. (2011). *Promoting employee wellbeing: Wellness strategies to improve health, performance and the bottom line.* Alexandria, Virginia: SHRM Foundation.

Chikotas, N. E., Parks, C. I., & Olszewski, K. A. (2012). Comprehensive review of the healthy people 2020 occupational safety and health objectives: Part 2. Tools for the occupational health nurse in goal attainment. *Workplace Health & Safety, 60*(2), 78–89.

Commission on Health & Safety & Worker's Compensation. (2010). *The whole worker: Guidelines for integrating occupational health and safety with workplace wellness programs.* Retrieved from http://www.lohp.org/docs/pubs/thewholeworker.pdf

Hochstadt, B., Kaplan, D., & Keyt, D. (2011). *Employer-sponsored worksite health: Offering solutions across the globe.* Retrieved from http://www.mercer.com/articles/employer-sponsored-worksite-health-1432910

Goetzel, R. Z. (2005a). *Examining the value of integrating occupational health and safety and health promotion programs in the workplace.* Retrieved from http://www.cdc.gov/niosh/steps/pdfs/BackgroundPaperGoetzelJan2005.pdf

Goetzel, R. Z. (2005b). *Policy and Practice Working Group examining the value of integrating occupational health and safety and health promotion programs in the workplace. Final report.* Retrieved from http://www.factsforhealthcare.com/management/Assets/NIOSH_Background_Paper_Goetzel.pdf

Goetzel, R. Z., Jacobson, B. H., Aldana, S. G., Vardell, K., & Yee, L. (1998). Health care costs of worksite health promotion participants and non-participants. *Journal of Occupational and Environmental Medicine, 40*(4), 341–346.

Goetzel R. Z., Long, S. R., Ozminkowski, R. J., Hawkins, K., Wang, S., & Lynch, W. (2004). Health, absence, disability, and presenteeism cost estimates of certain physical and mental health conditions affecting U.S. employers. *Journal of Occupational and Environmental Medicine, 46*(4), 398–412.

Goetzel, R. Z. & Ozminkowski, R. J. (2008). The health and cost benefits of work site health-promotion programs. *Annual Review of Public Health, 29*, 303–323.

Gorman, K. M, & Miller. R. M. (2011). Managing the risks of on-site health centers. *AAOHN Journal, 59*(11), 483–490.

Griffith, K. & Strasser, P. B. (2010). Integrating primary care with occupational health services: A success story. *AAOHN Journal, 58*(12), 519–523.

Health Savings Account Resource Center (HSA). (2003). What is an HSA. Retrieved from http://www.hsaresourcecenter.com/general/what.php

Hettler, B., National Wellness Institute. (1976). *Six dimensions of wellness model.* Retrieved from http://www.nationalwellness.org

Hodge, B. J. & Martin, M. (2008). Benefit design critical to protecting out-of-pocket costs for employees. *American Journal of Managed Care, 14*(8 Suppl), S246–251.

Hymel, P.A., Loeppke, R.R., Baase, C.M., Burton, W.N., Hartenbaum, N.P., Hudson, T.W., et al. (2011). Workplace health protection and promotion. A new pathway for a healthier—and safer—workforce. An ACOEM Guidance Statement. *Journal of Occupational and Environmental Medicine*, 53(6), 695–702.

Johnson, L. & Denham, S. A. (2008). Structuring successful interventions in employee health programs. *AAOHN Journal*, 56(6).

Kessler, R. C., Greenberg, P. E., Mickelson, K. D., Meneades, L. M., & Wang, P. S. (2001). The effects of chronic medical conditions on work loss and work cutback. *Journal of Occupational and Environmental Medicine*, 43, 218–225.

Lang, Y. C. (2009). Occupational health nursing in the driver's seat for health promotion. *AAOHN Journal*, 57(1), 9–11.

Linnan, L., Weiner, B., Graham, A., & Emmons, K. (2007). Manager beliefs regarding worksite health promotion: Findings from the working healthy project 2. *American Journal of Health Promotion*, 21(6), 521–528.

Loeppke R., Taitel M., Haufle, V., Parry, T., Kessler, R.C., & Jinnett, K. (2009). Health and productivity as a business strategy: A multi-employer study. *Journal of Occupational and Environmental Medicine*, 51, 411–428.

Loeppke, R., Taitel M., Richling D., et al. (2007). Health and productivity as a business strategy. *Journal of Occupational and Environmental Medicine*, 49, 712–721.

Main, T. (2008). *Health value solution: Addressing the coverage and affordability crisis.* Retrieved from http://www.oliverwyman.com/media/20081002_Affordabilty_Crisis.pdf

Marcy, Jessica. (2010). *Chronic disease expert: U.S. health care system needs to treat whole person.* Kaiser Health News. Retrieved from http://www.kaiserhealthnews.org/checking-in-with/lorig-chronic-disease.aspx?wwparam=1296495930.

Marinescu, L. G. (2007). Integrated approach for managing health risks at work- The role of occupational health nurses. *AAOHN Journal*, 55(2), 75–87.

Mayfield, M. Bureau of Labor Statistics. (2011). *Health, wellness, and employee assistance: A holistic approach to employee benefits.* Retrieved from http://www.bls.gov/opub/cwc/cm20110519ar01p1.htm

McClellan, R. K., Sherman, B., Loeppke, R. R., et al. (2012). ACOEM Position Statement. Optimizing health care delivery by integrating workplaces, homes, and communities: How occupational and environmental medicine can serve as a vital connecting link between accountable care organizations and the patient-centered medical home. *Journal of Occupational and Environmental Medicine*, 54(4), 504–512.

Mercer. (2011a). *Building a best-practice employee health management program.* Retrieved from http://www.mercer.com/hbperspective

Mercer. Mercer's National Survey of Employer Sponsored Health Plans. (2011b). *Latest survey finds health benefit cost growth for 2012 likely to be the lowest in 15 years.* Retrieved from http://www.mercer.us/press-releases/health-benefit-cost-growth-for-2012-likely-to-be-lowest-in-15-years-1425550

Mercer. (2011c). *Employers accelerate efforts to bring health benefit costs under control.* Retrieved from http://www.mercer.com/press-releases/national-survey-employer-sponsored-health-plans

Mills, P. R., Kessler, R. C., Cooper, J., & Sullivan, S. (2007). Impact of a health promotion program on employee health risks and work productivity. *American Journal of Health Promotion, 22*(1), 45–53.

National Institute for Occupational Safety and Health (NIOSH). (2008). *Essential elements of effective workplace programs and policies for improving worker health and well-being.* DHHS (NIOSH Publication No. 2010-140.) Retrieved from http://www.cdc.gov/niosh/docs/2010-140/pdfs/2010-140.pdf

National Institute for Occupational Safety and Health (NIOSH). (2012). *Total worker health: Essential elements of effective workplace programs.* Retrieved from http://www.cdc.gov/niosh/TWH/essentials.html

National Prevention, Health Promotion, and Public Health Council (NPHPPHC). (2011). *The National Prevention Strategy: America's plan for better health and wellness.* Retrieved from http://www.healthcare.gov/prevention/nphpphc/strategy/index.html#top

National Wellness Association. Defining Wellness. Retrieved from http://www.nationalwellness.org/index.php?id_tier=2&id_c=26

Naydeck B. L., Pearson, J. A., Ozminkowski, R. J., Day, B. T., & Goetzel, R. Z. (2008). The impact of the highmark employee wellness programs on 4-year health care costs. *Journal of Occupational and Environmental Medicine, 50*(2), 146–156.

Ozminkowski, R. J., Ling, D., Goetzel, R. Z., Bruno, J. A., Rutter, R. R., Isaac, F., & Wang, S. (2002). Long-term impact of Johnson & Johnson's Health & Wellness Program on health care utilization and expenditures. *Journal of Occupational and Environmental Medicine, 44*(1), 21–29.

Parks, C. I., Chikotas, N. E., & Olszewskim K. A (2012). Comprehensive review of the healthy people 2020 occupational safety and health objectives: Part 1. Tools for the occupational health nurse in goal attainment. *Workplace Health & Safety, 60*(1), 33–42.

Parks, C. I., Chikotas, N. E. & Olszewskim K. (2012). A comprehensive review of the healthy people 2020 occupational safety and health objectives: Part 2. Tools for the occupational health nurse in goal attainment. *Workplace Health & Safety, 60*(2), 90.

Redmond, M. S. & Kalina, C. M. (2009). A successful occupational health nurse-driven health promotion program to support corporate sustainability. *AAOHN Journal, 57*(12), 507–514.

Rogers, B., Marshall, J., Garth, K., Mopkins, D., Remington, J., Siemering, K., & Spivey, J. (2011). Focus on the aging worker. *AAOHN Journal, 59*(10), 447–457.

Serxner, S., Gold, D., Anderson, D., & Williams, D. (2001). The impact of a work-site health promotion program on short-term disability usage. *Journal of Occupational and Environmental Medicine, 43*(1), 25–29.

Sherman, B. & Click, E. (2007). Occupational and environmental health nursing in the era of consumer-directed health care. *AAOHN Journal*, *55*(5), 211–215.

Smith. G. S. 2001. Public health approaches to occupational injury prevention: Do they work? *Injury Prevention*, 7(Suppl 1). Retrieved from http://bmj-injuryprev.highwire.org/content/7/suppl_1/i3.full

Sullivan, S. (2004). Making the business case for health and productivity management. *Journal of Occupational and Environmental Medicine*, *46* (6 Supplement), S56–S61.

U.S. Department of Health and Human Services (USDHHS). (2006). *The health consequences of involuntary exposure to tobacco smoke: A report of the Surgeon General*. General. Atlanta, GA: Centers for Disease Control and Prevention National Center for Chronic Disease Prevention and Health Promotion.

U.S. Department of Health and Human Services (USDHHS). (2011a). *Healthy people 2020*. Retrieved from http://www.healthypeople.gov

U.S. Department of Health and Human Services (USDHHS). (2011b). Press Release: September 13, 2011. *New public-private sector initiative aims to prevent 1 million heart attacks and strokes in five years*. Retrieved from http://millionhearts.hhs.gov/index.html

U.S. Department of Health & Human Services (USDHHS). (2011). *The national prevention strategy: America's plan for better health and wellness*. Retrieved from http://www.healthcare.gov/prevention

U.S. Department of Health and Human Services (USDHHS). (2012). *National strategy for quality improvement in health care: Agency-specific quality strategic plans*. Retrieved from http://www.ahrq.gov/workingforquality/nqs/nqsplans.pdf

U.S. Department of Labor, Bureau of Labor Statistics. (2008). *Wellness program checklist*. (Field Assistance Bulletin No. 2008-02.) Retrieved from http://www.dol.gov/ebsa/regs/fab2008-2.html

U.S. Department of Labor, Bureau of Labor Statistics. (2010a). *National compensation survey: Employee benefits in the United States*. (Bulletin 2752). Retrieved from http://www.bls.gov/ncs/ebs/benefits/2010/ebbl0046.pdf.

U.S. Department of Labor, Bureau of Labor Statistics. (2010b). *American time use survey—2010 results*. Retrieved from http://www.bls.gov/news.release/pdf/atus.pdf

W.K. Kellogg Foundation. (2004). *Evaluation handbook*. Retrieved from http://www.wkkf.org/knowledge-center/resources/2010/W-K-Kellogg-Foundation-Evaluation-Handbook.aspx

World Health Organization, Whitaker, S. & Baranski. B., Eds. (2001). *The role of the occupational health nurse in workplace health management*. Retrieved from http://www.who.int/occupational_health/regions/en/oeheurnursing.pdf

Yen, L., Schultz, A., Schnueringer, E., & Edington, D.W. (2006). Financial costs due to excess health risks among active employees of a utility company. *Journal of Occupational and Environmental Medicine*, *48*(9), 896–905.

RESOURCES
Alcohol
Risk Factor Sponsoring Organization Website Alcohol Abuse The George Washington University Medical Center
http://www.alcoholcostcalculator

Asthma
Agency for Healthcare Research and Quality
http://statesnapshots.ahrq.gov/asthma/

Depression
Depression calculator
http://www.depressioncalculator.com

Diabetes
American Diabetes Association
http://www.diabetesarchive.net/advocacy-and-legalresources/cost-of-diabetes.jsp
Agency for Healthcare Research and Quality
http://www.ahrq.gov/populations/diabcostcalc/

Migraine
The Pharmaceutical Research and Manufacturers of America (PhRMA)
http://www.migrainecalculator.com

Obesity
Business Group on Health
http://www.businessgrouphealth.org/healthtopics/obesitycostcalculator.cfm

Physical inactivity
East Carolina University http://www.ecu.edu/picostcalc

Tobacco
American Health Insurance Plans
http://www.businesscaseroi.org/roi/default.aspx

ORGANIZATIONS
American College of Occupational & Environmental Medicine
http://www.acoem.org
American College of Sports Medicine
http://www.acsm.org
Institute for Health & Productivity Management
http://www.ihpm.org
Integrated Benefits Institute www.ibiweb.org
International Association of Worksite Health Promotion
http://www.acsm-iawhp.org

National Wellness Association
http://www.nationalwellness.org
Wellness Council of America
http://www.welcoa.org

Publications
Corporate Wellness magazine
http://www.corporatewellnessmagazine.com
Employee Benefit Adviser
http://eba.benefitnews.com/
Health Promotion Practitioner
http://www.hesonline.com
HR Magazine www.shrm.org

Healthcare Cost Drivers
U.S. Department of Health and Human Services. Public Health Service. (2006).
*The health consequences of involuntary exposure to tobacco smoke a report of the
Surgeon General.* Retrieved from http://www.cdc.gov/tobacco

Health Risk Assessment (HRA) Tools
Wellsource
http://www.wellsource.com
Wellstream
http://www.welcoa.org
Stay Well
http://www.staywellhealthmanagement.com
Summit Health
http://www.summithealth.com
Well Call
http://www.wellcall.com
Trale Inc.
http://www.trale.com
PreceptGroup
http://www.preceptgroup.com

Return on Investment (ROI) Calculators
Centers for Disease Control and Prevention
http://www.cdc.gov/leanworks/costcalculator/index.html
Well Steps http://new.wellsteps.com/resources/tools

Wellness Interest Survey
Wellness Proposals
http://www.wellnessproposals.com/pdfs/employee_interest_survey.pdf

Leadership and Change

14

"We must be the change we wish to see."

(Ghandi)

Today's business world is ever-changing, and an emphasis on health and well-being is seen as a core aspect of a productive workplace. Yet, we still struggle with ways to demonstrate the value of occupational health services, to demonstrate worth. In all business models, leaders analyze costs and look for clear evidence and proven benefits of investments. Too often, as healthcare professionals, we focus on the qualitative outcomes, those heartfelt stories, rather than on the outcomes that address the business objectives. Therefore, as leaders of the occupational health business unit, we must always strive to demonstrate our worth and our contribution to the business.

Ennals (2002) proposes that healthy work is accepted as a mainstream concern, integral to sustainable development, and it is now recognized as a key component to successful business operations. Yet, it remains difficult for the business accountants to evaluate the case for investments in workplace health, safety, and well-being. Often this is because outcomes have not been defined. When we fail to prove the business case for an investment in health without objective measures of return on investment, the proposal is often rejected. As we build proposals for programs, we must strive then to address reliable and measurable indicators of quality and continuous improvement that support business operations. This approach will elevate the occupational health strategies to a level commensurate with the mainstream of business benchmarking.

Essentials for Occupational Health Nursing, First Edition. Arlene Guzik.
© 2013 John Wiley & Sons, Inc. Published 2013 by John Wiley & Sons, Inc.

Case in Point

The OHN as health services manager had contracted with a service supplier to provide staffing for the on-site clinic with a nurse practitioner and medical assistant. The scope of services included all occupational health testing, medical surveillance, physical exams, treatment, case management of all workers' compensation cases, and medical direction. The OHN manager coordinated the service agreement with the company's sourcing (purchasing) manager, and a service delivery agreement was signed for a 3-year term. Each month, the service supplier manager provided the company's OHN manager with a monthly report of clinic activity, including volume of services rendered. The report included the typical market cost of those services. This was intended to demonstrate the value of services rendered as compared to the same cost that would have been incurred had they sent workers off-site for the same services. The report demonstrated the value of the on-site services as compared to the cost that would have been incurred in a community-based clinic. The aim of the service provider was to provide a report that demonstrated the cost savings of having services provided on-site. (See Appendix 25.)

At the time of the service agreement renewal, the service supplier manager was invited to attend a meeting with the OHN manager, the sourcing agent, and the environmental health and safety (EH&S) manager. Discussion ensued regarding the data the EH&S manager and sourcing manager needed to present to the executive management team (CEO, COO, and CFO) to support the intent to renew the service agreement for another 3-year period. After much discussion, the sourcing manager still did not think he had enough data to support the case. The service supplier manager asked the sourcing manager if he thought the monthly activity reports provided enough data to support the case. What was realized was that the OHN manager had never shared the monthly service reports with the EH&S manager (direct report) or the sourcing manager. For the 3-year term of service, the reports were being filed in the OHN manager's office and not communicated to corporate management to demonstrate the value of services being provided. Had this information been shared during the course of the service agreement, there would have been no question as to the value of the service and the cost savings it represented to the company. Once the reports were reviewed by the sourcing manager, he proclaimed: "This is exactly what I need."

The OHN must strategize with other leaders in the business when developing and evaluating occupational health programs. And this should be done at the inception of the program or service, deciding how the value of the program or service will be evaluated. Knave and Ennals (2002) propose that communication will not be successful if it is based on one-way exchange of information. The interaction with stakeholders provides various perspectives that lend credibility to the process and must be approached in a firm, fair, and consistent manner. The OHN is the central figure and must be open to garnering and understanding the various perspectives of the stakeholders (see Figure 14.1). Stakeholders include other healthcare professionals (physicians, nurses, and others involved in the delivery of healthcare services), safety professionals, human resources professionals, environmental and industrial

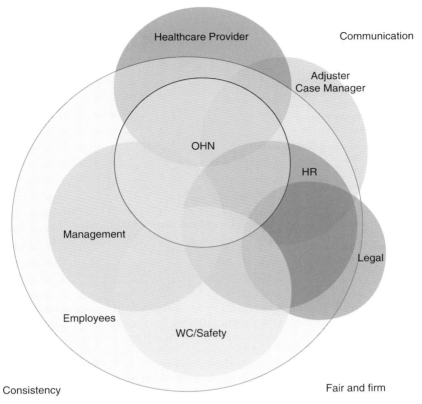

Healthcare Provider

Communication

Adjuster
Case Manager

OHN

HR

Management

Legal

Employees

WC/Safety

Consistency

Fair and firm

Figure 14.1 The OHN and stakeholder interaction.

engineers, business managers, risk managers, and health benefits professionals. The development of these partnerships leads to a culture of engagement, a heterogeneous approach with a vision for multidimensional outcomes (Miller, Rossiter, & Nuttall, 2002). Gaining visibility and knowing what management wants to hear are important attributes. Communicating financial information, such as cost savings and saved work time, as a financial value is an essential skill for the OHN (Gregory, Lukes, & Gregory, 2002). The OHN must be able to speak the language of business to make a meaningful impact As a result, the outcomes data or service delivery report will include data that is valued by the stakeholders and measured as a marker of program effectiveness. There will be no question as to what metrics or measures will be used for the evaluation and no question as to how and when the information will be communicated.

Measurable outcomes are described in a variety of fashions, depending on the program that is being measured. Although several outcomes have been

Table 14.1 Service metrics.

Quality Measures

- Best value for money spent
- Outcome oriented
- Safe, effective, appropriate
- Quality improvement strategies
  - Benchmarking
  - Service measures

Value Measures

- Cost of workers' compensation claims
- Disability costs
- Absenteeism

Outcome Measures

- OSHA recordable rate
- OSHA visits, fines
- Reduced lost time (days away from work, modified work days)
- Safe, effective, appropriate
- Cost of healthcare claims
- Length of healthcare claims
- Severity of healthcare claims

described in the literature, the OHN must establish a set of outcomes that are specific to the strategies of the program. Miller, Rossiter, and Nuttall (2002) propose measures that address maximizing the health and morale of employees, maximizing performance and increasing productivity, minimizing medicolegal costs, enhancing workplace safety, and reducing sickness absence. The World Development Report (World Bank, 2001) indicates that improved health can contribute to economic growth by reducing production losses caused by worker illness and through lower healthcare costs. The measures related to lowered healthcare costs can have an effect on economic, health, and social and environmental well-being. And as a result, this provides funds that that would otherwise be spent on treating illness that can now be allocated for other uses.

The World Health Organization (Whitaker & Baranski, 2001) proposes that program evaluation be based on improvements in company performance in the area of workplace health management, contribution of the occupational health and safety service to the business, and the individual contributions of the OHN. Evaluation criteria should be based on the structure, process, and outcome indicators (see Sample Occupational Health Services Delivery Evaluation Criteria in Appendix 26). Evaluating service delivery is accomplished by comparing the delivery of services against predetermined service agreement metrics, including quality standards for services, specific achieved metrics, through stakeholder satisfaction surveys, or by assessing the adequacy of service delivery. The services metrics of quality, value, and outcome measures provide a well-rounded view of program effectiveness (see Table 14.1). The aim of the service delivery analysis is to identify areas for potential intervention or improvement, establish priorities for modification or enhancement, quantify the value of the service, demonstrate accountability of the service, and address financial viability or return on investment. Table 14.2 provides a sample outcomes report that demonstrates the effectiveness of a safety and workers' compensation case management program over a continuum of time.

The four areas of intention that will demonstrate the best value are related to quality, utilization, access, and cost. In demonstrating quality, one must consider comparison to industry and professional standards; therefore, benchmarking becomes important. Are your services as effective as those of others in a like industry? Are workers receiving the best quality for the value of service? Are workers using the right provider, at the right place, at the right time? Is access to service timely and appropriate, and does it support the productivity of the worker? Are costs controlled? Are costs predictable? And are they benchmarked against defined standards? Are other cost-effective alternatives being explored?

Remember that outcome measures are unique to the perspective of the stakeholders and span a wide scope from reduction in costs and litigation to increased productivity, including the goal of having healthier workers and enhanced morale.

CHANGE FROM WITHIN

If we expect to influence change in our profession, it must start first with individuals. If we expect to influence change in our workplace, it must first start with ourselves. In all life there are sequential stages of growth and development, and each stage is important in leading to the next stage. Each stage requires a new level of thinking, an inside-out approach to personal and interpersonal effectiveness (Covey, 1989). As change evolves, you must first take a look at yourself, as a professional and as a person. Start with yourself, your character and your motives. Burgel and Childre (2012) propose that trusted partnerships between OHNs and workers are vital, and in order to achieve this engagement, the OHN must develop a professional, ethical practice base. The OHN must strive for a continual process of self-renewal, searching for higher levels of responsibility, independence, and effective interdependence with stakeholders, peers, and mentors. As a professional in the world of business, we must strive to develop strategic partnerships and think like a business leader.

Change must begin from the inside-out, by first creating a paradigm or personal worldview; a sort of lens through which you see the world and your role as a professional expert. Never be satisfied with the status quo. Continue to build your professional script and build positive relationships, achieving unity with others that will help achieve your paradigm. Build a character of integrity and know that internal change precedes external victories (Covey, 2004). Be involved with local, state, and national professional organizations that provide resources and opportunities for professional growth. And network with other professionals involved in the specialty.

Table 14.2 Outcomes report: effectiveness of a safety and workers' compensation case management program over time.

2012

Work Status Trend

Decrease in lost days and Increase in modified duty days

Worker's Compensation Comparisons

Lost days decreased

- 2009 lost days   112
- 2010 lost days   112   (no change)
- 2011 lost days   36   (decreased 68%)
- 2012 lost days   1   (decreased 99%)

Modified days increased

- 2009 modified days   442
- 2010 modified days   382   (decreased 14%)
- 2011 modified days   78   (decreased 82%)
- 2012 modified days   111   (decreased 75%)

There is a consistent trend in reducing lost work time evidenced by fewer lost work days and increased modified work days.

Injury Type Comparison

Injury Type

	2007	2009	2009	2010	2011	2012
Repetitive motion	7	5	2	1	0	0
Sprains/strains	13	1	9	10	1	3
Cuts/contusions	13	10	8	7	9	6
Dermatitis	0	0	0	0	1	0
Amputation	0	0	0	0	1	0
Fracture	3	2	3	3	1	3
Insect bites	0	0	0	0	0	2
TOTAL	36	34	22	21	14	14

Trend Analysis
- Top loss source for 2012 again was cuts/contusions.
- Sprains/stains are no longer presenting as an issue.
- 67% occurred on the third shift. Interesting since the first shift represents the larger headcount.
- The most frequently occurring severe injuries experiencing lost or modified days were related to falls. Additionally, we had other falls treated at the Health Services Clinic and not recorded on the OSHA log. Several of these would have resulted in OSHA recordable cases had the OHN intervention not been available.
- The highest incidence of claims continues to be experienced in areas where a higher incident rate was anticipated due to number of employees or job duties of those involved (i.e., Press and Machine Maintenance in 2012).

Table 14.2 (*Continued*)

Injury Recap

	2007	2008	2009	2010	2011	2012
Injuries	36	34	22	21	14	14
# Lost Work Days	3	3	3	2	3	1
# Modified Work Days	9	14	19	10	4	3
# Hours Worked	*2,540,949*	*2,577,875*	*2,412,650*	*2,442,114*	*3,455,289*	*2,825,364*
Incident Rate	2.60	2.66	2.64	1.58	.81	.99

Return on Investment of OHN

Providing occupational health services on site provides immediate injury care.
- In 2008, our OHN(s) provided healthcare triage eliminating the need for outpatient treatment resulting in savings of approximately $1,000 per incident.
- Total savings represented is $76,000.00

Additionally, due to intervention and case management by OHN(s), six (6) cases were denied by the claims adjuster or because of OHN's intervention were not required to be reported and hence were not work related. Avoided costs (not including potential costs of time away from work or modified duty) are estimated below:

1 Contusion (R) Middle finger	$ 5,000	No referral required
1 Lac (L) Hand	$ 5,000	Care on site
1 Complained of back/hand pain	$90,000	Preexisting/denied
1 Contusion/laceration finger	$ 5,000	Tx OTC meds
1 Soft tissue injury	$10,000	Not recordable
1 (R) Knee strain	$ 40,000	Preexisting
1 (R) Foot injury	$ 30,000	Preexisting
Total savings approximated at	$185,000	

Total savings to company
Result of on-site nurses
- Savings related to care on-site
  - $76,000.00
- Savings related to case management
  - $185,000
- Total net savings
  - $261,000

OUTCOMES
- Reduced healthcare costs
- Reduced litigation
- Healthier employees
- Increased productivity
- Enhanced morale
- Increased retention and recruitment

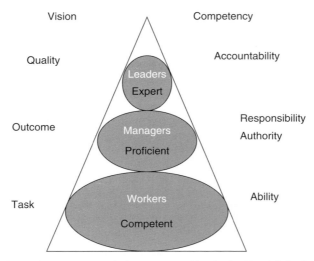

Figure 14.2 Guzik's Occupational Health Competency and Leadership Model. © Guzik, 2005.

BE A LEADER

As an occupational health professional, you must strive to achieve the core competencies expected of the profession and build expertise along the continuum of practice experience. Figure 14.2 depicts a model or framework on which to build your professional growth and development. The OHN's role is often defined as "manager"; however, it is important to acknowledge that you hold a breadth of content expertise in the specialty of occupational health. As a result, stakeholders and workers will look to you to be the content expert, providing the guidance and direction needed to propel the program forward, to maintain value, and to strive to not only maintain effectiveness, but also to bring new ideas and new initiatives to the business.

As a leader, you will be setting a path, goal, or vision for others. You will be the motivating force to pursue and eventually achieve the goal, and you must achieve the desired competencies commensurate with Guzik's Occupational Health Competency and Leadership Model. As the content expert, it is not sufficient to just be a worker who holds competent clinical nursing skills who will accomplish the healthcare tasks. Businesses look to the OHN to be much more, to provide greater value. This expectation is valid because, as the content expert, you will hold more responsibility, have more authority, and should be focused on program management and outcomes. This midlevel leadership is the level of performance most desired by company leaders because of the inherent value of not just having a nurse focused on tasks, but having a nurse who is focused on managing the occupational health services in a proficient manner.

Table 14.3 Traits of managers vs. leaders.

Issue	Manager	Leader
Planning	Detail oriented and time oriented	Provides overview and is focused on results
Thinking	Assesses risk and is rational	Challenges status quo, forward thinker, intuitive
People	Supervises and provides support	Motivates, encourages, and mentors
Change	Manages status quo	Seeks and affects change
Resources	Allocates and monitors	Looks for opportunities and seek out options
Focus	Detail oriented	Sees the big picture and looks to the future

A few OHNs strive to develop and hold a greater level of authority as they move to the top of Guzik's Occupational Health and Leadership Model, striving to be a leader, rather than a manager. At this level, the OHN has become an expert in a broad dimension of occupational health competencies and is viewed as a true leader, focused on quality. This level is associated with a high level of accountability and is often in a top-level position in the organization. In this role, the OHN sets the path, goal, or vision for the occupational health program and provides the motivation and aptitude to eventually achieve the established goals. This includes developing strategies, communicating, making decisions, and collecting data, along with sustaining the motivation and enthusiasm of all stakeholders. Table 14.3 depicts traits specific to managers versus leaders.

As a true leader, the OHN should never be satisfied with the status quo. Be an innovator and be willing to take risks. As an innovator of ideas, it is important to always look for better processes and opportunities. Seek challenging opportunities to change, grow, and improve, not only the program, but yourself. Look to the future. Remember that programs often reach a plateau, where they can no longer continue to increase in value. This is often a time when the program comes under scrutiny by executive leadership in regard to the resources being spent and the return on investment. Therefore, it is important to always strive to know what ideas and concepts are on the cutting edge in the profession and to develop and propose new, value-added services. Being a true leader requires self-confidence, honesty, integrity, and the desire to lead. It requires a comprehensive knowledge of the business. And most of all, it requires drive and ambition.

Power exists in all organizations and it is important to identify where the power lies that will provide value to decision making or support. Table 14.4 describes the various sources of power in business. Know your audience and know your stakeholders and what type of power they hold in relation to the program. By knowing the resources of power, you are then able to leverage relationships and support that will influence decision making. And know

Table 14.4 Source of power in business.

Office power	Associated with a particular managerial function
Expert power	Information, knowledge, skills, abilities, and experience
Referent power	Connection with other individuals and groups who possess influence
Reward/coercive power	In control of incentives
Charismatic power	The power of one's own persona

Table 14.5 Decision influencers in business.

Authoritarian	Decisions or mandates made by business leaders and executive
Financial	Decisions made by financiers or finance officers
Legal	Decisions made by company or consulting attorneys and legal counsel
Regulatory	Decisions influenced by regulatory statute or law
Human Resources	Decisions made by human resource professionals
Operations	Decisions made by operations management

what stakeholders will be involved in making decisions related to programs and services. Table 14.5 lists the various decision influencers who will lend input from their expert viewpoint. In business, there is often need to consider the input and decisions from a cross-section of various perspectives. Get to know these individuals well before their expertise and input is needed. Consider them mentors and get to know how they think. This will keep you one step ahead in anticipating the challenges that may be incurred from their perspectives.

SUMMARY
Occupational health nursing services vary from business to business. Every business holds its unique set of risks and challenges in relation to the health, safety, and well-being of its population. The OHN must strive to engage a variety of initiatives, both traditional and not so traditional, in order to meet those needs. A service that provides health resources and integrated health management programs focused on optimal health, regulatory compliance, and enhanced productivity will provide a value-added service.

The OHN provides a supportive and encouraging force for the business, and it is important to continue to reach for new opportunities. As a professional, you must learn from and share best practices. You must be a propeller of new ideas and think outside the box for new and innovative strategies to enhance the health and safety of the workplace.

Always strive to be professional, proactive, and helpful. Be knowledgeable and give stakeholders what they expect and need. Collaborate every step of the way. Practice what you preach. Be human, and be humane. Keep your promises, and provide a high-quality product. Develop loyalty and think long term in your endeavors. Customize, personalize, and hang over the leading edge. Be creative. Add value. Most of all, become an expert resource and trusted advisor ... and always be looking **Upstream**.

Wishing you success, every step of the way.

REFERENCES

Bergstrom, M. (2005). The potential-method—An economic evaluation tool. *Journal of Safety Research - ECON Proceedings, 36*, 237–240. Retrieved from http://www.who.int/occupational_health/topics/bergstrom.pdf

Bunn, W. B., Allen, H., Stave, G. M., & Naim, A.B. (2010). How to align evidence-based benefit design with the employer bottom-line: A case study. *Journal of Occupational and Environmental Medicine, 52*(10), 956–963.

Burgel, B. J. & Childre, F. (2012). The occupational health nurse as the trusted clinician in the 21st century. *Workplace Health and Safety, 60*(4), 143–150.

Carnegie, D. (Speaker). (2000). *The Dale Carnegie Leadership Mastery Course: How to challenge yourself and others to greatness.* [Sound recording] Chicago: Simon and Schuster Audio.

Centers for Disease Control and Prevention. (2011). *NIOSH Program: Global Collaborations.* Retrieved from http://www.cdc.gov/niosh/programs/global/economics.html

Covey, S. R. (1989). *The 7 habits of highly effective people.* New York: Fireside Press.

Covey, S. R. (2004). *The 8th habit. From effectiveness to greatness.* New York: Free Press.

Ennals, R. (2002). *Partnership for sustainable healthy workplaces.* (Warner Lecture). Sheffield: British Occupational Hygiene Society. Retrieved from http://annhyg.oxfordjournals.org/content/46/4/423.full

Goetzel, R. Z. (2005). *Examining the value of integrating occupational health and safety and health promotion programs in the workplace. Final report.* National Institute of Occupational Safety and Health (NIOSH) #211-2004-M-09393. Retrieved from www.factsforhealthcare.com/management/Assets/NIOSH_Background_Paper_Goetzel.pdf

Goetzel, R. Z., Anderson, D. R., Whitmer, R. W., Ozminkowski, R. J., Dunn, R. L., Wasserman, J., & Health Enhancement Research Organization (HERO) Research Committee. (1998). The relationship between modifiable health risks and health care expenditures. An analysis of the multi-employer HERO health risk and cost database. Journal of Occupational and Environmental Medicine. *40*(1), 843–854.

Goetzel, R. Z., Guindon, A. M., Turshen, I. J., & Ozminkowski, R. J. Health and productivity management – Establishing key performance measures, benchmarks and best practices. *Journal of Occupational and Environmental Medicine*, 43(1), 10–17.

Goetzel, R. Z., Hawkins, K., Ozminkowski, R. J., & Wang, S. (2003). The health and productivity cost burden of the "top 10" physical and mental health conditions affecting six large U.S. employers in 1999. *Journal of Occupational and Environmental Medicine*, 45(1), 5–14.

Goetzel, R. Z., Juday, T. R., & Ozminkowski, R. J. (1999). What's the ROI? A systematic review of return-on-investment studies of corporate health and productivity management initiatives. *AWHP's Worksite Health*, 6(3), 12–21.

Goetzel, R. Z. & Ozminkowski, R. J. (2008). The health and cost benefits of work site health-promotion programs. *Annual Review of Public Health*, 29, 303–323.

Goetzel, R. Z., Shechter, D., Ozminkowski, R. J., Marmet, P. F., Tabrizi, M.J., & Roemer, E. C. (2007). Promising practices in employer health and productivity management efforts: Findings from a benchmarking study. *Journal of Occupational and Environmental Medicine*, 49(2), 111–130.

Green-McKenzie, J., Rainer, S., Behrman, A., & Emmett, E. (2002). The effect of a health care management initiative on reducing workers' compensation costs. *Journal of Occupational and Environmental Medicine*, 44(12), 1100–1105.

Gregory J. W., Lukes, E., & Gregory, C. A. (2002). Using financial metrics to prove and communicate value to management: Occupational health nurses as key players on the management team. *AAOHN Journal*, 50(9), 143–150.

Guzik, A., Menzel, N. N., Fitzpatrick, J., & McNulty, R. (2009). Patient satisfaction with nurse practitioner and physician services in the occupational health setting. *AAOHN Journal*, 57(5), 191–197.

Harber, P., Rose, S., Bontemps, J., Saechao, K., Liu, Y., Elashoff, D., & Wu, S. (2010). Occupational medicine practice: One specialty or three? *Journal of Occupational and Environmental Medicine*, 52(7), 672–679.

Kaline, C. M., Haag, A. B., & Tourigan, R. (2004). What are some of the challenges in case management and how have you handled them? *AAOHN Journal*, 52(4), 143–145.

Knave, B. & Ennals, R. (2002). International trends in occupational health research and practice. *Industrial Health*, 40, 69–73.

Levine, S. (1993). The leader in you: How to win friends, influence people, and succeed in a changing world. New York: Simon & Schuster.

Linhard, J. B. (2005). Understanding the return on health, safety and environmental investments. *Journal of Safety Research - ECON Proceedings*, 36, 257–260. Retrieved from http://www.who.int/occupational_health/topics/linhard.pdf

Miller, P., Rossiter, P., & Nuttall, D. (2002). Demonstrating the economic value of occupational health services. *Occupational Medicine*, 52. Retrieved from http://occmed.oxfordjournals.org/content/52/8/477.full.pdf+html

Mellor, G. & St. John, W. (2009). Managers' Perceptions of the current and future role of occupational health nurses in Australia. *AAOHN Journal*, 57(2), 79–87.

Miller, P., Whynes, D., & Reidj, A. (2000). An economic evaluation of occupational health. *Occupational Medicine*, 50(3), 159–163.

Oxenburgh, M. & Marlow, P. (2005). The productivity assessment tool: Computer-based cost benefit analysis model for the economic assessment of occupational health and safety interventions in the workplace. *Journal of Safety Research – ECON Proceedings 36*, 209–214.

Randolph, S. A. (2006). Developing policies and procedures. *AAOHN Journal, 54*(11), 501–504.

Redmond, M. S., & Kalina, C. M. (2009). A successful occupational health nurse-driven health promotion program to support corporate sustainability. *AAOHN Journal, 57*(12), 507–514.

Robbins, Anthony. (1991). *Awaken the giant within*. New York: Fireside Press.

Rogers, B. (2012). Occupational and environmental health nursing: Ethics and professionalism. *Workplace Health & Safety, 60*(4), 177–181.

Weiss, M. D. (2009). Changing the conversation—The occupational health nurse's role in integrated Hs3™. *AAOHN Journal, 57*(7), 293–299.

Whitaker, S. & Baranski, B. (Eds.). (2001). The role of the occupational health nurse in workplace health management. Copenhagen: WHO Regional Office for Europe. Retrieved from http://www.who.int/occupational_health/regions/en/oeheurnursing.pdf

The World Bank. *World development report 2000/2001*. (2001). Retrieved from http://documents.worldbank.org/curated/en/2000/09/1561427/world-development-report-20002001-attacking-poverty

Williamson, G. (2007). Providing leadership in a culturally diverse workplace. *AAOHN Journal, 55*(8), 329–333.

General Definitions and Terms

A1

Absenteeism—the time an employee spends away from work. Absences can be scheduled (e.g., vacation time) or unscheduled (e.g., due to illness or injury).

Administrative controls—policies and practices that reduce work-related musculoskeletal disorders risk but they do not eliminate workplace hazards.

Biometric screening—the measurement of physical characteristics such as height, weight, body mass index, blood pressure, blood cholesterol, blood glucose, and aerobic fitness tests that can be taken at the worksite and used as part of a workplace health assessment to benchmark and evaluate changes in employee health status over time.

Community linkages—partnerships with organizations in the surrounding community such as YMCAs or local hospitals to offer health-related programs and services to employees when the employer does not have the capacity or expertise to do so or to provide support for healthy lifestyles to employees when not at the workplace.

Culture of health—the creation of a working environment where employee health and safety is valued, supported, and promoted through workplace health programs, policies, benefits, and environmental supports. Building a culture of health involves all levels of the organization and establishes the workplace health program as a routine part of business operations aligned with overall business goals. The results of this culture change include engaged and empowered employees, an impact on healthcare costs, and improved worker productivity.

Demographics—a statistic characterizing human population groups data such as age, sex, race/ethnicity, or vital statistics.

Disability—a physical or mental impairment that substantially limits one or more of the major life activities of an individual.

Essentials for Occupational Health Nursing, First Edition. Arlene Guzik.
© 2013 John Wiley & Sons, Inc. Published 2013 by John Wiley & Sons, Inc.

Employee health survey—a means to gain input from an employee on health-related issues. Survey items may include questions relating to health behavior (physical activity, dietary habits), use of preventive health services, and measures of health status (blood pressure and cholesterol levels). Additional items could include employees and management health promotion needs and interests as well as opportunities and barriers to participating in workplace health programs.

Engineering controls—the preferred approach to prevent and control work-related musculoskeletal disorders by designing job tasks to take account of the capabilities and limitations of the workforce.

Ergonomics—the science of designing the job and the workplace to suit the capabilities of the workers. Simply stated, ergonomics means "fitting the task to the worker." The aim of ergonomics is the evaluation and design of facilities, workstations, jobs, training methods, and equipment to match the capabilities of users and workers and thereby reduce stress and eliminate injuries and disorders associated with the overuse of muscles, bad posture, and repeated tasks.

Environmental assessment—a process to observe the workplace to understand more about the setting employees work in and the physical factors, such as the built environment, at and nearby the worksite that support or hinder employee health. The built environment includes all the physical parts of the worksite (building, workstations, open spaces, streets, and infrastructure) that can influence employee health. It considers such components as land use patterns, transportation systems, and design features.

Genetic Information Nondiscrimination Act (GINA) of 2008—a law that prohibits discrimination in health coverage and employment based on genetic information. It generally prohibits health insurers or health plan administrators from requesting or requiring an individual or individual's family member's genetic information or using the information for decisions regarding coverage such as determining premium rates or eligibility.

Health behavior—an action taken by an individual or group of individuals to change or maintain their health status or prevent illness or injury.

Health benefits—health insurance coverage conditions and other services or discounts regarding health provided as part of an employee benefits package.

Health education—learning opportunities designed to encourage or promote the adoption of healthy behaviors.

Health-related programs and services—opportunities available to employees at the workplace or through outside organizations to start, change, or maintain health behaviors. Programs and services can be (1) informational approaches directed at changing knowledge or attitudes about the benefits of and opportunities for healthy lifestyles or (2) behavior or social approaches designed to teach employees the behavioral management skills necessary for successful adaptation and maintenance of behavior change.

Health risk appraisal (HRA)—an assessment tool used to evaluate an individual's health. An HRA could include a health survey or questionnaire (*see* employee health survey); physical examination, or laboratory tests resulting in a profile of individual health risks, often with accompanying advice or strategies to reduce the risks.

Health and safety risk—a behavior or condition that influences the chance or probability of susceptibility to a specific health issue.

Health status—the state of health, such as the prevalence of diseases or health conditions of an individual, group, or population.

Incentives—a tangible commodity or service given to an employee for completion of a predetermined action or based upon achievement of goal or desired outcome.

Intervention—a generic term used in public health to describe a program or policy designed to have an impact on a health problem.

Job (work-related/occupational) stress—the harmful physical and emotional responses that occur when the requirements of the job do not match the capabilities, resources, or needs of the worker, which can lead to illness or injury.

Material safety data sheets—forms used to describe the short and long-term health effects, physical and chemical properties, flammability, safety hazards, and emergency response procedures of a particular substance or industrial product.

Personal protective equipment (PPE)—specialized gear or clothing worn by workers to protect them from job hazards.

Physical activity—an action that gets the body moving.

Presenteeism—the measurable extent to which health symptoms, conditions, and diseases adversely affect the work productivity of individuals who choose to remain at work.

Productivity (health-related)—a measure of worker output impacted by the worker's health status.

Program evaluation— the systematic investigation of the merit (e.g., quality), worth (e.g., effectiveness), and significance (e.g., importance) of an organized health promotion action/activity (e.g., workplace health program, policy, or environmental support) intended to improve employee health.

Program planning—a process to develop the components of a workplace health program including goal determination, implementation, and evaluation strategies.

Return on investment (ROI)—an analysis used to compare the investment costs to the magnitude and timing of expected gains. For workplace health programs, this usually refers to the medical savings or productivity gains associated with the employer's investment in employee health programs.

Self-management—the activities and skills (e.g., goal setting, decision making, self-monitoring) an individual with one or more chronic conditions learns and uses to improve quality of life. Education and support from healthcare or other providers can enhance an individual's self-confidence and self-management skills.

Social support—physical or emotional comfort given to an individual by family, friends, coworkers, or others. Groups of individuals can form social support networks to provide motivation or reassurance when making behavior changes such as increasing physical activity.

Wellness council or committee—a group of employees and managers who broadly represent (across departments, business units, or job categories) a worksite's workforce. The committee works with workplace health promotion program staff to advise, consult or make program decisions, promote and champion the program, and represent the needs and interests of employees.

Workers' compensation—a type of insurance paid by employers to provide benefits and medical care to employers in the event they become ill or are injured on the job.

Workplace governance—infrastructure at the workplace to lead and support employee health programs. The infrastructure includes the management and strategic direction of the program that runs through all levels of the organization, including leadership support, dedicated resources, a workplace health improvement plan, communications, and workplace health informatics and data.

Workplace health assessment—a process of gathering information about the factors that support and/or hinder the health of employees at a particular workplace and identifying potential opportunities to improve or address them.

Workplace health programs—a coordinated and comprehensive set of strategies that include programs, policies, benefits, environmental supports, and links to the surrounding community designed to meet the health and safety needs of all employees.

Adapted from: The Centers for Disease Control and Prevention. National Center for Chronic Disease Prevention and Health Promotion. Division of Population Health. http://www.cdc.gov/workplacehealthpromotion/glossary/index.html#W3

Sample Occupational Health Nurse Job Description

A2

Job Title: Occupational Health Registered Nurse

Department:

Reports To:

FLSA Status:

Prepared By:

Prepared Date:

Approved By:

Approved Date:

Summary Responsible for the development and administration of efficient and professional operations of occupational health services in accordance with company policies, practices, procedures, and applicable regulations to achieve the desired goals and objectives. Assists with all aspects of health services staffing, competency, processes, customer service, and quality improvement.

Essential Duties and Responsibilities Include, but are not limited to the following. Other duties may be assigned.

Oversee and manage the administrative and operational activities of occupational health services

- Assure compliance with regulatory requirements related to clinical operations
- Responsible for securing and developing all records, equipment, and programs related to occupational health services
- Collaborate with outside resources for program development, such as healthcare providers, third-party administrators, legal advisors, medical director, regulatory agencies, etc.

Essentials for Occupational Health Nursing, First Edition. Arlene Guzik.
© 2013 John Wiley & Sons, Inc. Published 2013 by John Wiley & Sons, Inc.

Responsible for assuring the appropriate access and utilization of healthcare services

- Evaluate and treat all injuries and illnesses in an efficient and professional manner within the scope of practice and consistent with clinical nursing guidelines
  - Guide and direct all referrals to outside healthcare providers and services

Provide or manage the required physical evaluation programs and services to meet regulatory requirement; such as OSHA, Department of Transportation, CDC, etc.

Train and lead ergonomic team to assess jobs and provide input regarding ergonomic improvements.

Administer the company's Drug-Free Workplace Program.

Assist with the accident investigation program to identify root cause analysis of all incidents and near misses.

Provide appropriate case management

- Manage all cases to facilitate productivity, assuring appropriate care and return to work
- Includes workers' compensation, short- and long-term disability cases
- Assess healthcare needs, then implement and manage healthcare programs to improve health and facilitate return to work, maintain OSHA records/ reports and worker medical files
- Assist departments with identifying, evaluating, and implementing accommodations and return to work options for workers with restricted duty.

Collaborate with Environmental Health and Safety, Operations, and Human Resources to develop operations, programs, and services by providing content expertise.

- Contribute in the design of controls for injury prevention and health surveillance related to actual and potential hazards in the work environment.
- Identify primary, secondary, and tertiary prevention and health promotion strategies to optimize health of the population.

Supervisory Responsibilities
Responsible for direct and indirect supervision of health services staff

Qualifications To perform this job successfully, an individual must be able to perform each essential duty satisfactorily. The requirements listed below are representative of the knowledge, skill, and/or ability required. Reasonable accommodations may be made to enable individuals with disabilities to perform the essential functions.

Education and/or Experience

Active state nursing license as registered nurse. Bachelor's degree and certification in occupational health nursing or case management preferred.

Basic understanding of federal and state regulations applicable to occupational and environmental health and safety.

Language Skills

Ability to read and interpret documents such as safety rules, operating and maintenance instructions, and procedure manuals. Ability to write routine reports and correspondence.

Mathematical Skills

Ability to add, subtract, multiply, and divide in all units of measure, using whole numbers, common fractions, and decimals.

Reasoning Ability

Ability to solve practical problems and deal with a variety of concrete variables in situations where only limited standardization exists. Ability to interpret a variety of instructions furnished in written, oral, diagram, or schedule form.

Computer Skills

Intermediate computer skills are essential in use of an electronic medical record.

Certificates, Licenses, Registrations

Active state license as registered nurse. Certified as occupational health nurse or case manager.

Other Skills and Abilities

Must be detail oriented, have ability to multitask and possess great interpersonal skills. Travel to other company locations is required.

Other Qualifications

Must be willing to travel to other locations to assist with audits, training, and setup of new facilitates. May require extended stay in remote location for brief period of time for new acquisitions or start-up facilities.

Physical Demands The physical demands described here are representative of those that must be met by any worker to successfully perform the essential functions of this job. Reasonable accommodations may be made to enable individuals with disabilities to perform the essential functions. While performing the duties of this Job, the worker is regularly required to talk and hear. The worker is frequently required to stand; walk; use hands to finger, handle, or feel and reach with hands and arms. The worker is occasionally required to sit and stoop, kneel, crouch, or crawl. The worker must frequently lift and/or move up to 50 pounds. Specific vision abilities required by this job include close vision, distance vision, color vision, peripheral vision, depth perception, and ability to adjust focus.

Work Environment The work environment characteristics described here are representative of those any worker encounters while performing the essential functions of this job. Reasonable accommodations may be made to enable individuals with disabilities to perform the essential functions. While performing the duties of this job, the worker is occasionally exposed to risk of communicable disease. The noise level in the work environment is usually moderate.

Sample Agreement for Professional Services

A3

Medical Direction and Program Oversight for Occupational Health Nurse

This Agreement is executed and made effective as of the _____ by and between COMPANY NAME (hereinafter referred to as the "Company") and, MEDICAL DIRECTOR NAME (hereinafter referred to as "Medical Director").

WHEREAS, the Company desires to provide its employees with occupational health services; and

WHEREAS, Medical Director is a provider of occupational health services;

The Company agrees to retain Medical Director to provide occupational health services for the Company's employees, and the parties further agree as follows:

I. COMPENSATION

Company agrees to pay Medical Director a fee in the amount of $xxx per month, paid at the time of execution and monthly thereafter.

II. PERFORMANCE AND PROFESSIONAL RESPONSIBILITIES

A. DUTIES OF MEDICAL DIRECTOR

Medical Director agrees to maintain full licensure to practice medicine in the State of _____ and remain in good standing with the Agency for Health Care Administration. Medical Director will maintain the required protocols for the Occupational Health Nurse(s)s and Nurse(s) Practitioners and provide proof of foregoing protocol renewal on an annual basis as desired by the Company.

Medical Direction and program oversight for Occupational Health Nurse(s)

Essentials for Occupational Health Nursing, First Edition. Arlene Guzik.
© 2013 John Wiley & Sons, Inc. Published 2013 by John Wiley & Sons, Inc.

Includes the following description of services

- Annual review of Occupational Health Nurse protocols
- Annual review and signature for Prescription Authorization Release
- AED Medical Direction
- Annual on-site Company walk-through
- Annual on-site Occupational Health Clinic inspection and audit
- Verbal consultation and guidance for cases regarding fitness for duty, FMLA, ADA, short-term disability, health concerns in the workplace

Medical Director hereby represents and warrants that he/she has had substantial prior experience in providing occupational health services that are the same or similar in design, function and complexity as the project to be performed under the Scope of Services and has the necessary expertise, skill, and ability to perform such Services. Medical Director agrees that he/she will perform its services in accordance with the standards of care and diligence normally practiced by recognized firms in performing services of a similar nature.

Medical Director represents that during Medical Director's performance of services hereunder, adequate provision shall be made to staff and retain the services of such competent personnel having sufficient qualification by education, experience, license and skill as may be appropriate or necessary for the performance of such services. The Company shall have the right to review the personnel assigned and Medical Director shall remove any personnel not acceptable to The Company.

B. DUTIES OF THE COMPANY AND COMPENSATION TO MEDICAL DIRECTOR

1. The Company agrees to retain Medical Director for a period of ___ years from the effective date of this contract, with an option to renew for an additional ___ year period thereafter. Medical Director shall be entitled to annual increases for its services on the anniversary date of each year of the original ___ year term. Such annual increases shall be a minimum of ___ percent but no more than ___ percent over the previous year's gross amount paid to Medical Director for his/her services, not including the cost of any additional services provided by Medical Director. The Company will provide adequate physical facilities and medical equipment to conduct the services described within the scope of services. Such annual increases shall be determined at the discretion of Medical Director within the parameters noted herein. Medical Director shall give the Company a minimum of ___ days prior written notice of the increase that will be in effect for the next annual period.

   The Company shall give written notification to Medical Director no sooner than XXX days prior to the expiration of the initial ___ year term of this agreement of its intention to not renew this agreement for an additional term.

Should Medical Director not seek to renew the agreement with the Company for an additional term, then he/she shall notify the Company in writing, at least ___ days prior to the expiration of the initial ___ year term, of its intentions not to renew this agreement, and the Company's right to renew the agreement for an additional ___ year period shall be terminated.

2. The Company shall provide Medical Director with copies of the professional license(s) of the Occupational Health Nurse(s).

3. The Company shall give written notification to Medical Director immediately upon any change in personnel staffing the occupational health services, specifically the Occupational Health Nurse(s).

4. The Company shall give written notification to Medical Director immediately upon any change in liability coverage for the Occupational Health Nurse(s).

5. The Company shall give written notification to Medical Director immediately upon any notice of professional, regulatory or liability issues regarding the Occupational Health Nurse(s).

6. The Company agrees to utilize Medical Director Clinics and Medical Providers as Provider of Choice for services listed in Duties of Medical Director (II. A.)

7. The Company agrees to maintain all pertinent licenses and permits as required by the State of practice. A copy of these permits will be provided to Medical Director before authorization for purchase of prescription drugs is given.

C. CONFIDENTIALITY

The parties agree that all patient records shall be treated as confidential so as to comply with all State, Federal, and ethical requirements regarding confidentiality of medical records.

III. ADDITIONAL SERVICES PROVIDED BY MEDICAL DIRECTOR

Medical Director will participate in quality monitoring and on-site clinic audits on an annual basis. Reports of these audits will be provided to The Company.

Additional medical on-site testing/screenings, specialty training, specialty evaluations provided by Medical Director employees, other than the Company's Occupational Health Nurse(s), or care provided in a community-based clinic, will be billed as a fee for service, in addition to this contract rate.

IV. INSURANCE

Medical Director shall, at his/her own expense, beginning with the date this Agreement commences and at all time during performance of this Agreement, carry and maintain, with an insurance carrier or carriers reasonably acceptable to The Company, policies acceptable to The Company as follows:

1. Workers' Compensation insurance in accordance with Workers' Compensation Act(s) of the state or states wherein work under this Agreement is to be performed.
2. Employers' Liability insurance with limits of liability of no less than $___ per accident or disease including death at any time resulting therefrom.
3. Medical Malpractice insurance will be maintained by Medical Director. $___ per occurrence, $___ aggregate.

    The Company shall, at its own expense, beginning with the date this Agreement commences and at all time during performance of this Agreement, carry and maintain, with an insurance carrier or carriers reasonably acceptable to The Company, policies acceptable to The Company as follows:

4. Medical Malpractice insurance to cover medical liability for all medical personnel employed by the Company: $___ per occurrence, $___ aggregate.

    Medical Director shall furnish The Company certificates of insurance evidencing the insurance coverages required in this Article III (1) through (3) above.

    The Company shall furnish Medical Director certificates of insurance evidencing the insurance coverages required in this Article III (4) through (5) above.

    The certificates shall stipulate that should any of the above insurance policies be canceled or materially altered before the termination of this Agreement, the issuing company shall mail a notice to other party of such change of termination (30) days prior to any such change or termination. Either party shall request to examine original policies issued in compliance with the requirements hereof.

V. OWNERSHIP AND MAINTENANCE OF DOCUMENTS AND TREATMENT OF PROPRIETARY AND CONFIDENTIAL MATERIALS

Medical Director shall maintain accurate and detailed financial records, books, and documents ("Records") in connection with the Work and all transactions related thereto.

Medical Director will use his/her proprietary forms, procedures, etc, which will remain the property of Medical Director. By signing this agreement, Medical Director does not relinquish ownership of or control over any of his/her proprietary property. Such proprietary property of Medical Director shall include, but shall not be limited to, policies (written or oral), procedures (written or oral), forms, and all systems including computer systems and procedures employed by Medical Director.

The Company or Medical Director may designate certain documents provided to Medical Director or the Company respectively as Confidential and/or subject to a legal privilege against disclosure. Each party to this Agreement shall safeguard and maintain these documents in confidence; shall disclose these documents to their employees only on a need-to-know basis and only after such employees have agreed to equivalent conditions pertaining to non-disclosure as contained herein; and shall not disclose such documents to any third party without prior written consent of the other Party to this Agreement.

The nondisclosure obligations of this Article shall not apply to:

a. such information as is or becomes a part of the public domain otherwise than by a wrongful act or omission of one of the parties;
b. such information that is subsequently available or becomes generally available to the public; or,
c. such information that was obtained from a third party on a nonconfidential basis; provided however, nothing in this Agreement shall prevent the parties from using information obtained from an independent third party consistent with the obligations, if any, imposed by such third party.

VI. MEDIATION AND ARBITRATION OF DISPUTES:

a. Mediation of Disputes: Except for disputes arising under paragraph 6(b) herein, the parties agree to mediate in good faith any disputes which may arise under this agreement or its termination.
b. Arbitration of Disputes: Except for disputes arising under paragraph 6(b) herein, Medical Director and (Company) agree to use final and binding arbitration to resolve any dispute not previously resolved by mediation, and that relates to or in any way arises from this agreement or its termination.
c. The Arbitration: Arbitration shall take place in (City, State) before an experienced arbitrator licensed to practice in (State) and selected in accordance with the Dispute Resolution Rules of the American Arbitration Association. The arbitrator may not modify or change this agreement in any way. The arbitrator shall apply the substantive law of the state in which the claim arose, or federal law where applicable. The arbitrator shall have the authority to grant any remedies provided under the substantive law of the state in which the claim arose, or federal law applicable, except for remedies and/or relief excluded by the agreement. The arbitrator, and not any federal, state or local court or agency, shall have exclusive authority to resolve any dispute relating to the interpretation, applicability, or enforceability of this agreement, including but not limited to, any claim that all or any part of this agreement is void or avoidable. The arbitration shall be final and binding upon the parties.
d. Fees and Expenses: Each party shall pay the fees of their respective attorneys, the expenses of their witnesses, and any other expenses connected with preparing for and attending mediation and arbitration,

but all other costs of the arbitration, including the fees of the arbitrator, cost of any record or transcript of the arbitration, administrative fees, and other fees of the arbitrator, cost of any record of transcript of the arbitration, administrative fees, and other fees and costs shall be paid in equal shares by the parties. The party losing the arbitration shall reimburse the party who prevailed for all expenses the prevailing party paid pursuant to the preceding sentence.

e. Exclusive Remedy: Mediation and arbitration in the manner described above shall be the exclusive remedy for any dispute between us arising under this agreement. Should either party attempt to resolve such a dispute by any method other than mediation and arbitration pursuant to this section, the responding party shall be entitled to recover from the initiating party all damages, expenses, and attorneys' fees incurred as a result of that breach.

VII. TERMINATION

A. Either The Company or Medical Director may terminate the services provided under this Agreement, in whole or in part, with ___ days written notice to the other party that services are to be terminated. Upon Medical Director's receipt of such notice from the Company, Medical Director shall cease performance of the services to the extent specified by the Company in the notice. Medical Director shall thereafter perform only such portion of the services (if any) that have not been terminated by the Company. In the event of termination, Medical Director shall be paid for all services actually performed and all expenses actually incurred by Medical Director in compliance with the Agreement prior to such termination and all costs and expenses which are necessary to effect the termination of this Agreement, or to protect the Company's interests. In addition, Medical Director will be paid for any identifiable cost commitments incurred by Medical Director as a result of the Company's Agreement, provided the commitments are of no value to Medical Director. Except those matters that are required to be maintained by Medical Director as confidential, all work completed by Medical Director and paid for by the Company shall become the property of the Company.

VIII. NOTICES AND INVOICING

A. All notices referenced in this agreement shall be sent by the sending party to the receiving party by certified mail, return receipt requested as well as a copy by first class mail to the representative and address listed below for each of the parties to this agreement. Notice shall be deemed received on the date indicated by the return receipt of the certified mailing, or within five (5) days of mailing, whichever occurs first.

COMPANY NAME   Medical Director:

ADDRESS   ADDRESS

Key Contact: _____   Key Contact: _____

B. All invoices for the services covered by this agreement shall be addressed as follows:

Company Name

Address

Attention: _____

All invoices are due and payable within thirty (30) days. Overdue invoices will be charged 3% interest per month.

IX. GENERAL PROVISIONS

The parties agree that in the event of Court action regarding this agreement, that the venue of such action shall solely be _____ County, State, and the laws of the State of _____ shall govern the interpretation and enforcement of this agreement. This agreement may not be modified except by further written agreement executed by both parties.

Medical Director   COMPANY

By: _____   By: _____

Title: _____   Title: _____

Date: _____   Date: _____

NOTE: CONTRACT SHOULD BE REVIEWED AND APPROVED BY COMPANY's LEGAL REPRESENTATIVE

Sample Practice Guidelines for the Registered Occupational Health Nurse

The following guidelines are provided to assist the registered professional nurse in the day-to-day care of the adult patient in an on-site occupational health setting.

Under the consultant medical direction of (MEDICAL DIRECTOR'S NAME AND CREDENTIALS) the registered nurse shall practice within the scope of practice established by the (STATE) Board of Nursing. The nurse is also expected to maintain the appropriate licensure for the practice setting.

The consultant medical director supports the actions of the registered occupational health nurse who uses prudent judgment while rendering care within these guidelines. Any care that deviates from these guidelines should be discussed with the medical director and documented as such in the medical record.

Any care or treatment not covered within these guidelines must be discussed with the medical director.

These guidelines must be reviewed and signed annually.

(NAME)   Date

Medical Director

(NAME)   Date

OHN

Essentials for Occupational Health Nursing, First Edition. Arlene Guzik.
© 2013 John Wiley & Sons, Inc. Published 2013 by John Wiley & Sons, Inc.

Sample: Anaphylaxis, Adults

EVALUATION/ASSESSMENT PROTOCOL
Subjective
History: This is a medical emergency. Focus immediately on treatment. When able, ascertain likely etiology, bee sting, wasp sting, hornet sting, fire ant bite, adverse drug reaction (oral or injectable), occasionally food or other ingestant.

Objective
Physical Examination: General appearance (pallor), vital signs (decreased blood pressure, increased pulse), respiratory distress.

Assessment: Note that this is a life-threatening emergency if patient has severe bronchospasm, airway obstruction, cyanosis.

PLAN/MANAGEMENT PROTOCOL
General Measures:

• Summon emergency medical services.

Specific Measures:

• Call 911
• Maintain airway
• Aqueous epinephrine* 1:1,000 0.3–0.5 mL subcutaneously or administer via Epipen
• Administer oxygen, 4 L/NC

Physician Consultation: Immediate.

Referral:

Immediate Transfer to: Nearest emergency facility

Follow-up Plan:

Patient Education:

• Avoidance of allergen.
• Self treatment.

* Unless allergic, contraindicated, or pregnant/lactating

Sample: Minor Lacerations

EVALUATION/ASSESSMENT PROTOCOL

Subjective

History: Obtain details of circumstances surrounding the injury. Any under-lying conditions that might have predisposed the patient toward the injury? Any medications (over-the-counter, prescription, illicit) being used? If head wound, then document any alteration in sensorium.

Objective

Physical Examination: General appearance, vital signs, wound location and description with attention to whether or not there is any functional impair-ment. Consider diagramming, with the anatomic location showing, also the wound pre- and post-repair when you record the physical examination.

Assessment: Characterize the wound as abrasion (with or without embedded foreign matter), simple laceration, avulsion/flap-type laceration. Do not close lacerations that are more than 6 hours old.

Differential Diagnosis: differentiate minor lacerations from the more significant injury with ligament, tendon, or nerve damage by considering mechanism of injury, depth of wound and range of motion.

Complications: secondary wound infection and/or disruption of repair.

PLAN/MANAGEMENT PROTOCOL

General Measures:

- Soak in normal saline solution
- Cleanse with topical antiseptic (if not allergic)*
- Explore wound to be certain all foreign material is removed
- Irrigate and recleanse
- Complete Incident Report, if work-related

Specific Measures:

- For abrasions and very minor lacerations, consider closing with adhesive strips
- Use antibiotic ointment, if indicated
- For wounds needing sutures, cover with sterile dressing and refer to physician
- Consider tetanus prophylaxis,* and for animal bites rabies precautions and/or rabies prophylaxis.*

Physician Consultation: For all wounds over 6 hours old, penetrating or puncture wound, those resulting from an altercation, those suspicious of or reflecting abuse or neglect, those by a contaminated object, those occurring in non-chlorinated fresh water.

Referral: Consider referring facial wounds to plastic surgeon (in particular if desired by patient or parent), eyelid and wounds to plastic surgeon or ophthalmologist, wounds with functional impairment to the appropriate plastic or orthopedic surgeon.

Immediate Transfer: Indicated if suspicion of internal organ damage, functional impairment (in some instances), and for bleeding not easily brought under control.

Follow-up Plan: Recheck as indicated in 2 day(s).

Patient Education:

- Teach wound care
- Teach signs and symptoms of infection

* Unless allergic, contraindicated, or pregnant/lactating

Sample: Sore Throat

EVALUATION/ASSESSMENT PROTOCOL
Subjective
History: Onset and course of symptoms. Predisposing factors or underlying conditions. General medical history.

Objective
Physical Examination: General appearance, vital signs, ENT, neck for nodes, liver and spleen.

Assessment: severity and degree of tonsillar enlargement.

Differential Diagnosis: Consider viral pharyngitis, mycoplasma, aphthous stomatitis, mononucleosis, bacterial tonsillitis.

Complications: Peritonsillar abscess, rheumatic fever is a complication of strep.

PLAN/MANAGEMENT PROTOCOL
General Measures:

- Guaifenesin DM (Robitussin DM) 2 tsp. TID for moisture (Use sugar-free/ alcohol free for persons with diabetes)
- Consider warm saline gargles.
- For pain, aspirin or acetaminophen
- For particular painful throats or marked tonsillitis with dysphagia, encourage extra nutritious and nonirritating liquids such as cold juices or nutritional drinks (e.g., Gatorade).
- Zinc throat lozenges
- Echinacea, 2 capsules TID × 7–10 days
- Cool, soothing liquids may be helpful.

Specific Measures:

- For viral, no treatment necessary.
- If severe pharyngeal inflammation or pustular drainage, refer to personal healthcare provider

Physician Consultation: Consider for severe, recurrent, or prolonged symptoms; peritonsillar abscess; severe cervical lymphadenitis.

Referral:

Immediate Transfer: May be necessary for peritonsillar abscess.

Follow-up- Plan: As needed or if persistent symptoms after 3 days or sooner if worsening.

Patient Education:
Signs and symptoms to report

* Unless allergic, contraindicated, or pregnant/lactating

Sample: Ankle Sprain

EVALUATION/ASSESSMENT PROTOCOL
Subjective
History: Description of injury and symptoms (acute, chronic, or recurrent). Frequency of sports activity/exercise program.

Objective
Physical Examination: Complete joint exam, pulses, and appropriate neurological exam.

Lab: Consider need for x-ray

Assessment: Ankle sprains may be classified into three grades: grade I, stretching of involved ligaments; grade II, partial tearing of involved ligaments with slight joint instability; grade III, severe ligament tearing with loss of stability.

Differential Diagnosis: is essentially among the types of sprains, but be careful to evaluate for predisposing conditions.

Complications: Instability.

PLAN/MANAGEMENT PROTOCOL
General Measures:

- RICE (Rest, Ice, Compression bandage, Elevate)
- Ice pack to ankle for 20 minutes every 2–4 hours for 24 hours.
- Elastic bandage to control swelling and provide stability.
- Elevate lower extremity.

Specific Measures:

- Analgesic or nonsteroidal anti-inflammatory drug:
  Ibuprofen 400 mg QID × 10 days*

Physician Consultation: Consider for grade II or grade III sprains or when in doubt about severity or need for x-ray. When an eversion injury due to increased risk for bony damage and tearing of deltoid and inferior tibiofibular ligaments if not significantly improved in 24 hours.

Referral: Orthopedic referral for persistent or severe pain, joint instability, or fracture. Consider physical therapy and rehabilitation program.

Immediate Transfer: If the joint is unstable and fracture is suspected.

Follow-up Plan: Follow up in 24 hour(s) or as indicated, or if not significantly improved after initial follow-up visit. Additional follow-up every 1 week(s) as indicated.

Patient Education:

- Teach RICE treatment
- Teach range of motion exercises (write alphabet with foot while it is elevated)
- Patient education regarding type of injury and healing time, strengthening exercises, and prevention.

* Unless allergic, contraindicated, or pregnant/lactating

Sample Medical Direction Prescription Release Authorization

Company: _____

Street Address: _____

City, State, Zip: _____

Phone: _____ Fax: _____

Authorized Agents:
(NAME(s) OF OHN) _____

Authorizing Physician Name: MEDICAL DIRECTOR NAME AND
                                       CREDENTIALS
                                       ADDRESS
                                       PHONE

State License #   0000000000

DEA #   0000000000

RX Prescriptions:
(LIST ALL PRESCRIPTION MEDICATIONS THAT ARE AUTHORIZED FOR USE IN THE OCCUPATIONAL HEALTH CLINIC)

Vaccinations	**Prescription Medications**
Tetanus Toxoid	Benadryl (Diphenhydramine) 25 mg po
Hepatitis A	Hydrocortisone Cream 1%
Hepatitis B	Epipen (Adrenalin)
Twinrix	
Varicella	
Flu	

MEDICAL DIRECTOR NAME   Date
Medical Director

Essentials for Occupational Health Nursing, First Edition. Arlene Guzik.
© 2013 John Wiley & Sons, Inc. Published 2013 by John Wiley & Sons, Inc.

Sample Program Development Checklist

A6

Priority	Description	Responsible Party	Target Date for Completion	Completion Date

Establish priority by assigning: A-High Prioirty B = Medium Priority
C = Low Prioirty

Staff Recruitment

Occupational Health Nurse

Administrative Support Staff

Business Partnerships

Human Resources

Benefits

Employee Relations

Purchasing

Operations/ Management

Safety

Workers' Compensation Insurer/TPA

Adjuster(s)

Case Manager(s)

(continued)

Essentials for Occupational Health Nursing, First Edition. Arlene Guzik.
© 2013 John Wiley & Sons, Inc. Published 2013 by John Wiley & Sons, Inc.

Priority	Description	Responsible Party	Target Date for Completion	Completion Date
	Group Health Insurer/ TPA			
	Employee Assistant Program Provider			
	Legal Advisors			
	Corporate Legal Department			
	Workers' Compensation Defense Attorney(s)			
	Labor Law Attorney			
Referral Partners				
	Develop Provider Referral Network			
	Occupational Medicine Specialtist			
	Primary Treating Providers			
	Specialty Physicians			
	Diagnostic Testing			
	Physical Therapy			
	Emergency Department			
	Other Community Health Resources			
Marketing				
	Internal Announcement to Employees			
	Meet and Greet			
	Announcement to Community EMS			
Policies and Procedures				
	Clinical			

Priority	Description	Responsible Party	Target Date for Completion	Completion Date
	Health Benefits (ADA, FMLA, etc.)			
	Safety			
	Professional Issues			
	OHN			
	Malpractice Insurance Secured			
	Professional License			
	Medical Director			
	Professional License			
	Curriculum vitae			
	DEA License			
	Agreement Signed			
	Practice Guidelines Signed			
	Prescriptive Authority Signed			
	Nurse Practitioner			
	Malpractice Insurance Secured			
	License			
	Curriculum Vitae			
	Nurse Practitioner Practice Protocol Secured (if applicable)			
	Licenses			
	Laboratory CLIA			
	Pharmacy License (if applicable)			
	Technology			
	Computer System			

(*continued*)

Priority	Description	Responsible Party	Target Date for Completion	Completion Date
	Phone System			
	Fax Machine			
	Electronic Medical Record Software			
	Cell Phone (for after-hours on-call)			
Forms				
	Patient Registration			
	Health History			
	Drug Screen Consent			
	Specific Testing Forms			
	Patient Education Material			
Laboratory				
	Requisitions			
	Printer			
	Tubes			
	Needles			
	Drug Screen Chain of Custody Forms			
Clinical Certifications				
	COHN			
	Breath Alcohol Technician			
	Certified Drug Screen Collector			
	Hearing Conservation			
	NIOSH Certified Spirometry Course			
Set up Vendors				
	Medical Supplies			
	Office Supplies			

Priority	Description	Responsible Party	Target Date for Completion	Completion Date
	Pharmaceuticals			
	Oxygen			
	Biohazard Waste Disposal			
	Laboratory Services			
	Document Shredding			
	Housekeeping			
Signage				
	Occupational Health Clinic Signage			
	Patient Education Signs			
	Safety Education Signs			
Clinic Equipment				
	Audiometer			
	Audiometric Booth			
	EKG Machine			
	Spirometer			
	Breath Alcohol Machine			
	Titmus Vision Tester			
	Oto/Ophthalmoscope			
	MedicationRrefrigerator			
	Specimen Refrigerator			
	Exam Table(s)			
	Exam Stool(s)			
	Automatic External Defibrillator			
Facility				
	Drug Screen Compliant Restroom			
	ADA Compliant			

Sample Documentation of
Health Services Visits

Documentation for a work injury/illness initial visit

Subjective	• Patient's subjective statement of how injury/illness occurred
	  ○ Time of onset
	  ○ Duration of symptoms
	• Specific complaints
	  ○ Specify affected body parts
	• History of similar injury
	• Any preexisting conditions or comorbid factors
	• Current medications
	• Allergies
	• Past/current medical and surgical history
	• Social history
	• Use of tobacco, alcohol, or illicit drugs
	• Last tetanus immunization
	• Family history
	• Hobbies
	• Details of incident investigation

Objective	• Vital signs, height, weight
	• Physical assessment findings
	  ○ Overall assessment
	  ○ Focused assessment of injury/illness

Assessment	• Physical, emotional, behavioral assessment
Plan	• Decision statement regarding work-relatedness of findings • Recommendations for nursing interventions, referrals, or resources • Interventions and actions • Follow-up plan ○ Include appropriate referrals for further evaluation or treatment

---

Essentials for Occupational Health Nursing, First Edition. Arlene Guzik.
© 2013 John Wiley & Sons, Inc. Published 2013 by John Wiley & Sons, Inc.

Documentation of a Work-Related Injury/Illness Follow-up Visit

Subjective
- Patient's progress as compared to expectations
- Status since last encounter
- Patient's response to treatment
- Tolerance to assigned work status

Objective
- Vital signs, if applicable
- Focused assessment of injury/illness

Assessment
- Physical, emotional, behavioral assessment

Plan
- Recommendations for nursing interventions, referrals, or resources
- Interventions and actions
- Follow-up plan
  - Include appropriate referrals for further evaluation or treatment

Documentation of Personal Health Visit

Subjective
- Patient's subjective statement of the heath problem
  - Specific complaints/injuries
- History of similar health problems
- Any current health conditions or comorbid, contributing, or risk factors
- Current medications
- Allergies
- Past medical and surgical history
- Social history
  - Use of tobacco, alcohol or illicit drugs
- Immunization history
- Family history
- Hobbies

Objective
- Vital signs, height, weight
- Focused assessment of health problem

Assessment
- Physical, emotional, behavioral assessment

Plan
- Recommendations for nursing interventions, referrals, or resources
- Interventions and actions
- Follow-up plan
  - Include appropriate referrals for further evaluation or treatment

Documentation for a Physical Examination

- Patient's completed medical and surgical history questionnaire
- Current medications
- Physical exam findings
- Diagnostic results
- Fitness for duty statement as related to the job description
- Any physical limitations or restrictions
- Recommendations for follow-up with personal healthcare provider

Things to Consider

A8

Occupational Health Clinic

Clinic Checklist

Location:_____   Date:_____

		Completed	Comments
Licenses			
	CLIA (Lab Waiver)	☐	_____
	Biomedical Waste Permit	☐	_____
	State Healthcare Clinic Permit (Pharmacy)	☐	_____
	Nursing License(s)	☐	_____
	Radiology Facility License		
Medical Direction			
	Medical Director License	☐	_____
	Medical Director DEA License	☐	_____
	Medical Director Agreement	☐	_____
	Clinical Guidelines	☐	_____
	Prescribing Authority Agreement	☐	_____

Essentials for Occupational Health Nursing, First Edition. Arlene Guzik.
© 2013 John Wiley & Sons, Inc. Published 2013 by John Wiley & Sons, Inc.

Certificates

Professional	☐	_____
Breath Alcohol Technician	☐	_____
Hearing Conservation	☐	_____
Drug Screen Collection	☐	_____

Calibrations

Audiometric Calibration Certificate (Annual)	☐	_____
Breath Alcohol Machine	☐	_____
Spirometer	☐	_____

Inspection Records

Biomedical Waste Pickup Records	☐	_____
Pharmacy	☐	_____

Medications

Expiration Dates	☐	_____
Patient Information Sheets	☐	_____
Daily Medication Count	☐	_____

Cleanliness

Trash	☐	_____
Restrooms	☐	_____
Break area / Appliances	☐	_____
Walls and Doors	☐	_____
General Appearance	☐	_____
Reception Area	☐	_____
Waiting Room	☐	_____
Exam Rooms	☐	_____
Storage room	☐	_____
X-ray	☐	_____

Instruments

Sterile Product Expiration Dates	☐	_____
General Condition	☐	_____

Equipment:

Audiometer	☐	_____
ECG Machine	☐	_____
Spirometer	☐	_____
Nebulizer	☐	_____
Titmus Vision Tester	☐	_____
Breath Alcohol Testing Machine	☐	_____
Computers/Keyboards	☐	_____
Specimen Refrigerator	☐	_____
Phones	☐	_____

Emergency Cart

Supply Expiration Dates	☐	_____
Easily Accessible	☐	_____
Oxygen Tank & Mask/Cannula	☐	_____
Ambubag	☐	_____
Monthly Cheklist	☐	_____

Lab

Lab Tubes and Expiration Dates	☐	_____

Logs

Blood Draw	☐	_____
Spirometer Calibration	☐	_____
Audiometer Calibration	☐	_____
Drug Screen Courier Log	☐	_____
Housekeeping	☐	_____
Breath Alcohol Machine Calibration	☐	_____
Refrigerator Tenperature	☐	_____
Maintenance and Repair	☐	_____
Clinical Testing	☐	
Instant HIV	☐	_____
Accucheck	☐	_____
HbA1C Test	☐	_____
Other	☐	_____

Resource and Procedure Manuals

    Exposure Control Plan ☐ _____

    Substance Testing ☐ _____

    Clinical Resource ☐ _____

    PDR or Prescribing Reference ☐ _____

    Pocket Guide to Chemical Hazards ☐ _____

    Equipment Manuals ☐ _____

Recordkeeping

    Audiometer Calibration ☐ _____

    Biohazard Pickup ☐ _____

    Breath Alcohol Testing Reports ☐ _____

    Chain of Custody Forms ☐ _____

Calibrations

    Audiometer ☐ _____

    Breath Alcohol Testing Machine ☐ _____

    Spirometer ☐ _____

Clinical Charts

    Chart Order

      Occupational ☐ _____

      Nonoccupational

    Filing

      Occupational ☐ _____

      Nonoccupational ☐ _____

    Electronic Medical Record ☐ _____

Observations: _____

_____

_____

Sample Mobile Equipment Operator Health Evaluation

A9

Policy & Procedure:

1. Workers who operate mobile equipment (e.g., forklifts, motorized man-lifts, tractors, company-owned vehicles) as part of their normal job function must have a health evaluation every two years. In addition, whenever a worker's health condition changes that may interfere with their safety regarding mobile equipment operation, the worker will be sent for reevaluation.
2. The worker will be required to:
   - Complete the "Mobile Equipment Operator Health Questionnaire"
   - Complete a health evaluation including:
     a. vision screen for acuity (near and far), peripheral fields, and color (red, green and yellow)
     b. blood pressure check
     c. whisper hearing test
3. The results of the health testing will be reviewed along with the health questionnaire.
   a. Based on these results, the following recommendations may be made:
      i. Decision rendered that no further evaluation is needed and the worker will be deemed qualified.
   b. If there are concerns about the workers ability to safely perform their duties as a mobile equipment operator based on available test results or health history, recommendations will be made for one or more of the following:
      i. Complete physical exam
      ii. Electrocardiogram
      iii. Lab tests (e.g., urine dip, CBC, chemistry profile)
      iv. Audiogram
4. If the healthcare provider recommends further evaluation or testing in regard to the aforementioned, the company contact will be notified for discussion of the case and for authorization before proceeding.

Essentials for Occupational Health Nursing, First Edition. Arlene Guzik.
© 2013 John Wiley & Sons, Inc. Published 2013 by John Wiley & Sons, Inc.

Health Questionnaire for
Mobile Equipment Operators

Worker Name: _____ **Date:** _____

Company Name: _____ **Date of Birth:** _____

1. Do you have a history of seizures? ☐ Yes ☐ No
   a. If yes, have you had a seizure in the past 6 months? ☐ Yes ☐ No
   b. If yes, when _____

2. Do you have a health condition (e.g. heart problem) that causes you temporary impairment or loss of consciousness without warning? ☐ Yes ☐ No
   a. If yes, please explain _____

3. Do you have diabetes? ☐ Yes ☐ No
   a. Do you take oral medication to control your blood sugar? ☐ Yes ☐ No
      List medications: _____
   b. If yes, are you currently taking insulin to control your blood sugar?
      What _____ ☐ Yes ☐ No
   c. If yes, have you in the past 3 years had an "insulin reaction," episode of
      dizziness, impairment or loss of consciousness that has interfered with
      normal, daily activities or interfered with the safe operation of a car or
      motorized equipment. ☐ Yes ☐ No
      i. If yes, how many episodes _____
      ii. When was the last one _____

4. Do you have problems with vision (e.g., blurred, color, useful vision in one
   eye) that impairs or interferes with your ability to operate a motorized
   equipment? ☐ Yes ☐ No

5. Do you require distant vision correction (glasses, contacts) in order to safely
   see and operate motorized equipments? ☐ Yes ☐ No
   a. If yes, when was your last eye exam? _____
   b. What correction do you use? ☐ Contacts ☐ Glasses

6. Do you have problems with hearing that impairs your ability to operate a
   motorized equipment or hear warning alarms or horns? ☐ Yes ☐ No

7. Do you have an impairment or disability of your leg(s)/feet that may interfere with the use of foot pedals/brakes/controls in the operation of motorized equipments? ☐ Yes ☐ No
   a. If yes, please explain _____

Health Questionnaire for
Mobile Equipment Operators
Page 2

Worker Name: _____ **Date:** _____

Company Name: _____ **Date of Birth**: _____

8. Do you have an impairment or disability of your arm(s)/hand(s) that may interfere with the use of hand controls and/or steering devices in the operation of motorized equipments? ☐ Yes ☐ No

   a. If yes, please explain _____

9. Have you in the past 5 years been involved in a motor equipment accident in which a health condition of yours was the cause or a contributing factor to the accident? ☐ Yes ☐ No

   a. If yes, please explain _____

10. Are you currently taking any medications that make you drowsy, sleepy or interfere with your ability to operate a motor equipment? ☐ Yes ☐ No

11. List all medications (prescription or over the counter) that you are currently taking. _____
   _____
   _____

12. Have you in the past 2 years taken or used illegal or illicit drugs?
   ☐ Yes ☐ No

If you answered yes to any of the above questions, can you offer or suggest a way that an accommodation could be made which would allow you to safely operate motorized equipment? _____
_____
_____

I, the undersigned applicant for employment, hereby state that I have examined the above questionnaire after its completion, and the answers are true and correct to the best of my knowledge and belief. I understand that falsification of answers, misleading answers or any relevant information which I have not disclosed, may result in my dismissal from employment. I give permission to release all necessary information as it relates to my fitness for duty or for payment of services to my prospective or current employer as it relates to the purpose of this examination.

_____   _____

Signature of worker   Date

Health Evaluation for
Mobile Equipment Operators

BLOOD PRESSURE and PULSE

Systolic _____ Diastolic _____   Pulse: _____ ▦ regular ▦ irregular
Recheck: Systolic _____   Diastolic _____

VISION
Eyeglasses required for:
___ Far Vision   ___ Near Vision   ___ None Required

1. FAR VISION: Snellen Chart (must be 20/40 or better):
   Without correction: 20/ ___ Right   20/___ Left
   With correction: 20/ ___ Right   20/___ Left
            ___ Pass   ___ Fail

2. COLOR PERCEPTION: Ability to distinguish red, green, blue, and yellow colors as determined by standard color plates:
            ___ Pass   ___ Fail

3. PERIPHERAL VISION: (must be 85 degrees bilaterally)
            ___ degrees left   ___ degrees right
            ___ Pass   ___ Fail

HEARING
1. Forced, whispered voice in the better ear at not less than 5 feet with or without a hearing aid.
            ___ With hearing aid   ___ Without a hearing aid
            ___ Pass   ___ Fail

Recommendations:
▦ No current health conditions   ▦ No current medications
_____
_____
_____

I have reviewed the health questionnaire and health testing for mobile equipment operators and find this person:
▦ Fit for operating mobile equipment for 2 years
▦ Meets standard but requires periodic monitoring due to: _____
   Fit for: ▦ 3 months   ▦ 1 year
▦ Not fit for mobile equipment operation

_____   _____
Health Provider Signature   Date

Nationally Notifiable Infectious Conditions

A10

Summary of Notifiable Diseases, United States, 2010

- Anthrax
- Arboviral neuroinvasive and non-neuroinvasive diseases
  - California serogroup virus disease
  - Eastern equine encephalitis virus disease
  - Powassan virus disease
  - St. Louis encephalitis virus disease
  - West Nile virus disease
  - Western equine encephalitis virus disease
- Babesiosis
- Botulism
  - Botulism, foodborne
  - Botulism, infant
  - Botulism, other (wound & unspecified)
- Brucellosis
- Chancroid
- *Chlamydia trachomatis* infection
- Cholera
- Coccidioidomycosis
- Cryptosporidiosis
- Cyclosporiasis
- Dengue
  - Dengue Fever
  - Dengue hemorrhagic fever
  - Dengue shock syndrome
- Diphtheria
- Ehrlichiosis/Anaplasmosis
  - *Ehrlichia chaffeensis*
  - *Ehrlichia ewingi*i

Essentials for Occupational Health Nursing, First Edition. Arlene Guzik.
© 2013 John Wiley & Sons, Inc. Published 2013 by John Wiley & Sons, Inc.

- ○ *Anaplasma phagocytophilum*
- ○ Undetermined
- Giardiasis
- Gonorrhea
- *Haemophilus influenzae*, invasive disease
- Hansen disease (leprosy)
- Hantavirus pulmonary syndrome
- Hemolytic uremic syndrome, post-diarrheal
- Hepatitis
  - ○ Hepatitis A, acute
  - ○ Hepatitis B, acute
  - ○ Hepatitis B, chronic
  - ○ Hepatitis B virus, perinatal infection
  - ○ Hepatitis C, acute
  - ○ Hepatitis C, past or present
- HIV infection *(AIDS has been reclassified as HIV stage III)*
  - ○ HIV infection, adult/adolescent (age >= 13 years)
  - ○ HIV infection, child (age >= 18 months and < 13 years)
  - ○ HIV infection, pediatric (age < 18 months)
- Influenza-associated pediatric mortality
- Legionellosis
- Listeriosis
- Lyme disease
- Malaria
- Measles
- Meningococcal disease
- Mumps
- Novel influenza A virus infections
- Pertussis
- Plague
- Poliomyelitis, paralytic
- Poliovirus infection, nonparalytic
- Psittacosis
- Q Fever
  - ○ Acute
  - ○ Chronic
- Rabies
  - ○ Rabies, animal
  - ○ Rabies, human
- Rubella (German measles)
- Rubella, congenital syndrome
- Salmonellosis
- Severe acute respiratory syndrome-associated coronavirus (SARS-CoV) disease

- Shiga toxin-producing *Escherichia coli* (STEC)
- Shigellosis
- Smallpox
- Spotted fever rickettsiosis
- Streptococcal toxic-shock syndrome
- *Streptococcus pneumoniae*, invasive disease
- Syphilis
- Tetanus
- Toxic-shock syndrome (other than streptococcal)
- Trichinellosis (Trichinosis)
- Tuberculosis
- Tularemia
- Typhoid fever
- Vancomycin-intermediate *Staphylococcus aureus* (VISA)
- Vancomycin-resistant *Staphylococcus aureus* (VRSA)
- Varicella (morbidity)
- Varicella (deaths only)
- Vibriosis

Viral hemorrhagic fevers, due to:
- Ebola virus
- Marburg virus
- Crimean-Congo hemorrhagic fever virus
- Lassa virus
- Lujo virus
- New world arenaviruses (Guanarito, Machupo, Junin, and Sabia viruses)

Yellow fever

From: http://wwwn.cdc.gov/nndss/document/2012_Case%20Definitions.pdf

Sample Safety Policy

A11

WORKPLACE SAFETY POLICY

The safety of the workplace and of our workers is of top concern to (Company Name), and every precaution will be taken to provide a safe work environment. The company will comply with all applicable workplace health and safety regulations and will strive to maintain operations that meet or exceed best practice. Workers will never be required to do a job or work in an environment that is perceived as unsafe.

(Company name) maintains the Safety Committee, comprised of workers representing all levels of the organization and all departments. The chair of the Safety Committee is responsible for conducting regular safety meetings. Recommendations that flow from the Safety Committee will be presented by the Safety Committee chair to management for implementation.

The commitment of every worker is needed in order to achieve our safety mission. Everyone's voice counts. We look to our workers to immediately report unsafe conditions or hazards to their supervisor or to a member of the Safety Committee. We expect workers to look out for their own safety, and to also look out for the safety of their coworkers and our visitors. Safety begins with each worker thinking of how he or she can perform their job in a safe manner.

Every worker is expected to participate in the safety program by immediately reporting incidents, hazards, and unsafe work practices to a supervisor or safety committee representative. Workers are also expected to comply with requirements for wearing applicable personal protective equipment and complying with all safety and health standards. And, workers are expected to participate in and support all safety committee activities and training. Supervisors are responsible for ensuring a safe workplace, which includes enforcing safety policies and procedures, and by providing the appropriate training and supervision of workers and by observing work practices.

Essentials for Occupational Health Nursing, First Edition. Arlene Guzik.
© 2013 John Wiley & Sons, Inc. Published 2013 by John Wiley & Sons, Inc.

Incident Reporting

Incidents lead to injuries. Therefore we expect every worker to report any incident that occurs, large or small, including near-misses. All incidents will be investigated, looking at root cause, in order to prevent future occurrence and to reduce the risk of injury to workers. All incident reports and investigations will be reviewed by the Safety Committee.

Injury/Illness Reporting

Workers are required to report all injuries and/or illnesses that occur as a result of one's work or work environment. The worker is required to notify a member of management immediately at the time of the injury or illness. Any injury at work—no matter how simple—must be reported immediately to your supervisor to assure appropriate evaluation and intervention.

Good Hygiene and Housekeeping

All work environments must be clean and orderly. All equipment must be cleaned daily. Walkways are to be free from obstruction. Spills and wet walking surfaces must be cleaned or contained in order to avoid slips and falls. Place trash in the appropriate receptacles. Good personal hygiene is expected of all workers.

Safety Equipment

Workers are requirement to keep safety and personal protective equipment clean and in good condition. The worker is responsible for notifying their supervisor of any equipment failure or malfunction.

Safety Restraints

The use of safety belts by all occupants is required in all company vehicles and on all mobile equipment. Failure to comply with the use of safety restraints will be considered a violation of this policy and subject to disciplinary action.

Commitment to Safety

Management's commitment to safety can only be achieved when each individual worker is committed. Management commitment will be demonstrated by training all workers in safe work practices and procedures in order to achieve the goal of zero incidents and injuries. Management will provide the necessary safeguards and interventions when applicable, including engineering and administrative controls, and personal protective equipment.

Routine safety and health inspections will be conducted in order to validate safe working conditions and safe work practices, to control and eliminate risks and hazards, and to assure compliance with all applicable health and safety regulations.

Safety is our Number One Priority.

OSHA's Strategic Map for Change and Continuous Improvement for Safety and Health

A12

1. **Obtain Top Management "Buy-in**." This is the very first step that needs to be accomplished. Top managers must be on board. If they are not, safety and health will compete against core business issues such as production and profitability, a battle that will almost always be lost. Management needs to understand the need for change and be willing to support it. Showing the costs to the organization in terms of dollars (direct and indirect costs of accidents) that are being lost, and the organizational costs (fear, lack of trust, feeling of being used, etc.) can be compelling reasons for doing something differently. Because losses due to accidents are bottom line costs to the organization, controlling these will more than pay for the needed changes. In addition, as you are successful you will eliminate organizational barriers such as fear and lack of trust—issues that typically get in the way of all of the organization's goals. A safety and health change process can very effectively drive change and bring an organization together due to the ability to get buy-in from all levels. This stems from the fact that most people place a high personal value on their own safety. They view the change efforts as things that are truly being done for them.

2. **Continue Building "Buy-in**." Get support for the needed changes by building an alliance or partnership between management, your union (if one exists), and employees. A compelling reason for the change must be spelled out to everyone. People have to understand WHY they are being asked to change what they normally do and what it will look like when they are successful. This needs to be done upfront. If people get wind that something "is going down" and haven't been formally told anything, they will tend to naturally resist and opt out.Identify key personnel to champion the change. These people must be visible and are the ones to articulate the reasons for the changes. The reasons need to be compelling and motivational. People frequently respond when they realize how many of their coworkers or subordinates are being injured and that they may be next. Management and

Essentials for Occupational Health Nursing, First Edition. Arlene Guzik.
© 2013 John Wiley & Sons, Inc. Published 2013 by John Wiley & Sons, Inc.

supervisors also respond when they see the money being lost due to accidents and they realize that their actions toward safety truly influence and define the employee safety culture.

3. **Build Trust**. Trusting is a critical part of accepting change and management needs to know that this is the bigger picture, outside of all the details. Trust will occur as different levels within the organization work together and begin to see success.

4. **Conduct Self Assessments/Benchmarking**. In order to get where you want to go, it is essential to know where you are starting from. You can use a variety of self-audit mechanisms to compare your site processes with other recognized models of excellence such as Star VPP sites. Visiting other sites to gain first-hand information is also invaluable. You can use perception surveys to measure the strengths and weaknesses of your site safety culture. These surveys can give you data from various viewpoints within the organization. For instance, you can measure differences in employees' and managers' perceptions on various issues. This is an excellent way to determine whether alignment issues exist and, if so, what they are. One example is the Safety and Health Program Check-Up. At this stage, it is important to look at issues that surface as symptoms of larger system failures. For example, ask what major system failed to detect the unguarded machine, or why the system failed to notice that incident investigations are not being performed on time, or if workers are being blamed for the failures. Your greatest level of success will come when these larger system failures are recognized and addressed.

5. **Initial Training**. Train management-supervisory staff, union leadership (if present), and safety and health committee members, and a representative number of hourly employees. This may include both safety and health training and any needed management, team building, hazard recognition, or communication training. This provides you with a core group of people to draw upon as resources and also gets key personnel on board with needed changes.

6. **Establish a Steering Committee**. Create a committee made up of management, employees, union (if present), and safety staff. This group's purpose is to facilitate, support, and direct the change processes. This will provide overall guidance and direction and avoid duplication of efforts. To be effective, the group must have the authority to get things done.

7. **Develop Site Safety Vision**. This vision should include key policies, goals, measures, and strategic and operational plans. These policies provide guidance and serve as a check-in that can be used to ask yourself if the decision you're about to make supports or detracts from your intended safety and health improvement process.

8. **Align the Organization**. Establish a shared vision of safety and health goals and objectives versus production. Upper management must be willing to

support by providing resources (time) and holding managers and supervisors accountable for doing the same. The entire management and supervisory staff needs to set the example and lead the change. It's more about leadership than management.

9. **Define Specific Roles.** Roles and responsibilities for safety and health should be assigned at all levels of the organization. Safety and health must be viewed as everyone's responsibility. Clearly spell out how the organization deals with competing pressures and priorities, i.e., production versus safety and health.

10. **Develop a System of Accountability.** All levels of the organization are accountable. Everyone must play by the same rules and be held accountable for their areas of responsibility. The sign of a strong culture is when the individuals hold themselves accountable.

11. **Develop Measures.** Measures and an ongoing measurement and feedback system should be developed. Drive the system with upstream activity measures that encourage positive change. Examples include: the number of hazards reported or corrected, numbers of inspections, number of equipment checks, Job Safety Analysis (JSA), prestart-up reviews conducted, etc. While it is always nice to know what the bottom line performance is, i.e., accident rates, overemphasis on rates and using them to drive the system typically only drives accident reporting under the table. It is all too easy to manipulate accident rates, which will only result in risk issues remaining unresolved and a probability for future, more serious events to occur.

12. **Develop Policies for Recognition.** Provide recognition with rewards, incentives, and ceremonies. Reward employees for doing the right things and encourage participation in the upstream activities. Continually re-evaluate these policies to ensure their effectiveness and to ensure that they do not become entitlement programs.

13. **Awareness Training and Kick-off for all employees.** It's not enough for a part of the organization to be involved and know about the change effort. The entire site needs to know and be involved in some manner. A kick-off celebration can be used to announce "It's a new day," and seek buy-in for any new procedures and programs.

14. **Implement Process Changes.** Implement change via involvement of management, union (if one is present) and employees using a "Plan To Act" process such as total quality management (TQM).

15. **Continually Measure Performance, Communicate Results, and Celebrate Successes.** Publicizing results is very important to sustaining efforts and keeping everyone motivated. Everyone needs to be updated throughout the process. Progress reports during normal shift meetings (allowing time for comments back to the steering committee) opens communications, but also allows for input. Everybody needs to have a voice, otherwise, they will

be reluctant to buy-in. A system can be as simple as using current meetings, a bulletin board, or a comment box.

16. **On-going Support**. Reinforcement, feedback, reassessment, mid-course corrections, and on-going training is vital to sustaining continuous improvement.

Source: http://www.osha.gov/SLTC/etools/safetyhealth/mod4_strategicmap. html

OSHA's Responsibility, Authority, and Accountability Checklist

A13

Essentials for Occupational Health Nursing, First Edition. Arlene Guzik.
© 2013 John Wiley & Sons, Inc. Published 2013 by John Wiley & Sons, Inc.

Task	Is this your responsibility? ... Yes!	Is this your responsibility? ... No!	Do you have COMPLETE authority?	Do you have the authority to DECIDE; BUT TELL?	Is your authority limited to DECIDE; BUT CHECK FIRST?	Do you have NO authority	Are you measured for accountability? ... Yes!	Are you measured for accountability? ... No!	Is this issue of key importance? ... Yes!	Is this issue of key importance? ... No!
Ensure equipment, materials, facilities, and conditions are safe.										
Provide for safety and health training										
Require employee compliance with safety requirements and rules.										
Recognize and reinforce safe behaviors.										
Make safety and health part of job standards and procedures.										
Request safety and health technical assistance.										
Obtain safe work permits										
Investigate accidents and take appropriate corrective action.										
Conduct inspections, audits and surveys.										
Establish emergency procedures for area.										
Hold safety meetings and workshops										
Correct unsafe conditions and behaviors.										
Stop production for safety reasons.										
Delegate authority for safety to others.										

From: http://www.osha.gov/SLTC/etools/safetyhealth/mod4_tools_checklist.html

Common Hazards and Descriptions

A14

Hazards	Hazard Descriptions
Chemical (Toxic)	A chemical that exposes a person by absorption through the skin, inhalation, or through the bloodstream that causes illness, disease, or death. The amount of chemical exposure is critical in determining hazardous effects. Check Material Safety Data Sheets (MSDS), and/or OSHA 1910.1000 for chemical hazard information.
Chemical (Flammable)	A chemical that, when exposed to a heat ignition source, results in combustion. Typically, the lower a chemical's flash point and boiling point, the more flammable the chemical. Check MSDS for flammability information.
Chemical (Corrosive)	A chemical that, when it comes into contact with skin, metal, or other materials, damages the materials. Acids and bases are examples of corrosives.
Explosion (Chemical Reaction)	Self-explanatory.
Explosion (OverPressurization)	Sudden and violent release of a large amount of gas/energy due to a significant pressure difference such as rupture in a boiler or compressed gas cylinder.
Electrical (Shock/Short Circuit)	Contact with exposed conductors or a device that is incorrectly or inadvertently grounded, such as when a metal ladder comes into contact with power lines. 60 Hz alternating current (common house current) is very dangerous because it can stop the heart.
Electrical (Fire)	Use of electrical power that results in electrical overheating or arcing to the point of combustion or ignition of flammables, or electrical component damage.
Electrical (Static/ESD)	The moving or rubbing of wool, nylon, other synthetic fibers, and even flowing liquids can generate static electricity. This creates an excess or deficiency of electrons on the surface of material that discharges (spark) to the ground resulting in the ignition of flammables or damage to electronics or the body's nervous system.

(Continued)

Essentials for Occupational Health Nursing, First Edition. Arlene Guzik.
© 2013 John Wiley & Sons, Inc. Published 2013 by John Wiley & Sons, Inc.

Hazards	Hazard Descriptions
Electrical (Loss of Power)	Safety-critical equipment failure as a result of loss of power.
Ergonomics (Strain)	Damage of tissue due to over exertion (strains and sprains) or repetitive motion.
Ergonomics (Human Error)	A system design, procedure, or equipment that is error-provocative. (A switch goes up to turn something off).
Excavation (Collapse)	Soil collapse in a trench or excavation as a result of improper or inadequate shoring. Soil type is critical in determining the hazard likelihood.
Fall (Slip, Trip)	Conditions that result in falls (impacts) from height or traditional walking surfaces (such as slippery floors, poor housekeeping, uneven walking surfaces, exposed ledges, etc.)
Fire/Heat	Temperatures that can cause burns to the skin or damage to other organs. Fires require a heat source, fuel, and oxygen.
Mechanical/Vibration (Chaffing/ Fatigue)	Vibration that can cause damage to nerve endings, or material fatigue that results in a safety-critical failure. (Examples are abraded slings and ropes, weakened hoses and belts.)
Mechanical Failure	Self-explanatory; typically occurs when devices exceed designed capacity or are inadequately maintained.
Mechanical	Skin, muscle, or body part exposed to crushing, caught-between, cutting, tearing, shearing items or equipment.
Noise	Noise levels (>85 dBA 8 hr TWA) that result in hearing damage or inability to communicate safety-critical information.
Radiation (Ionizing)	Alpha, beta, gamma, neutral particles, and X-rays that cause injury (tissue damage) by ionization of cellular components.
Radiation (Non-Ionizing)	Ultraviolet, visible light, infrared, and microwaves that cause injury to tissue by thermal or photochemical means.
Struck By (Mass Acceleration)	Accelerated mass that strikes the body causing injury or death. (Examples are falling objects and projectiles.)
Struck Against	Injury to a body part as a result of coming into contact of a surface in which action was initiated by the person. (An example is when a screwdriver slips.)
Temperature Extreme (Heat/Cold)	Temperatures that result in heat stress, exhaustion, or metabolic slow down such as hypothermia.
Visibility	Lack of lighting or obstructed vision that results in an error or other hazard.
Weather Phenomena (Snow/Rain/Wind/Ice)	Self-explanatory.

Source: http://www.osha.gov/Publications/osha3071.html

Guide to Recordability of Cases under OSHA

A15

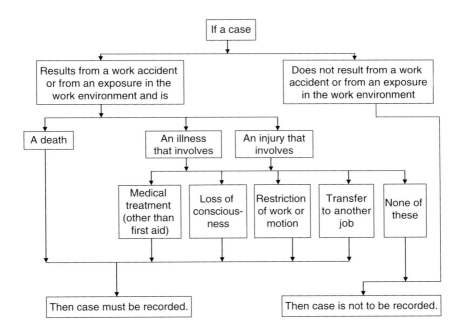

Flowchart:

If a case

- **Results from a work accident or from an exposure in the work environment and is**
  - **A death**
  - **An illness that involves**
  - **An injury that involves**
    - **Medical treatment (other than first aid)**
    - **Loss of consciousness**
    - **Restriction of work or motion**
    - **Transfer to another job**
    - **None of these**

- **Does not result from a work accident or from an exposure in the work environment**

Then case must be recorded.

Then case is not to be recorded.

Essentials for Occupational Health Nursing, First Edition. Arlene Guzik.
© 2013 John Wiley & Sons, Inc. Published 2013 by John Wiley & Sons, Inc.

OSHA Recordable Reference

A16

First Aid vs. Medical Treatment

Category	First Aid (If first aid, not OSHA)	Medical Treatment (If medical treatment, OSHA)
Medication	Over-the-counter	Prescription medication Nonprescription medication at prescription dosage
Immunizations	Tetanus Hepatitis (preventive)	Hepatitis (in response to an exposure incident) Rabies (to treat a specific injury)
Cleaning or soaking wounds on the surface of the skin	Always first aid even if multiple applications	Not applicable
Wound coverings	Adhesive bandages Steri-Strips Butterfly adhesives	Sutures Staples Glues and tapes for closure of the wound
Hot or cold therapy	Always first aid even if administered by medical personnel	Not applicable
Supports	Wraps Wristlets Elastic bandages Nonrigid supports	Cast Splints Orthopedic devices for immobilization

(Continued)

Essentials for Occupational Health Nursing, First Edition. Arlene Guzik.
© 2013 John Wiley & Sons, Inc. Published 2013 by John Wiley & Sons, Inc.

First Aid vs. Medical Treatment

Category	First Aid (If first aid, not OSHA)	Medical Treatment (If medical treatment, OSHA)
Immobilization devices	During Initial transport: Backboard Neck collar Air splint	Rigid back belts The use of cast splints or orthopedic devices (generally with stays or nonbinding support) designed to immobilize a body part to permit it to rest and recover is medical treatment since they are typically prescribed by a PLHCP and are for long-term use for serious injuries or illnesses. Splints and other devices after initial transport.
Drilling a fingernail or toenail or lancing a blister	Always first aid	Not applicable
Eye patches	Always first aid	Not applicable
Removal of foreign bodies from the eye	Irrigation Cotton swab	Embedded or adhered objects which require more complicated procedures
Removal of foreign bodies (other than the eye)	Irrigation Tweezers Cotton swabs Other simple means	Complicated procedures Excision of tissue
Finger guards	Always first aid	Not applicable
Massages	Always first aid	Physical therapy Chiropractic manipulation
Drinking fluids for heat stress relief	Always first aid	Intravenous injections Diagnosis of heat syncope (fainting)

Source: Based on Revised OSHA Guidelines 2002.
PLHCP, physician or licensed healthcare provider.

Health History Form

A17

PRINT ALL INFORMATION: Job Position: _____

NAME: _____ Date of Birth _____

      FIRST   **MIDDLE**   **LAST**

AGE: _____   **SEX: M or F**   **PHONE:** _____

ADDRESS: _____ CITY-STATE-ZIP: _____

Do you have any health conditions for which you are currently being treated?
         ☐ No ☐ Yes

If yes, date last seen: _____

List all health condition(s) _____

Name(s) of treating healthcare provider(s): _____

List all medications you are currently taking, including prescription and over-the-counter: _____
_____
_____

Do you currently have a disability?   ☐ No ☐ Yes
Explain: _____

Do you require an accommodation because of your disability? ☐ No ☐ Yes
Explain: _____

Do you require the use of any special appliances (e.g., splints, crutches, wheelchair, artificial limbs, etc.)?   ☐ No ☐ Yes
Explain: _____

Essentials for Occupational Health Nursing, First Edition. Arlene Guzik.
© 2013 John Wiley & Sons, Inc. Published 2013 by John Wiley & Sons, Inc.

Do you have any limitations to your physical activities?　　　☐ No ☐ Yes
Explain: _____

Have you ever been assigned a permanent "impairment rating" or "disability rating"?　　　　　　　　　　　　　　　　　　　☐ No ☐ Yes
Explain: _____

Are you allergic to any medications?　　　　　　　　☐ No ☐ Yes
List: _____

Do you have environmental allergies?　　　　　　　　☐ No ☐ Yes
List: _____

Do you wear eye glasses:
　　　For far vision:　　☐ No ☐ Yes　　For near vision:　☐ No ☐ Yes

Do you wear contact lenses? ☐ No ☐ Yes

Do you wear a hearing aid? ☐ No ☐ Yes　(circle one)　Right　Left　Both

Do you drink alcoholic beverages? ☐ No ☐ Yes
　　　(circle one)　　< 1 per week　　3-7 per week　　> 7 per week

Do you or have you ever smoked cigarettes or cigars?　　☐ No ☐ Yes

How many cigarettes/cigars per day? _____
　　　For how many years? _____　Quit when: _____

Do you use other tobacco products?　　　　　　　　☐ No ☐ Yes

Do you use marijuana, any illicit or "street" drugs?　　☐ No ☐ Yes
Explain: _____

Have you ever participated in an alcohol or drug treatment/rehabilitation program?　　　　　　　　☐ No　　☐ Now　　☐ In the past

Females Only: Are you pregnant?　　　　　　　　☐ No ☐ Yes
When was your last menstrual period? _____

NAME: _____ Date of Birth _____

OCCUPATIONAL HISTORY

Have you ever been injured on the job?　　　　　　　☐ No ☐ Yes
When? _____　　Explain: _____

Have you ever been refused employment or forced to give up a job because of
your health?　　　　　　　　　　　　　　　　　☐ No ☐ Yes
When _____ Reason _____

Have you ever been rejected for or discharged from military duty because of
your health?　　　　　　　　　　　　　　　　　☐ No ☐ Yes
When _____ Reason _____

Have you ever received pension for disability?　　　☐ No ☐ Yes
If yes, when _____

Have you ever had excessive absences from work?　　☐ No ☐ Yes

Have you been exposed to loud noise at work?　　　☐ No ☐ Yes

Have you ever had a hearing problem because of work?　☐ No ☐ Yes

Have you ever been exposed to (check all that apply):

☐ Arsenic
☐ Asbestos
☐ Benzene
☐ Beryllium
☐ Biological/blood-
　borne pathogens
☐ Cadmium
☐ Epoxy/resin

☐ Excessive noise
☐ Fiberglass
☐ Fluorides
☐ Formaldehyde
☐ Lead
☐ Mercury
☐ PCBs
☐ Pesticides

☐ Plastics
☐ Radioactive
　substances
☐ Solvents
☐ Spray paints
☐ Vibration
☐ Welding/soldering
　fumes

PAST HEALTH HISTORY

List below any past hospitalizations or operations, including out-patient
procedures:

YEAR	HEALTH CONDITION	OPERATION/PROCEDURE
____	_____	_____
____	_____	_____
____	_____	_____

VACCINATION HISTORY

Check all vaccinations you have received:

☐ Normal Childhood Vaccinations   ☐ Pneumonia   Year: _____
☐ Influenza   Year: _____   ☐ Rabies   Year: _____
☐ Hepatitis A   Year: _____   ☐ Tetanus   Year: _____
☐ Hepatitis B   Year: _____

TB HISTORY

Have you ever had a positive reaction to a TB skin test?
     When _____   ☐ No   ☐ Yes

Have you ever received the TB vaccination (BCG)?
     When _____   ☐ No   ☐ Yes

Have you ever been exposed to someone with active TB?
     When _____   ☐ No   ☐ Yes

Have you ever taken drug therapy (INH) because of a positive TB test?
     When _____   ☐ No   ☐ Yes

Have you ever been treated for active, infectious TB?
     When _____   ☐ No   ☐ Yes

HEALTH HISTORY

Have you been diagnosed with any of the following (check all that apply):

☐ Anemia   ☐ Hearing deficit   ☐ Psychiatric/mental
☐ Asthma/bronchitis/   ☐ Heart attack/disease   disorder
    COPD   ☐ Heart murmur   ☐ Seizure/epilepsy
☐ Bleeding disorder   ☐ Hepatitis   ☐ Stroke/TIA
☐ Cancer   ☐ Hernia   ☐ TB
☐ Depression/anxiety   ☐ High blood pressure   ☐ Other: _____
☐ Diabetes   ☐ Kidney disease   ☐ Other: _____
☐ Eye disorder   ☐ Liver disease

NAME: _____ **Date of Birth** _____

Have you been diagnosed with or experienced any of the following:

General

Excessive tiredness/fatigue	▢ No ▢ Yes	Explain: _____
Loss of consciousness/head injury	▢ No ▢ Yes	Explain: _____
Unexplained weight loss	▢ No ▢ Yes	Explain: _____
Communicable disease	▢ No ▢ Yes	Explain: _____
Snoring/sleep disorder/apnea	▢ No ▢ Yes	Explain: _____

Eyes/Ears/Nose/Throat

Blindness	▢ No ▢ Yes	Explain: _____
Ringing in ears	▢ No ▢ Yes	Explain: _____
Sneezing/allergies	▢ No ▢ Yes	Explain: _____
Thyroid disorder	▢ No ▢ Yes	Explain: _____

Heart/Lung

Chest pain/pressure	▢ No ▢ Yes	Explain: _____
Irregular heart beat/palpitations	▢ No ▢ Yes	Explain: _____
Shortness of breath	▢ No ▢ Yes	Explain: _____
Wheezing	▢ No ▢ Yes	Explain: _____

Musculoskeletal

Arthritis	▢ No ▢ Yes	Explain: _____
Back pain/strain	▢ No ▢ Yes	Explain: _____
Back/neck surgery	▢ No ▢ Yes	Explain: _____
Foot/ankle surgery	▢ No ▢ Yes	Explain: _____
Fractures/broken bones	▢ No ▢ Yes	Explain: _____
Hand/wrist surgery	▢ No ▢ Yes	Explain: _____
Knee/hip surgery	▢ No ▢ Yes	Explain: _____
Loss of arm/leg/finger/toe	▢ No ▢ Yes	Explain: _____
Muscle aches/pains	▢ No ▢ Yes	Explain: _____
Neck pain/strain	▢ No ▢ Yes	Explain: _____

Painful/swollen joints   ☐ No   ☐ Yes   Explain: _____

Shoulder/elbow surgery   ☐ No   ☐ Yes   Explain: _____

Spinal disorder   ☐ No   ☐ Yes   Explain: _____

Weakness of arms/legs   ☐ No   ☐ Yes   Explain: _____

Neurological

Claustrophobia   ☐ No   ☐ Yes   Explain: _____

Fainting/dizziness   ☐ No   ☐ Yes   Explain: _____

Headaches/migraine   ☐ No   ☐ Yes   Explain: _____

Memory loss   ☐ No   ☐ Yes   Explain: _____

Skin

Cancer   ☐ No   ☐ Yes   Explain: _____

Excessive itching   ☐ No   ☐ Yes   Explain: _____

Moles/growths   ☐ No   ☐ Yes   Explain: _____

Rash   ☐ No   ☐ Yes   Explain: _____

Skin infections   ☐ No   ☐ Yes   Explain: _____

Digestive/Genitourinary

Blood in urine   ☐ No   ☐ Yes   Explain: _____

Constipation   ☐ No   ☐ Yes   Explain: _____

Difficult/painful urination   ☐ No   ☐ Yes   Explain: _____

Excessive diarrhea   ☐ No   ☐ Yes   Explain: _____

Heartburn/indigestion   ☐ No   ☐ Yes   Explain: _____

Kidney stones   ☐ No   ☐ Yes   Explain: _____

Any other major accidents or illnesses: ☐ No   ☐ Yes   Explain: _____

_____

_____

_____

NAME: _____ **Date of Birth** _____

Permission to Interview, Examine, and Disclose

I, the undersigned, consent to be interviewed and physically examined. I understand that this interview/physical examination is not designed nor intended to replace a comprehensive health examination by my private health-care provider. I understand that this examination is fully intended to determine my fitness for duty to perform certain job tasks/punctions related to my current or prospective employment. I also understand that this examination is not intended to diagnose any current or potential health conditions, and is job-specific.

I hereby attest that the answers to all questions and statements on this health history are true and correct to the best of my knowledge and belief. I understand that falsification of answers, misleading answers, or any relevant information which I have not disclosed may have implications leading to physical harm on the job or potential loss of employment. I give (THE EXAMINER) permission to release all necessary information as it relates to my fitness for duty, or for payment of services, to my current or prospective employer as it relates to the purpose of this examination.

_____   _____
Signature   Date

_____
Print Name

Healthcare Provider Review of Health History

The Healthcare Provider must review & discuss all "Yes" answers.

Document status of past and existing health conditions, including the potential risk of medications and treatment modalities.

☐ There are no current health conditions   ☐ No current medications

_____
_____
_____

_____   _____
Healthcare Provider Signature   Date

Policy & Procedure

A18

Title: **Fitness for Duty**	Policy #:
Original Issue: ____ Review Dates: _____ Revision Date: _____	Approved by: _____ Approved by: _____

Purpose: To protect the physical health and well being of (Company) workers and to provide guidelines that will assist in the determination of a worker's ability to safely perform the essential functions of the assigned job.

Policy: The (Company) is committed to providing a safe work environment, protecting the health of workers, and to providing reasonable accommodations in accordance with the Americans with Disabilities Act.

Procedure: The (Company) reserves the right to determine a worker's fitness for duty by requiring a medical evaluation by the Company's selected medical provider.

MEDICAL EVALUATIONS

A. Preplacement

A preplacement fitness for duty evaluation is required prior to the first day of work for individuals in the following job categories:

(LIST JOB CATEGORIES HERE)

Essentials for Occupational Health Nursing, First Edition. Arlene Guzik.
© 2013 John Wiley & Sons, Inc. Published 2013 by John Wiley & Sons, Inc.

The purpose of the fitness for duty evaluation is to determine if the individual is physically capable of performing the essential job functions. The fitness for duty evaluation will include a physical examination with review of the medical history. Job specific medical testing may also be required, based on the job risks or requirements.

B. Change in Health Status

The Company may require an individual who occupies a position that has medical standards or physical requirements to undergo a fitness-for-duty medical examination whenever there is a direct question about the worker's continued capacity to meet the physical or medical requirements of the position. Such an examination may be requested for instances of job-related injuries/illnesses and for those injuries/illnesses that are not job-related. A fitness for duty evaluation may also be required if there is evidence of a job performance or safety problem, or if an examination is required by federal regulation to determine fitness for duty.

C. Return-to-work

A medical statement from the worker's treating healthcare provider, including dates of necessary absence, nature of the illness and work restrictions, if any, must be provided to Human Resources **prior** to returning to work for any of the following reasons:

- Medical Leave of Absence
- Absenteeism due to illness or injury which exceeds three (3) days
- Any surgical procedure
- Conditions requiring restrictions or limitations of work activities or job accommodations
- At the request of the Human Resources, Department Manager or Occupational Health Professional
- After treatment of chemical dependency

A fitness for duty evaluation may be conducted to evaluate any change in the worker's health status that might require a change in the worker's duties and to assure proper placement to prevent further illness and injury. A return to work evaluation may be requested:

- To evaluate a worker after a severe illness or injury
- To evaluate an worker after an absence from work for an extended duration

D. Benefits Eligibility or Regulatory Entitlement – A fitness for duty evaluation may also be indicated in order to determine worker's eligibility for benefits entitlement, such as disability insurance or requests for accommodation under the American's With Disabilities Act.

E. Reasonable Suspicion

A fitness-for-duty evaluation may also be ordered before management takes disciplinary and/or adverse action against a worker for unacceptable conduct or behavior if it appears that a medical condition may be at the root of the problem.

F. Periodic Health Monitoring

Periodic health evaluations, conducted at intervals during employment, are performed for preventive and health surveillance purposes and to meet required federal regulations and standards.

General Considerations:

Medical Decisions: Decisions related to fitness for duty are made by a medical examiner selected by the Company who has an understanding of the performance requirements of the position.

Confidentiality: All information obtained during the preplacement medical evaluation or during the course of employment will be maintained in a confidential medical file. The supervisor will be informed only of the restrictions and accommodations needed.

Safety: Members of the safety/first responder team will be notified if the individual has a condition that may require emergency treatment.

REASONABLE ACCOMMODATIONS

It is the responsibility of the disabled individual to inform the Company of the need for an accommodation, unless that need is obvious.

The Company's Occupational Health Professional will evaluate the potential for job modifications, to include modification of work environment and/or tasks performed.

Preplacement: Human Resources will review candidates who are determined "not fit-for-duty" following preplacement medical evaluation.

- If the condition is temporary, determine if the position can be held with a delayed start date until the condition is controlled or corrected.
- If the condition is permanent, in consultation with the Occupational Health Professional, determine if reasonable accommodation can be provided.
- If reasonable accommodation is not feasible, determine if there is another position for which the candidate may qualify. The candidate will then be given the opportunity to apply for an alternate position with the Company, in which they can perform the essential job functions.

Current worker: Workers who are determined "not fit-for-duty" during the course of their employment will be referred to Human Resources. The role of Human Resources, in consultation with the Occupational Health Professional, is:

- If the condition is permanent, determine if reasonable accommodations can be provided in the current position by temporarily or permanently modifying essential functions and/or work environment

- If reasonable accommodation is not feasible, determine if there is another position for which the candidate may qualify. The candidate will then be given the opportunity to apply for an alternate position with the Company, in which they can perform the essential job functions
- If the condition is temporary, place the worker on medical leave until the condition is controlled or corrected. A medical evaluation by a medical provider selected by the Company will be required before the worker returns to work.
- If accommodation is not feasible and the condition cannot be corrected, action may be taken to remove the worker from employment for failure to meet the elements and standards of the assigned position.

Job Transfer Assessments

Job transfer assessment may be conducted when there has been a change in the health status of the worker or when working conditions change, thereby placing the worker at risk of work-related injury or illness. The Occupational Health Professional and a representative from Human Resources will conduct the job transfer assessment. The focus is to determine the availability of a job for which the worker is qualified.

Collective Bargaining Agreement Statement

(if indicated)

Sample: Drug-Free Workplace Policy

A19

PURPOSE AND GOAL

(COMPANY NAME) is committed to protecting the safety, health, and well-being of all workers and other individuals in our workplace. (COMPANY NAME) also strives to maintain a workforce free from the influences of illegal drugs and substance abuse, recognizing that alcohol abuse and drug use pose a significant threat to our goals. We have established a drug-free workplace program that balances our respect for individuals with the need to maintain an alcohol- and drug-free environment.

It is, therefore, a violation of company policy for any worker to possess, sell, trade, or offer for sale illegal drugs or otherwise engage in the use of illegal drugs, intoxicants, or alcohol on the job. (COMPANY NAME) encourages workers to voluntarily seek help with drug and substance abuse problems.

DEFINITIONS

- **"Legal Drug"**: includes prescribed drugs and over-the-counter drugs that have been legally obtained and are being used solely for the purpose for which they were prescribed or manufactured.
- **"Illegal Drugs"**: any drug that is not legally obtainable, which may be legally obtainable but has not been legally obtained, or is being used in a manner or for a purpose other than as prescribed.
- **"Intoxicant"**: a substance that leads to marked impairment of physical and mental control.

COVERED WORKERS

Any individual who conducts business for the organization, is applying for a position, or is conducting business on the organization's property is covered by our drug-free workplace policy. Our policy includes, but is not limited to, CEO, executive management, managers, full-time workers, part-time workers, off-site workers, volunteers, interns, and applicants.

Essentials for Occupational Health Nursing, First Edition. Arlene Guzik.
© 2013 John Wiley & Sons, Inc. Published 2013 by John Wiley & Sons, Inc.

APPLICABILITY
Our drug-free workplace policy is intended to apply whenever anyone is representing or conducting business for the organization. Therefore, this policy applies during all working hours, whenever conducting business or representing the organization, while on call or paid standby, while on organization property, and at company-sponsored events.

PROHIBITED BEHAVIOR
It is a violation of our drug-free workplace policy to use, possess, sell, trade, and/or offer for sale alcohol, illegal drugs, or intoxicants. The illegal or unauthorized use of prescription drugs is also prohibited. It is a violation of (COMPANY NAME)'s drug-free workplace policy to intentionally misuse and/or abuse prescription medications.

Prescription and over-the-counter drugs, when taken as prescribed, are not prohibited. Any worker taking prescribed or over-the-counter medications should consult with the prescribing healthcare provider and/or pharmacist to determine if the drug may interfere with safe performance on the job. If the use of a drug is determined to interfere with the ability to perform the essential functions of the job, or has an effect on the safety of the worker or workplace, it is the worker's responsibility to take the appropriate interventions to avoid unsafe workplace practices. This includes taking appropriate work leave or seeking alternatives to the use of the prescribed drug.

A worker reporting to work visibly impaired will be deemed unable to properly perform the essential duties of the job and will not be allowed to work until further evaluated. If, in the opinion of the supervisor, the worker is considered impaired, the worker should be sent home or to a medical facility by taxi or other safe transportation alternative, depending on the determination of the observed impairment, and accompanied by the supervisor, if necessary. An impaired worker should not be allowed to drive.

NOTIFICATION OF CONVICTIONS
Any worker who is convicted of a criminal drug violation in the workplace must notify the organization in writing within 5 calendar days of the conviction. The organization will take appropriate action within 30 days of notification. Federal contracting agencies will be notified when appropriate.

SEARCHES
Entering the organization's property constitutes consent to searches and inspections. If an individual is suspected of violating the drug-free workplace policy, he or she may be asked to submit to a search or inspection at any time. Searches can be conducted of pockets and clothing, lockers, desks and work stations, and vehicles and equipment.

DRUG TESTING

To ensure the accuracy and fairness of our testing program, all testing will be conducted according to Substance Abuse and Mental Health Services Administration (SAMHSA) guidelines where applicable and will include a screening test; a confirmation test; the opportunity for a split sample; review by a Medical Review Officer, including the opportunity for workers who test positive to provide a legitimate medical explanation, such as a physician's prescription, for the positive result; and a documented chain of custody.

All drug-testing information will be maintained in separate confidential records.

Testing will take place in the following situations: pre-placement, random, post-accident, reasonable suspicion, fitness-for-duty, and follow-up testing.

- **Postoffer, Preplacement Testing**: All final candidates for jobs to which employment or job transfer has been offered will be tested.
- **Random**: Workers may be selected for drug testing through a verifiable and tamper-proof method without prior notification and for no particular reason.
- **Postaccident**: Workers who have caused, contributed to, or are involved in an on-the-job incident or accident involving injury, illness, or property damage will be tested.
- **Reasonable Suspicion Testing**: Drug tests will be conducted following any observed behavior creating "reasonable suspicion", such as:
  - Direct observation of the use of drugs or alcohol or the behavior consistent with being under the influence of a drug, substance, or alcohol.
  - Abnormal behavior while at work or a significant deterioration in performance.
  - A report of drug use, provided by a reliable and credible source.
  - Evidence that an individual has tampered with a drug test.
  - Evidence that an employee has used, possessed, sold, or solicited drugs while working or while on company premises or in a company vehicle.
- **Fitness-For-Duty**: Testing may be conducted during annual evaluations for fitness-for-duty.
- **Follow-up Testing**: Random, unannounced drug testing will be required for workers who have participated in a substance abuse rehabilitation program after completion of the program.

The substances that will be tested for are: Amphetamines, Cannabinoids (THC), Cocaine, Opiates, Phencyclidine (PCP), Alcohol, Barbiturates, Benzodiazepines, Methaqualone, Methadone and Propoxyphene.

Testing for the presence of alcohol will be conducted by analysis of breath.

Testing for the presence of the metabolites of drugs will be conducted by the analysis of urine.

Any worker who tests positive will be immediately removed from duty and referred to a substance abuse professional for assessment and recommendations.

The individual will be required to successfully complete recommended rehabilitation including continuing care, and will be required to pass a Return-to-Duty test and sign a Return-to-Work Agreement, and be subject to random, unannounced drug tests at the employer's discretion. Any individual, if tested positive a second time or violates the Return-to-Work Agreement, will be terminated immediately. (OPTIONAL WORDING: A zero-tolerance policy would include: "If a worker violates this policy, the worker will be terminated from employment").

A worker will be terminated immediately if he/she refuses the screening or the test, adulterates or dilutes the specimen, substitutes the specimen with that from another person or sends an imposter, will not sign the required forms or refuses to cooperate in the testing process in such a way that prevents completion of the test.

CONSEQUENCES

One of the goals of our drug-free workplace program is to encourage workers to voluntarily seek help with alcohol and/or drug problems. If, however, an individual violates the policy, the consequences are serious.

In the case of applicants, if he or she violates the drug-free workplace policy, the offer of employment can be withdrawn. The applicant may not reapply.

If a worker violates the conditions of this policy, he or she will be terminated from employment.

ASSISTANCE

(COMPANY NAME) recognizes that alcohol and drug abuse and addiction are treatable illnesses. We also realize that early intervention and support improve the success of rehabilitation. To support our workers, our drug-free workplace policy:

- Encourages workers to seek help if they are concerned that they or their family members may have a drug and/or alcohol problem.
- Encourages workers to use the services of qualified professionals in the community to assess the seriousness of suspected drug or alcohol problems and identify appropriate sources of help.
- Ensures the availability of a current list of qualified community professionals.
- Offers all workers and their family members assistance with alcohol and drug problems through the Employee Assistance Program (EAP).
- Allows the use of accrued paid leave while seeking treatment for alcohol and other drug problems.

Treatment for alcoholism and/or other drug use disorders may be covered by the worker benefit plan. However, the ultimate financial responsibility for recommended treatment belongs to the worker.

CONFIDENTIALITY

All information received by the organization through the drug-free workplace program is confidential communication. Access to this information is limited to those who have a legitimate need to know in compliance with relevant laws and management policies.

SHARED RESPONSIBILITY

A safe and productive drug-free workplace is achieved through cooperation and shared responsibility. Both workers and management have important roles to play.

All workers are required to not report to work or be subject to duty while their ability to perform job duties is impaired due to on- or off-duty use of alcohol or other drugs.

In addition, workers are encouraged to:

- Be concerned about working in a safe environment.
- Support fellow workers in seeking help.
- Use the Employee Assistance Program.
- Report dangerous behavior to their supervisor.

It is the supervisor's responsibility to:

- Inform workers of the drug-free workplace policy.
- Observe worker performance.
- Document negative changes and problems in performance.
- Counsel workers as to expected performance improvement.
- Refer workers to the Employee Assistance Program.
- Clearly state consequences of policy violations.

COMMUNICATION

Communicating our drug-free workplace policy to both supervisors and workers is critical to our success. To ensure all workers are aware of their role in supporting our drug-free workplace program:

- All workers will receive a written copy of the policy.
- The policy will be reviewed in orientation sessions with new workers.
- The policy and assistance programs will be reviewed at safety meetings.
- Posters and brochures will be available at all locations.
- Worker education about the dangers of alcohol and drug use and the availability of help will be provided to all workers.
- Every supervisor will receive training to help him/her recognize and manage workers with alcohol and other drug problems.

Certificate of Agreement

I do hereby certify that I have received and read (COMPANY NAME) Drug-Free Workplace Program and Policies regarding substance abuse and substance abuse testing, have had the entire program explained to me, and have had the opportunity to ask questions.

I understand that if conditions as specified in the policy indicate it is necessary, I will submit to substance abuse testing.

I also understand that failure to comply with a request or a positive result may lead to termination of employment.

_____

Employee's Name (Please Print)

_____

Signature

_____

Date

(To be a permanent part of worker's personnel file.)

SAMPLE LETTER TO WORKERS

Dear Worker:

We have come to recognize that substance abuse is a problem in the workplace, as well as a social problem. We believe abuse of illegal drugs, alcohol or other substances may endanger the health and safety of the workplace.

(COMPANY NAME) is committed to creating and maintaining a drug-free workplace. Our policy will not jeopardize valued but troubled workers' job security, providing they are prepared to help us help them.

Our policy now formally states it is a condition of employment to refrain from substance abuse on or off the job. This prohibition includes the possession, use, or sale of illegal drugs.

Workers who are found to be under the influence of illegal drugs or alcohol or who violate this policy in other ways are subject to disciplinary action which may include termination. Because of the serious nature of these violations, each individual case will be thoroughly investigated to determine the appropriate course of action.

It is important that we all work together to deal with substance abuse and other personal problems to make (COMPANY NAME) a safer and more rewarding place to work.

A copy of the complete (COMPANY NAME) policy is attached for your use along with a certificate of agreement. Sign and return the certificate to _____. The policy will be effective on _____.

Sincerely,

_____

COMPANY OFFICIAL

Urine Drug Screen Collection Checklist

A20

Before Doing Any Urine Drug Screen Collection

1. Is collection area clean and ready for a collection?
   Yes   No

2. Are there enough kits and chain of custodies for collections that day?
   Yes   No

Performing a Urine Drug Screen Collection

1. Has the collector put on gloves?
   Yes   No

2. Has the collector obtained the correct Custody and Control Form?
   Yes   No

3. Has the collector checked the donor's photo identification against the donor to make sure they match?
   Yes   No

4. Has the collector asked the donor to pick out a drug collection kit?
   Yes   No

5. Has the collector verified to assure the appropriate type of drug screen to be collected?
   Yes   No

6. Has the collector put the donors I.D. # on the Custody and Control Form?
   Yes   No

Essentials for Occupational Health Nursing, First Edition. Arlene Guzik.
© 2013 John Wiley & Sons, Inc. Published 2013 by John Wiley & Sons, Inc.

7. Has the collector marked the reason for the drug screen on the Custody and Control Form?
Yes   No

8. Has the collector marked the drug screen panel to be used on the Custody and Control Form?
Yes   No

9. Has the collector asked the donor to empty out his/her pockets?
Yes   No

10. Has the collector asked the donor to remove any hats or bulky clothing?
Yes   No

11. Has the collector opened the drug screen kit in front of the donor?
Yes   No

12. Has the collector instructed the donor to rinse his/her hands with cold water? (no soap)
Yes   No

13. Has the collector instructed the donor how much specimen he/she is to provide?
Yes   No

14. Has the collector instructed the donor to bring the specimen out to him/her when finished?
Yes   No

15. Has the collector told the donor not to flush toilet when finished?
Yes   No

16. Has the collector closed bathroom door to give donor privacy?
Yes   No

17. Has the collector turned off the water supply to bathroom?
Yes   No

After Performing a Urine Drug Screen Collection

1. Has the collector noted the temperature of the specimen?
Yes   No

2. Has the collector marked the temperature on the Custody and Control Form?
Yes   No

3. Has the collector poured specimen into specimen tube and sealed it?
Yes   No

4. Has the collector removed the seal from the Custody and Control Form and placed it over the lid of the specimen tube?
Yes   No

5. Has the collector had the donor initial the seal on the specimen tube?
Yes   No

6. Has the collector initialed the seal on the specimen tube?
Yes   No

7. Has the donor verified the correct ID# on the Custody and Control Form?
Yes   No

8. Has the donor signed all the appropriate places on the Custody and Control Form?
Yes   No

9. Has the donor provided a phone number where he/she may be reached if there is a need to discuss results?
Yes   No

10. Has the collector signed all the appropriate places on the Custody and Control Form?
Yes   No

11. Has the collector placed the lab copy of the Custody and Control Form in the specimen bag?
Yes   No

12. Has the collector placed the specimen tube in the specimen bag and sealed it in the presence of the donor?
Yes   No

13. Has the collector given the donor the donor copy of the Custody and Control Form?
Yes   No

14. Has the collector told donor that he/she may now wash his/her hands?
Yes   No

15. Has the collector turned the water supply back on?
Yes   No

16. Has the collector told donor that they may retrieve personal belongings?
    Yes   No

17. Has the collector told the donor the anticipated time frame for the results to be reported?
    Yes   No

18. Has the collector informed donor that drug screen is over?
    Yes   No

19. Has the collector inspected the bathroom to inspect for signs of specimen tampering?
    Yes   No

20. Has the collector cleaned the bathroom for the next drug screen?
    Yes   No

21. Has the collector thrown away residual specimen and collection cup?
    Yes   No

22. Has the collector removed gloves and washed his/her hands?
    Yes   No

23. Has the collector written down COC # and or donor ID on courier collection sheet?
    Yes   No

24. Has the collector cleaned the collection area so that it is ready for the next drug screen?
    Yes   No

25. Has the collector checked supplies and ensured enough are available for future collections?
    Yes   No

26. Has the collector mailed the MRO copy of the Custody and Control Form to the MRO Office?
    Yes   No

Sample Request for Workplace Accommodation	**A21**

TO BE COMPLETED BY WORKER:

Worker Name (PRINT): _____ Date of Birth _____

In order to evaluate the medical necessity of this accommodation, I hereby give consent for the release of medical records from the healthcare provider stated below to (COMPANY) and/or (Medical Advisor) such healthcare records and information concerning the current medical condition of the patient identified above as is necessary to support the request of the worker for the following work restriction(s)/accommodation(s).

Requested restriction or accommodation: _____

Worker Signature: _____ **Date**: _____

****

Healthcare Provider Name (PRINT): _____

Address: _____ Phone: _____Fax: _____

HEALTHCARE PROVIDER: Please complete the following information. This information will be maintained in the worker's confidential medical file and used to support the need for medical accommodation, as requested. A copy of the job description, including essential functions of the job, has been provided.

TO BE COMPLETED BY PHYSICIAN/HEALTHCARE PROVIDER
Medical Disposition

_____ Released to regular duty on (date)
_____ Released to work with restrictions/accommodation on (date)

Essentials for Occupational Health Nursing, First Edition. Arlene Guzik.
© 2013 John Wiley & Sons, Inc. Published 2013 by John Wiley & Sons, Inc.

_____ **Temporary** restrictions/accommodation   * state length of time _____
                                                      * reevaluation date _____
_____ **Permanent** disability as defined by the American's With Disabilities Act as substantially limiting one or more life activity (define below)

Statement of disability (if applicable): _____
_____

RESTRICTIONS/PHYSICAL LIMITATIONS

1. No lifting or carrying > _____ lbs.
2. No lifting above shoulder > _____ lbs.
3. No lifting over _____ lbs. More then _____ times per hour
4. Limited use of _____ hand/arm
5. Limit pulling, grasping, twisting more than _____ times per hour
6. No pushing or pulling > _____ lbs.
7. No bending or stooping
8. No crawling or kneeling
9. No standing/walking > _____ minutes
10. No sitting > _____ minutes
11. No climbing ladder/stairs
12. No exposure to _____ because of _____
13. Avoid temperatures < _____ degrees or > _____ degrees
14. Other _____

USE OF MEDICAL DEVICES:

_____ splint   _____ brace   _____ eye patch   _____ wheelchair

_____ sling   _____ dressing   _____ walker

_____ crutches   _____ cane   _____ other: _____

Type of Accommodation recommended: _____

Comments: _____

PHYSICIAN/HEALTHCARE PROVIDER SIGNATURE: _____DATE: _____

Fax form to: _____

Attention: _____

Notice of Intermittent FMLA Absence

A22

NOTICE OF INTERMITTENT FMLA ABSENCE

MUST BE COMPLETED BY THE EMPLOYEE AND SUBMITTED WITHIN
TWO (2) BUSINESS DAYS OF RETURNING TO WORK FROM <u>EACH</u> FMLA ABSENCE.

This is to certify that the following absence(s) should be covered under the terms of the approved intermittent family or medical leave for:

Employee Name (PRINT): _____ Employee # _____

DATE: _____ HOURS WORKED: _____ HOURS MISSED: _____

DATE: _____ HOURS WORKED: _____ HOURS MISSED: _____

DATE: _____ HOURS WORKED: _____ HOURS MISSED: _____

Employee Signature: _____ Date: _____

Failure to submit this notice may not provide protection for this absence under the Family and Medical Leave Act and the absence may be handled per corporate attendance policy.

    White: OHN office   Yellow: Employee   Pink: Supervisor

Essentials for Occupational Health Nursing, First Edition. Arlene Guzik.
© 2013 John Wiley & Sons, Inc. Published 2013 by John Wiley & Sons, Inc.

Sample Fitness for Duty Form

A23

Worker Name (PRINT): _____ Date of Birth _____

Healthcare Provider Name (PRINT): _____

Address: _____ Phone: _____ Fax: _____

HEALTHCARE PROVIDER: Please complete the following information. This information will be maintained in the worker's confidential medical file and used to support the need for medical accommodation, as requested. A copy of the job description, including essential functions of the job, has been provided.

TO BE COMPLETED BY PHYSICIAN/HEALTHCARE PROVIDER
Medical Disposition

_____ Released to regular duty on (date) _____

_____ Released to work with restrictions/accommodation on (date) _____

_____ **Temporary** restrictions/accommodation   * state length of time ____
                                                        * reevaluation date _____

_____ **Permanent** disability as defined by the American's with Disabilities Act as substantially limiting one or more life activity (define below)

Statement of disability (if applicable): _____
_____

RESTRICTIONS/PHYSICAL LIMITATIONS

1. No lifting or carrying > _____lbs.
2. No lifting above shoulder >_____ lbs.
3. No lifting over _____lbs. More then _____ times per hour

Essentials for Occupational Health Nursing, First Edition. Arlene Guzik.
© 2013 John Wiley & Sons, Inc. Published 2013 by John Wiley & Sons, Inc.

4. Limited use of _____ hand/arm
5. Limit pulling, grasping, twisting more than _____ times per hour
6. No pushing or pulling > _____ lbs.
7. No bending or stooping
8. No crawling or kneeling
9. No standing/walking > _____ minutes
10. No sitting > _____ minutes
11. No climbing ladder/stairs
12. No exposure to _____ because of _____
13. Avoid temperatures < _____ degrees or > _____ degrees
14. Other _____

USE OF MEDICAL DEVICES:

_____ splint   _____ brace   _____ eye patch   _____ wheelchair

_____ sling   _____ dressing   _____ walker

_____ crutches   _____ cane   _____ other: _____

Type of Accommodation recommended: _____

Comments: _____

PHYSICIAN/HEALTHCARE PROVIDER SIGNATURE: _____ DATE: _____

Fax form to: _____

Attention: _____

MILLION HEARTS: PREVENTION AT WORK

As an Employer we strive to:

- **EMPOWER** our workers by supporting activities that help people access high-quality healthcare, manage their conditions effectively, get active, eat healthy, and stay smoke-free.
- **INCREASE** awareness of heart disease and stroke and their risk factors to empower workers to take control of their heart health.
- **PROVIDE** convenient and simple blood pressure monitoring in the workplace.
- **IMPLEMENT** smoke-free air policies at worksites to help smokers quit and protect nonsmokers from the hazardous effects of second hand smoke exposure.
- **SUPPORT** efforts to reduce sodium and eliminate trans fats in the food supply

We encourage workers to:

- **PREVENT** heart disease and stroke by **UNDERSTANDING** the risks.
- **GET UP** and **GET ACTIVE** by exercising for 30 minutes on most days of the week.
- **KNOW** the **ABCs**:
  - Appropriate Aspirin Therapy
  - Blood Pressure Control
  - Cholesterol Management
  - Smoking Cessation
- **STAY STRONG** by eating a heart-healthy diet that is high in fresh fruits and vegetables and low in sodium, saturated and trans fats, and cholesterol.
- **TAKE CONTROL** of your heart health by following your healthcare provider's recommendations

Essentials for Occupational Health Nursing, First Edition. Arlene Guzik.
© 2013 John Wiley & Sons, Inc. Published 2013 by John Wiley & Sons, Inc.

MILLION HEARTS: PREVENTION AT WORK

Leading Health Indicator	Worksite Initiatives	First Year Worker Participation Goal
Health education related to aspirin use	• Article in company newsletter and on company website • Article in payroll stuffer • Article by email to all workers • Provide written information at company's annual health fair	100%

Blood pressure control	• Article in company newsletter and on company website
	• Article in payroll stuffer
	• Article by email to all workers
	• Initiate "Know Your Numbers" campaign
	  ○ Provide quarterly blood pressure screening events in various worksite locations
	  ○ Provide participants with written information regarding the meaning of the numbers
	  ○ Provide appropriate guidance and referral information for healthcare resources to workers
	• Provide blood pressure screening as part of company's annual health fair
		30%

Cholesterol control	• Article in company newsletter and on company website
	• Article in payroll stuffer
	• Article by email to all workers
	• Initiate "Know Your Numbers" campaign
	  ○ Provide quarterly cholesterol screening events in various worksite locations
	  ○ Provide participants with written information regarding the meaning of the numbers
	  ○ Provide appropriate guidance and referral information for healthcare resources to workers
	• Provide cholesterol screening as part of company's annual health fair
		20%

Tobacco cessation	• Article in company newsletter and on company website
	• Article in payroll stuffer
	• Articles by email to all workers
	• Initiate Tobacco Cessation Campaign
	  ○ Provide tobacco cessation program
	  ○ Establish a tobacco-free campus
	  ○ Provide appropriate guidance and referral information for healthcare resources to workers
	• Provide information and resources as part of company's annual health fair
		5%

| Nutritional Awareness | • Article in company newsletter and on company website
• Article in payroll stuffer
• Articles by email to all workers
• Nutritional awareness to include:
  ○ Sodium intake
  ○ Artificial trans fats
  ○ Healthy heating and portion control
• Work with company cafeteria vendor and vending machine supplier to offer only healthy meal and food choices | 20% |

Source: http://millionhearts.hhs.gov/partners.shtml. For more information about Million Hearts visit http://millionhearts.hhs.gov.

Service Provider
Service Delivery
Activity Report
May 2012

A25

Essentials for Occupational Health Nursing, First Edition. Arlene Guzik.
© 2013 John Wiley & Sons, Inc. Published 2013 by John Wiley & Sons, Inc.

DATE	New Injury		Follow-up		New Hire Physical		Regulatory Physical		Personal Health Visit		Medical Surveillance Testing		Substance Testing		TOTAL
	#	$	#	$	#	$	#	$	#	$	#	$	#	$	$
1		0.00		0.00		0.00		0.00		0.00		0.00		0.00	0.00
2		0.00		0.00	1	115.00	1	125.00	3	112.50		0.00	1	25.00	377.50
3	1	189.00	4	356.00		0.00		0.00	4	150.00	4	100.00		0.00	795.00
4		0.00		0.00		0.00	1	125.00	1	37.50		0.00		0.00	162.50
5	1	189.00	2	178.00	2	230.00	3	375.00		0.00		0.00	2	50.00	1,022.00
6	1	189.00	3	267.00		0.00	3	375.00	3	112.50		0.00		0.00	943.50
7		0.00		0.00		0.00		0.00		0.00		0.00	1	25.00	25.00
8		0.00		0.00		0.00		0.00		0.00		0.00		0.00	0.00
9	1	189.00		0.00		0.00	2	250.00	1	37.50		0.00		0.00	476.50
10	2	378.00	4	356.00	3	345.00		0.00	2	75.00	2	50.00		0.00	1,204.00
11	2	378.00	4	356.00		0.00	4	500.00	4	150.00		0.00		0.00	1,384.00
12	1	189.00	6	534.00		0.00	1	125.00	1	37.50		0.00		0.00	885.50
13	2	378.00	6	534.00		0.00	1	125.00		0.00		0.00		0.00	1,037.00
14		0.00		0.00		0.00		0.00		0.00		0.00		0.00	0.00
15		0.00		0.00		0.00		0.00		0.00		0.00		0.00	0.00
16	1	189.00	5	445.00		0.00	1	125.00	1	37.50	6	150.00	1	25.00	971.50
17		0.00	4	356.00	2	230.00		0.00	1	37.50	5	125.00		0.00	748.50
18	1	189.00	2	178.00		0.00	1	125.00	1	37.50		0.00		0.00	529.50
19		0.00	3	267.00	1	115.00		0.00	2	75.00	2	50.00	1	25.00	532.00
20	2	378.00	2	178.00		0.00	1	125.00	4	150.00		0.00		0.00	831.00
21		0.00		0.00		0.00		0.00		0.00		0.00		0.00	0.00

															Value
22		0.00		0.00		0.00		0.00		0.00		0.00		0.00	0.00
23		0.00	5	445.00		0.00		0.00	2	75.00		0.00		0.00	520.00
24	1	189.00	2	178.00		0.00	1	125.00	4	150.00	10	250.00	1	25.00	917.00
25	1	189.00	1	89.00	1	115.00	2	250.00	1	37.50	5	125.00		0.00	805.50
26		0.00	2	178.00		0.00	3	375.00	2	75.00	6	150.00		0.00	778.00
27		0.00		0.00	2	230.00	3	375.00	2	75.00	4	100.00	1	25.00	805.00
28		0.00		0.00		0.00		0.00		0.00		0.00		0.00	0.00
29		0.00		0.00		0.00		0.00		0.00		0.00		0.00	0.00
30		0.00		0.00		0.00		0.00		0.00		0.00		0.00	0.00
31	2	378.00	4	356.00	1	0.00	1	125.00	2	75.00		0.00	8	200.00	934.00
	19	3,591.00	59	5,251.00	12	1,380.00	29	3,625.00	41	1,537.50	44	1,100.00	8	200.00	16,684.50

Value of Service Rendered	16,684.50
Monthly Service Contract Cost	15,000.00
Difference	1,684.50

Occupational Health Services Service Delivery Evaluation Criteria

Structure	Process	Outcome

Roles and Responsibilities
• Job descriptions for all workers employed in occupational health clinic
  ○ Match with daily functions of role
• Roles clearly defined
  ○ Qualifications equate to role
• Established goals and objectives are in place.
	Service Delivery
	• Clinic encounter data
	• Analysis of current services rendered
	  ○ Health promotion
	  ○ Health protection
	  ○ Health restoration
	  ○ Training and education
	  ○ Record keeping
	• Participation in committees and task force events
	• Involvement in multidisciplinary meetings (safety, HR, etc.)
		Customer Service
		• Evaluation of customer service
		  ○ Who
		  ○ How often
		  ○ What is feedback loop for process improvement
		  ○ Addresses internal and external customer service
		  ○ Involves multidisciplinary stakeholders

Reporting Structure
• Current organizational chart and reporting relationships
  ○ Corporate
  ○ By division
  ○ By location
	Scope of Practice
	• Written practice guidelines in place
	• Appropriate medical direction
	  ○ Medical director site visit
	• Clinical competencies are validated
	• Performance is evaluated
		Stakeholder Interaction
		Interdepartmental
		• Safety
		• Human Resources/Benefits
		• Risk management
		• Operations
		
		Service Providers
		• Diagnostic service
		• Medical services (clinics, PT, hospitals, etc)
		• Vendor relations
		• Community involvement

(Continued)

Essentials for Occupational Health Nursing, First Edition. Arlene Guzik.
© 2013 John Wiley & Sons, Inc. Published 2013 by John Wiley & Sons, Inc.

Structure	Process	Outcome
Policies and Procedures • Written clinical policies and procedures are in place • Written documentation of medical direction and oversight	Communication Evaluate current process and methods of communication • What is communicated • To whom • In what format • How often	Financial Metrics • Healthcare costs • Reduction in lost time • Reduced sickness absence • Cost savings on services
Regulatory and Business Compliance • All licenses (business and professional) are consistent with state requirements. • Regulatory permits and certificates are up to date • Clinic is in full HIPAA compliance	Privacy and Confidentiality Facility • Assurance of privacy • Health records maintenance HIPAA • Consents • What information is shared, with whom, and in what format	Benchmark data • Decrease incidents, injuries • Decrease OSHA recordables • Decrease lost time • Decrease severity of claims • Decreased length of claims • Reduced litigation • Risk reduction
Facility • Meets regulatory and professional standards • Supplies and equipment up-to-date and appropriate for services • Inventory adequate for volume of services • Accountability for inventory management		

Professional Resources Related to Occupational Health

A27

Organization	Description	Web Address
Agency for Toxic Substances and Disease Registry (ATSDR)	The ATSDR is a federal public health agency of the U.S. Department of Health and Human Services. ATSDR serves the public by using the best science, taking responsive public health actions, and providing trusted health information to prevent harmful exposures and diseases related to toxic substances.	www.atsdr.cdc.gov/
American Association of Occupational Health Nurses (AAOHN)	The AAOHN is the primary professional association for occupational health nurses and other healthcare professionals serving the workplace. AAOHN is "dedicated to advancing and maximizing the health, safety and productivity of domestic and global workforces by providing education, research, public policy and practice resources for occupational and environmental health nurses.	www.aaohn.org
American Cancer Society	The American Cancer Society is a nationwide, community-based voluntary health organization dedicated to eliminating cancer as a major health problem.	www.cancer.org
American College of Occupational and Environmental Medicine (ACOEM)	ACOEM is the nation's largest medical society and is dedicated to promoting the health of workers through preventive medicine, clinical care, research, and education. ACOEM focuses efforts on enhancing "the health and safety of workers, workplaces, and environments."	www.acoem.org
American Heart Association	The mission of the American Heart Association is to build healthier lives, free of cardiovascular diseases and stroke.	www.americanheart.org

(Continued)

Essentials for Occupational Health Nursing, First Edition. Arlene Guzik.
© 2013 John Wiley & Sons, Inc. Published 2013 by John Wiley & Sons, Inc.

Organization	Description	Web Address
American Industrial Hygiene Association (AIHA)	AIHA is a professional association for scientists and engineers, with an emphasis on the health and safety of workers and workplaces in the community. AIHA is "devoted to the anticipation, recognition, evaluation, prevention, and control of those environmental factors or stresses arising in or from the workplace which may cause sickness, impaired health and well-being, or significant discomfort among workers or among citizens of the community."	www.aiha.org
American Public Health Association	The American Public Health Association represents a broad array of health professionals and others who care about their own health and the health of their communities. The association aims to protect all Americans, their families, and their communities from preventable serious health threats and strives to ensure that community-based health promotion and disease prevention activities and preventive health services are universally accessible in the United States.	www.apha.org
America Society of Safety Engineers (ASSE)	ASSE, the oldest professional safety society, is "committed to protecting people, property, and the environment, providing key information and action on occupational safety, health and environmental issues and practices." Members focus on creating a safer, healthier workplace and developing safer products in order to prevent workplace injuries and illnesses.	www.asse.org
Americans with Disabilities (ADA) home page	Information and technical assistance on the Americans with Disabilities Act	www.ada.gov
Bureau of Labor Statistics	The Bureau of Labor Statistics of the U.S. Department of Labor is the principal federal agency responsible for measuring labor market activity, working conditions, and price changes in the economy. Its mission is to collect, analyze, and disseminate essential economic information to support public and private decision making.	www.bls/gov
E-laws Employment Law Guide	The guide describes the major statutes and regulations administered by the U.S. Department of Labor (DOL) that affect businesses and workers. The guide is designed mainly for those needing "hands-on" information to develop wage, benefit, safety and health, and nondiscrimination policies for businesses.	www.dol.gov/ compliance
Environmental Protection Agency (EPA)	The mission of the EPA's is to protect human health and the environment.	www.epa.gov

Organization	Description	Web Address
Federal Aviation Administration (FAA)	The FAA provides resources and information related to the aerospace industry.	www.faa.gov
Federal Motor Carrier Safety Administration (FMCSA)	The FMCSA develops and enforces data-driven regulations that balance motor carrier (truck and bus companies) safety with efficiency; targets educational messages to carriers, commercial drivers, and the public; and partners with stakeholders including federal, state, and local enforcement agencies, the motor carrier industry, safety groups, and organized labor on efforts to reduce bus and truck-related crashes.	www.fmcsa.dot.gov
Haz-Map	An occupational health database designed for health and safety professionals and for consumers seeking information about the adverse effects of workplace exposures to chemical and biological agents.	www.hazmap.nlm. nih.gov/index.php
Healthy People	The Healthy People program provides science-based, 10-year national objectives for improving the health of all Americans.	www.healthypeople. gov
HR-Guide	This website contains information related to human resources. Provide links to other websites in the HR field and provides guides to HR-related topics.	www.hr-guide.com
Institute for Health and Productivity Management	The Institute for Health and Productivity Management (IHPM) is a global nonprofit enterprise created in 1997 to establish the full value of employee health as an investment in workplace productivity and business performance. The Institute champions the idea of health as human capital and the greatest untapped source of competitive advantage in a global marketplace.	www.ihpm.org
Mine Safety and Health Administration (MSHA)	The mission of the MSHA is to administer the provisions of the Federal Mine Safety and Health Act of 1977 (Mine Act) and to enforce compliance with mandatory safety and health standards as a means to eliminate fatal accidents, to reduce the frequency and severity of nonfatal accidents, to minimize health hazards, and to promote improved safety and health conditions in U.S.mines.	www.msha.gov/
Morbidity and Mortality Weekly (*MMWR*)	The *MMWR* series is prepared by the Centers for Disease Control and Prevention (CDC). Often called "the voice of CDC," the *MMWR* series is the agency's primary vehicle for scientific publication of timely, reliable, authoritative, accurate, objective, and useful public health information and recommendations.	www.cdc.gov/mmwr/

(Continued)

411

Organization	Description	Web Address
National Center for Environmental Health (NCEH)	The CDC's National Center for Environmental Health plans, directs, and coordinates a national program to maintain and improve the health of the American people by promoting a healthy environment and by preventing premature death and avoidable illness and disability caused by noninfectious, nonoccupational environmental and related factors.	www.cdc.gov/nceh/
National Fire Protection Association (NFPA)	The mission of the international nonprofit NFPA is to reduce the worldwide burden of fire and other hazards on the quality of life by providing and advocating consensus codes and standards, research, training, and education.	www.nfpa.org
National Hearing Conservation Association (NHCA)	The mission of the NHCA is to "prevent hearing loss due to noise and other environmental factors in all sectors of society." The NHCA provides an avenue for education and exchange of information that promotes the development of "improved and more effective occupational hearing conservation programs."	www.hearingconservation.org
National Institute for Occupational Safety and Health (NIOSH)	NIOSH is the federal agency "responsible for conducting research and making recommendations for the prevention of work-related injury and illness." The efforts of research and practice, NIOSH serves to "generate new knowledge in the field of occupational safety and health and to transfer that knowledge into practice for the betterment of workers."	www.niosh.gov
National Institute of Environmental Health Science (NIEHS)	The mission of the NIEHS is to discover how the environment affects people in order to promote healthier lives.	www.niehs.nih.gov/
National Library of Medicine (NLM)	The NLM is the world's largest biomedical library. NLM maintains and makes available a vast print collection and produces electronic information resources on a wide range of topics that are searched billions of times each year by millions of people around the globe. It also supports and conducts research, development, and training in biomedical informatics and health information technology.	www.nlm.nih.gov/
National Safety Council (NSC)	The NSC is committed to the prevention of "injuries and deaths at work, in homes and communities, and on the roads through leadership, research, education and advocacy." Initially established to focus on workplace safety, the NSC has expanded focus to also include transportation safety and safety of homes and communities.	www.nsc.org

Organization	Description	Web Address
Occupational Safety and Health Administration (OSHA)	OSHA's mission is to "ensure safe and healthful working conditions for working men and women by setting and enforcing standards and by providing training, outreach, education, and assistance." OSHA publishes a set of regulatory standards applicable to specific workplaces and work hazards.	www.osha.gov
Substance Abuse and Mental Health Services Administration (SAMHSA)	SAMHSA provides oversight for the federal Drug-Free Workplace Program, which aims to eliminate illicit drug use in the federal workforce, and for the National Laboratory Certification Program, which certifies laboratories to conduct forensic drug testing for the federal agencies and for some federally regulated industries.	www.drugfreeworkplace.gov
The Centers for Disease Control (CDC)	The CDC is one of the major operating components of the Department of Health and Human Services created to provide the "expertise, information, and tools that people and communities need to protect their health—through health promotion, prevention of disease, injury and disability, and preparedness for new health threats."	www.cdc.gov
U.S. Department of Labor (DOL)	The DOL is charged with fostering, promoting, and developing the welfare of the wage earners, job seekers, and retirees of the United States. The mission is to improve working conditions, advance opportunities for profitable employment, and ensure work-related benefits and rights. The DOL enforces federal statutes, which cover a wide variety of workplace activities protecting workers' wages, health, safety, employment, and pension rights; promoting equal employment opportunity; and administering job training, unemployment insurance, and workers' compensation programs.	www.dol.gov
U.S. Department of Transportation (DOT)	This arm of the U.S. government is charged with ensuring a fast, safe, efficient, accessible, and convenient transportation system that meets the vital national interests and enhances the quality of life of the American people.	www.dot.gov
U.S. Department of Health and Human Services (DHHS)	The DHHS is the U.S. government's principal agency for protecting the health of all Americans and providing essential human services, especially for those who are least able to help themselves.	www.hhs.gov

Index

AAOHN. *See* American Association
of Occupational Health
Nurses
Abilities, fitness for duty and,
156–157
Absence management, integrated,
239, 241–242
Absenteeism, 241
defined, 309
factors related to, 220, 220*t*
health-related, costs related to,
219–220
lower, workplace health and
wellness program and, 287
overall costs of, 240
Accelerated mass hazard,
description of, 364
Access to care
service delivery analysis and, 299
through workplace, 265–266
Accident reporting, 359
Accommodation requests, fitness for
duty evaluations and, 163
Accountability, wellness guiding
principles and, 270–271
ACOEM. *See* American College of
Occupational and
Environmental Medicine
ADA. *See* Americans with
Disabilities Act
Adjusters, 201, 206
Administrative assistants, job
demands for, 156–157

Administrative controls
defined, 309
hazard control measures, *140*
Administrators, occupational health
nurses as, 6–7
Adoption, FMLA and, 254–255
Advance practice registered nurses
in occupational health, 8–9
statutory requirements for, 20
*Advisory on Over-the-Counter
Medications,* 85–86
AED. *See* Automatic external
defibrillator
After-hours appointments, 88
Age, of workforce, 36
Agency for Healthcare Research &
Quality, Prevention and
Chronic Care Program, 273
Agency for Toxic Substances and
Disease Registry, description
and web address, 409
Aging workers, 44
fitness for duty and, 167
injuries on the job and,
214–215
Agreement for Professional Services
compensation, 317
confidentiality, 319
general provisions, 323
insurance, 319–320
mediation and arbitration of
disputes, 321–322
notices and invoicing, 322

Essentials for Occupational Health Nursing, First Edition. Arlene Guzik.
© 2013 John Wiley & Sons, Inc. Published 2013 by John Wiley & Sons, Inc.

Agreement for Professional Services
(*cont'd*)
  ownership and maintenance of
    documents, 320–321
  performance and professional
    responsibilities, 317–319
  sample, 317–323
  termination, 322
Agriculture industry standards, 100*t*
AHRQ. *See* Agency for Healthcare
    Research & Quality
AIHA. *See* American Industrial
    Hygiene Association
Airborne contaminants, Respiratory
    Protection Standard and,
    110–112
Air-supplied respirators, 112
Alarm systems, 139
Alcohol, testing for, 173, 183–185, 383
Alcohol abuse, prevalence of, 172
Alcoholism
  as covered disability, 247
  treatment, coverage for, 384
Allergies, noting on health record, 91
AMA. *See* American Medical
    Association
*AMA Guides to the Evaluation of
    Permanent Injury,* 232–233
American Association of
    Occupational Health Nurses,
    5, 27, 224
  *Advisory on Over-the-Counter
    Medications,* 85–86
  core competencies for occupational
    health nurse, 26*t*
  description and/or web address
    for, 64*t*, 217, 238, 409
  Position Statement on Delivery of
    Occupational and
    Environmental Health
    Services, 6
  vision of, 16
American Board of Occupational
    Health Nursing, 27

American Cancer Society, description
    and web address for, 409
American College of Occupational
    and Environmental Medicine,
    2, 3, 108, 223
  confidentiality recommendations, 29
  description and/or web address
    for, 64*t*, 217, 238, 409
  vision of, 16
American Conference of
    Governmental Industrial
    Hygienists' Biological
    Exposure Committee, 141
American Heart Association, 108
  description and web address
    for, 409
American Industrial Hygiene
    Association, description and
    web address for, 410
American Medical Association, 232
American National Standards
    Institute
  first aid kit standards, 107
  minimum standard
    supplies, 107*t*
American Nurses Association,
    Nursing's Social Policy
    Statement, 3
American Public Health Association,
    description and web address
    for, 410
American Red Cross, 108
American Society of Safety
    Engineers, description and
    web address for, 64*t*, 410
Americans with Disabilities,
    description and web address
    for, 410
Americans with Disabilities Act, 30,
    155, 160, 174, 240, 242–248,
    256, 257
  case in point, 244
  confidentiality and, 247–248
  covered workers under, 243

disability defined by, 243
enactment and amendments to, 242
essential job functions defined
by, 245
major life activities defined by, 244
physical or mental impairment
defined by, 243–244
providing reasonable
accommodation according to,
245, 246
substantially limits defined by, 244
Amphetamines, 383
5-panel test for, 183
hair drug test for, 182
preemployment and random
testing of workers for, 158
saliva tests for, 182
urine drug testing and, 181
Anaphylaxis, adult, sample practice
guidelines for, 326
Ankle sprain, sample practice
guidelines for, 330–331
Annual Survey of Occupational
Injuries and Illnesses, 145
ANSI. *See* American National
Standards Institute
Appointments, after-hours, 88
Asbestos, 139
ASSE. *See* American Society of Safety
Engineers
Assessment of workplace, 54–59
Assigned risk pool, workers'
compensation insurance, 195
ATSDR. *See* Agency for Toxic
Substances and Disease
Registry
Attitudes toward workplace safety,
129, 135–136
Audiograms, 113, 142, 164
Audits, routine and exhaustive, 92
Automated external defibrillators, 77,
107–108
Aviation pilots, FAA medical
qualifications for, 161

Baby Boomers
characteristics of, 37, 38
training and development for, 39*t*
Barbiturates, 383
drug panel tests for, 183
urine drug testing and, 181
Bath salts, 187
BBP. *See* Bloodborne pathogens
Behavioral sciences, occupational
health and, 9
Behavior-based safety approach,
134–135, 136
Behavior-based safety incentives, 134
Benefit entitlement, integrated
absence management and, 241
Benefits eligibility, requirements
for, 163
Benzene exposure, 138
Benzodiazepines, 383
drug panel tests for, 183
saliva tests for, 182
urine drug testing and, 181
Best practices, 16, 167, 304
Biohazardous waste, storage and
disposal of, 87
Biological exposure indices, 141
Biological hazards, 138, 139
Biological monitoring, 141
Biologic or physical stimulus, triad of
intervention and, 226
Biometric screening, 268, 309
Biopsychosocial holistic approach, to
health, 233
Births, FMLA and, 254–255
Blaze, 187
Bloodborne pathogens, 114–115, 139
Bloodborne Pathogens Standard
(OSHA), 114–115
Board certificates, 79
Botulism, 139
Breath alcohol analysis, 184
Budget
facilities and resources, 75
occupational health program, 60